NEUROLOGY for NON-NEUROLOGISTS

NEUROLOGY for NON-NEUROLOGISTS
Third Edition

Wigbert C. Wiederholt, M.D
Professor of Neurosciences
Department of Neurosciences
University of California, San Diego
La Jolla, California

W.B. Saunders Company
A Division of Harcourt Brace & Company
Philadelphia   London   Toronto   Montreal   Sydney   Tokyo

W.B. SAUNDERS COMPANY

A Division of Harcourt Brace & Company

The Curtis Center
Independence Square West
Philadelphia, Pennsylvania 19106

Library of Congress Cataloging-in-Publication Data

NEUROLOGY FOR NON-NEUROLOGISTS / Wigbert C. Wiederholt. — 3rd ed.
    p.   cm.
   ISBN 0-7216-4191-1
   1. Nervous system—Diseases. 2. Neurology. I. Wiederholt, Wigbert C.
   [DNLM: 1. Nervous System Diseases. WL 140 N4935 1995]
   RC346.N452   1995
   616.8—dc20
   DNLM/DLC
                                                               95-11485

NEUROLOGY FOR NON-NEUROLOGISTS   ISBN   0-7216-4191-1

Copyright © 1995, 1988, 1982 by W.B. Saunders Company

All rights reserved. No part of this publication may be reproduced or transmitted in any form or by any means, electronic or mechanical, including photocopy, recording, or any information storage and retrieval system, without permission in writing from the publisher.

Printed in the United States of America

Last digit is the print number: 9   8   7   6   5   4   3   2   1

To Sven, Karen, and Kristin

Preface

This is the first appearance of *Neurology for Non-Neurologists* as a book that can be carried in a pocket. That is where it belongs, because it should be readily available as a guide in the daily encounter with patients suffering from neurologic diseases. The third edition has been revised and updated. Decisions had to be made about what to select, leave out, change, and emphasize. The final product is the result of the author's experience, judgment, and perceptions and thus reflects one physician's approach to clinical neurology. With this caveat, nevertheless, the author believes that the book can be of help to students, residents, and practicing physicians whose primary interest is not neurology.

I am indebted to the patients I have cared for because they have taught me about nature and humanity, to my colleagues who have kept me honest and stimulated, and to the students and residents who have kept my mind open and my heart young. Janie Fay, my able assistant of many years, deserves a special thank you for her unwavering support.

W. C. Wiederholt

NOTICE

Research and clinical experience lead to changes in patient assessment, treatment, and drug therapy. The author believes that the information provided is complete, current, and generally in accord with the standards accepted at the time of publication. However, human errors occur, and neither the author nor the publisher involved in the preparation of this publication warrant that the information obtained here is in every respect accurate or complete, and they are not responsible for any errors or omissions, or for the results obtained from the use of such information. Readers are urged to confirm the information contained herein with other sources. Specifically, readers should consult the production information sheet included in the package of each drug they plan to administer or prescribe in order to be absolutely certain that the information contained in the book is accurate and that changes have not been made in the recommended dose or in the contraindications for administration. This information is particularly important for antibiotics, new drugs, and infrequently used drugs.

Contents

1
Review of Clinical Neuroanatomy — 1

2
Neurologic History and Examination — 23

3
Ancillary Methods of Study — 43

4
Headache — 57

5
Cerebrovascular Disease — 81

6
Dementias — 95

7
Demyelinating Diseases — 109

8
Amyotrophic Lateral Sclerosis and Other Motor System Diseases — 125

9
Toxic–Metabolic Encephalopathies and Coma — 133

10
Muscle Diseases and Disorders of Neuromuscular Transmission   159

11
Diseases of Peripheral and Cranial Nerves   179

12
Radiculopathies   203

13
Seizure Disorders   211

14
Parkinson's Disease and Other Movement Disorders   233

15
Infections of the Nervous System   249

16
Dizziness and Vertigo   269

17
Tumors   285

18
Craniospinal Trauma   297

19
Congenital Anomalies and Inherited Disorders   305

Index   329

1
Review of Clinical Neuroanatomy

Some working knowledge of neuroanatomy is essential to interpret the results of a neurologic examination. The nervous system is organized in a logical fashion, and although certain facts must be remembered, many others can be deducted by reasoning, using basic anatomical information. The following discussion of neuroanatomy is limited to those aspects of it that are of direct clinical relevance. Neuroanatomy is best learned by repetition. Unless one deals with neurologic problems daily, one cannot expect to remember, for example, all the muscles that are innervated by a certain root or a certain peripheral nerve. Therefore, the findings on neurologic examination should always be compared with appropriate illustrations and tables.

GENERAL FEATURES OF THE NEURON AND NERVOUS SYSTEM

The basic building blocks of the nervous system are the neurons, with their axons and dendrites. Axons terminate on cell bodies or dendrites of other neurons or in the periphery, on striated muscle, smooth muscle, or glands. Sensory axons either terminate as bare endings or are surrounded by specialized structures that allow activation of the terminal axon by specific sensory stimuli.

The space between neurons is filled with glial elements and their processes. In the central nervous system (CNS), processes of oligdendroglia wrap around several axons to form a myelin sheath. In the periphery, one Schwann cell wraps its process around a segment of one axon to form a myelin sheath. Peripheral nonmyelinated fibers are embedded in processes from Schwann cells, but these processes are not wrapped several times around the axon.

Electrical impulses are generated in the neuronal cell body and travel nondecrementally along axons away from the cell body. When such a nervous impulse reaches the axon terminal, the axon terminal releases a chemical transmitter, which in turn produces a depolarization of the postsynaptic membrane; in some instances, the postsynaptic membrane is excited by electric coupling. Postsynaptic excitatory and inhibitory potentials are small localized potentials of relatively long duration that are not propagated away from their site of origin. If a sufficient area of the postsynaptic membrane is depolarized by many relatively synchronous synaptic excitatory potentials, the neuronal cell body will be depolarized, and an electric impulse will travel in a nondecremental fashion along the axon away from the cell body. At any given time, the net total of excitatory and inhibitory input to a neuron and its dendrites will determine the firing level of that particular cell. In addition to propagating impulses for fast communication between different parts of the nervous system, axons and dendrites transport chemicals from the cell body to the periphery and vice versa.

PERIPHERAL NERVOUS SYSTEM

The final common pathway for CNS output is from somatic, branchial, and visceral efferent nuclei in the brainstem and from somatic and visceral efferent nuclei in the spinal cord. Sensory input from the entire body is through the brainstem and spinal cord, with the cell body of the primary sensory neuron located in the neural foramina of the spinal column (posterior root ganglia) or at bony openings in the skull. All output (somatic and visceral) from the spinal cord is through the anterior roots, and all sensory input (somatic and visceral) is through the posterior roots (Fig. 1–1). Anterior and posterior roots always fuse at their respective neural foramina. Sympathetic visceral efferents exit anteriorly and leave the spinal canal from T-1 through L-2. These fibers enter the sympathetic chain ganglia from C-1 through S-4, with some of the ganglia fused into larger groups; in the cervical area, for example, only three ganglia exist instead of eight. Some fibers pass through the chain ganglia to form visceral ganglia. Other fibers synapse in the chain ganglia, and the postsynaptic nonmyelinated fibers reenter the peripheral nerve to reach their ultimate destination in the periphery. It is beyond the point where the postsynaptic sympathetic fibers rejoin the peripheral nerve that the mixed peripheral nerve is complete. This mixed peripheral nerve consists of large myelinated somatic motor fibers that make contact with striated muscle, medium-sized myelinated gamma

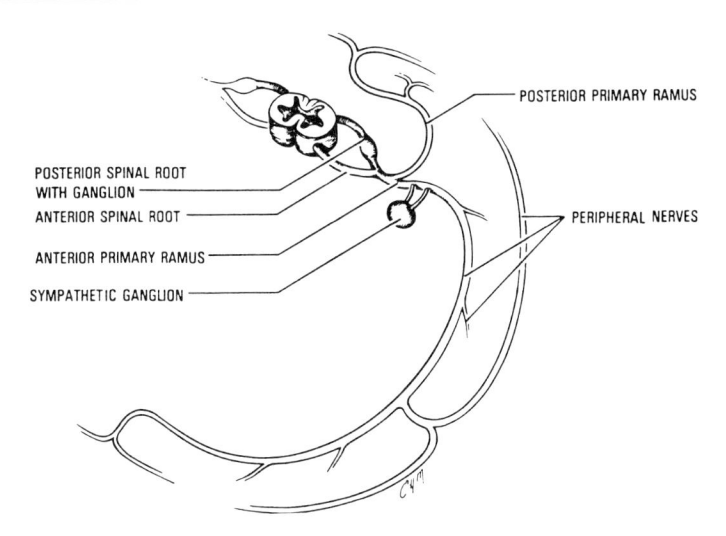

FIGURE 1–1. Components of a radicular nerve. Anterior and posterior spinal roots fuse at their respective bony neural foramina. Distal to the fusion of the two roots, the fused nerve and its branches are referred to as the *radicular nerve.* Each branch distal to the splitting of the radicular nerve into an anterior and a posterior primary ramus is referred to as a peripheral nerve.

motor fibers that terminate on intrafusal muscle fibers in striated muscle, nonmyelinated visceral efferent fibers that terminate on smooth muscle or glands, large myelinated afferent fibers that serve proprioception, medium-sized myelinated afferent fibers that serve touch and other sensory modalities, small myelinated fibers that serve epicritic pain and temperature sensation, and nonmyelinated visceral afferent fibers that transmit sensory input from the viscera.

Conduction velocity is directly proportional to the diameter of each axon. All axons branch into multiple axons. For example, an axon originating from an anterior horn cell may form several hundred subaxons in the periphery that make contact with many muscle fibers. This anterior horn cell—with its main axon, its subaxons, the neuromuscular synapses, and their muscle fibers—constitutes the lower motor neuron (Fig. 1–2). On the sensory side, one sensory axon entering the spinal cord divides into subaxons that make contact with many other neurons on the same side, on the opposite side, below the level of entry, and above the level of entry. Such contacts extend upstream as far as the cerebellum and the brainstem, including the thalamus. In general, the fewer subaxons, the more precise the function.

After anterior and posterior roots have joined at the neural foramina, the mixed peripheral nerve breaks up into an anterior and posterior pri-

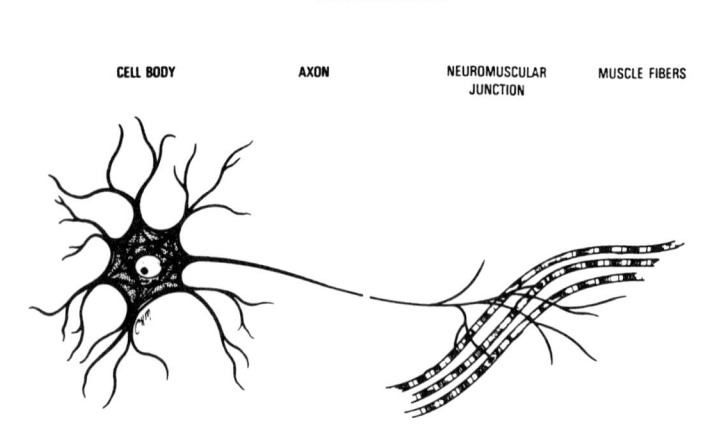

FIGURE 1–2. Schematic presentation of the lower motor neuron. The number of branching axons and muscle fibers innervated by one anterior horn cell is variable and dependent on functional requirements.

mary ramus. In the cervical and lumbosacral areas, the anterior primary rami innervate the extremities. Distal to the point where anterior and posterior primary rami branch, the radicular nerves form complex plexi in the cervical and lumbosacral areas. Each anterior and posterior root innervates certain muscles and certain areas of the skin and bone. This innervation is called segmental or radicular. Therefore, any lesion proximal to where the anterior and posterior roots fuse will produce a radicular or segmental deficit, whereas any lesion distal to it will produce a motor and/or sensory deficit that corresponds in a nonradicular or nonsegmental fashion to the distribution of the specific branch of the peripheral nerve. This anatomical distinction between segmental and peripheral innervation is important, because it allows the precise localization of lesions on the basis of clinical findings (Fig. 1–3).

If a peripheral nerve is injured, myelin may degenerate in a circumscribed area or diffusely. In either case, remyelination may take place, restoring function within weeks to months. If, on the other hand, the axon is degenerating, which also implies destruction of the myelin sheath, regeneration occurs over many months. Regeneration occurs from the neuronal cell body and proceeds distally at a rate of approximately 1 mm per day. In some instances a peripheral nerve is nonfunctioning either because of pressure on the nerve without degeneration of the axon or myelin sheath or because of toxic metabolic disturbances. In such a situation, recovery is prompt if the mechanical pressure or toxic insult is removed.

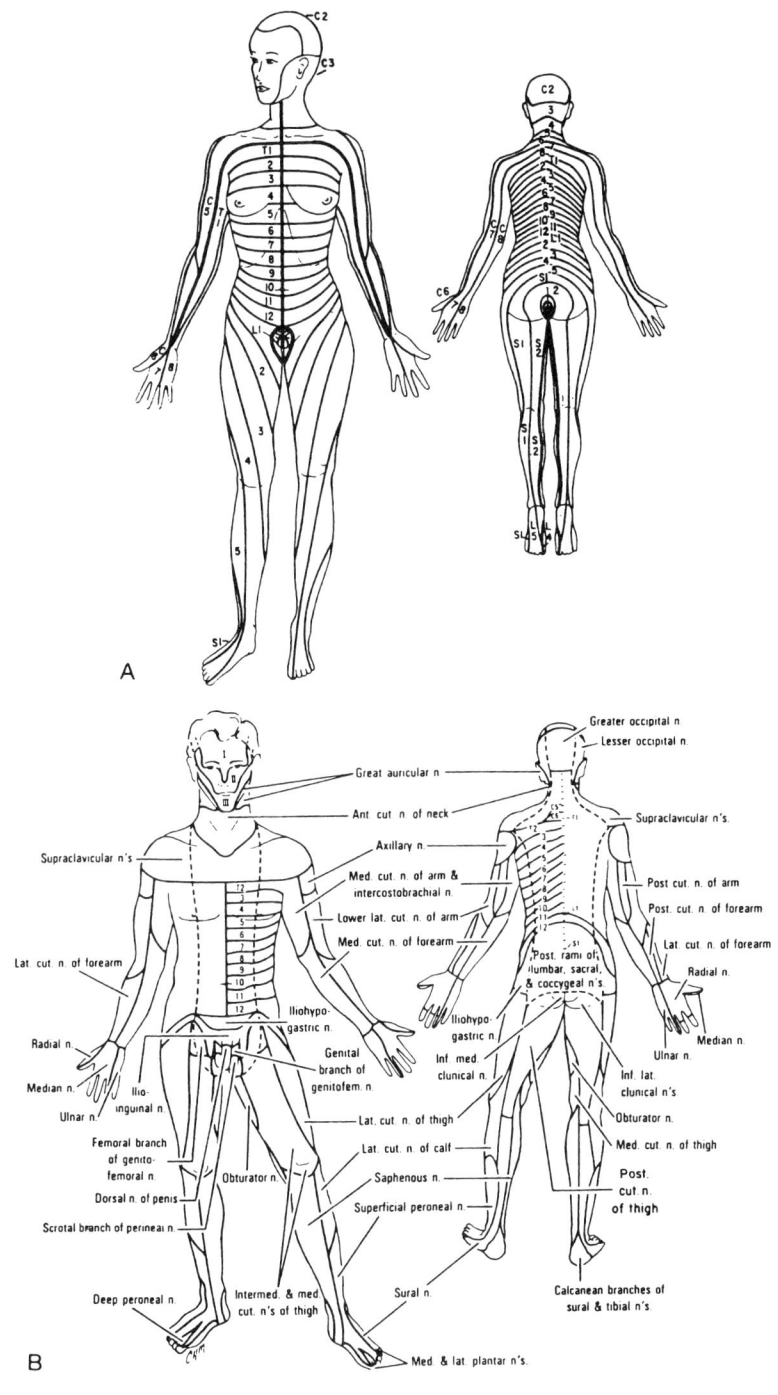

FIGURE 1-3. Radicular (A) and peripheral (B) cutaneous fields.

The simplest interaction between the sensory and motor systems occurs as the stretch reflex. Stretching a muscle activates a stretch receptor in that muscle, which produces an electrical impulse that travels via large myelinated fibers toward the spinal cord and enters via the posterior root entry zone. A subaxon of this sensory axon makes synaptic contact with an anterior horn cell, giving rise to a motor axon to the same muscle in which the sensory activity originated. If stretch activates enough afferent sensory axons to depolarize the anterior horn cell, a propagated nerve impulse will produce muscle contraction. Given this knowledge of the anatomy and physiology of the muscle stretch reflex, it is apparent that an interpretation of a stretch reflex can be made only after assessment of the sensory and motor systems.

SPINAL CORD

The spinal cord contains neurons, which form the gray matter, located centrally, with an anterior and a posterior horn. The gray matter is surrounded by white matter consisting of myelinated nerve fibers going up and down the spinal cord. Since all output and input to the CNS is through the spinal cord, except for the cranial nerves, the white matter is largest in the uppermost cervical area and gradually decreases as more caudal segments are reached. The size of the gray matter depends on the number of structures innervated at a given segment. Therefore, the gray matter is larger in the cervical and lumbosacral segments because the upper and lower extremities are innervated at these levels. The anterior horn of the gray matter contains large alpha motor neurons and smaller gamma motor neurons. Axons from the anterior horn leave the spinal cord as the anterior roots. Adjacent and posterior to the motor neurons are both visceral sympathetic efferent cells (T-1 through L-2) and parasympathetic efferent neurons (S-2 through S-4). Their axons also exit anteriorly. All somatic and visceral sensory neurons are located at the neural foramina as the posterior root ganglia. Central processes of some of these cells make synaptic contact with second-order sensory neurons in the posterior portion of the intermediolateral cell column for the visceral system and in the posterior horn for the somatic sensory system. Other fibers course to more caudal and rostral structures without interposed synapses. All sensory fibers enter the spinal cord posteriorly as the posterior roots. In summary, the organization of the gray matter in the spinal cord, from anterior to posterior, is as follows: somatic efferent, visceral efferent, visceral afferent, and somatic afferent. A similar arrangement is seen throughout the brainstem except that the orientation, instead of anterior-posterior, is from midline to lateral areas. Somatic and visceral efferents do not cross in the spinal cord but leave on the side of their origin. On the sensory side, some fibers synapse at the level of entry or one or two segments above and below, then ascend and descend either on the same side and/or the opposite side of entry. Other fibers do not synapse at the level of entry but ascend and descend to synapse at a considerable distance from their site of entry.

Supranuclear or upper motor neuron fibers descend in the spinal cord in a lateral position as the lateral corticospinal tract. This pathway generally contains crossed corticospinal tract fibers, except for a small anterior area that contains uncrossed corticospinal tract fibers (Fig. 1–4). Most of the nonpyramidal upper motor neuron axons originate in the basal ganglia and various levels of the brainstem and descend in a location anterior to the lateral corticospinal tract. These latter systems

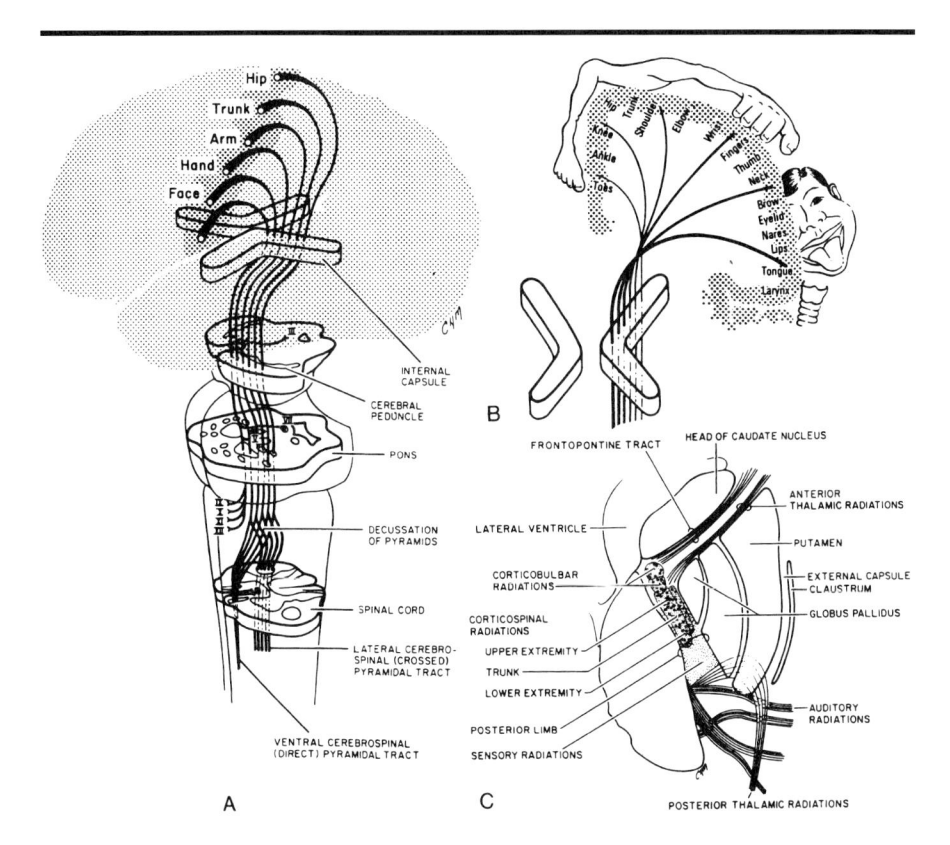

FIGURE 1–4. Diagram showing the course of corticobulbar and corticospinal pyramidal tracts (A), detail of cortical origin of fibers (B), and location of fiber tracts that pass through the internal capsule (C).

may contain fibers that are crossed, uncrossed, or both. Descending visceral pathways originating in the hypothalamus and brainstem travel on both sides in close proximity to the gray matter; other subdivisions descend in the peripheral field of the spinal cord. All descending fibers eventually impinge on alpha or gamma motor neurons and on visceral efferent neurons.

Sensory fibers subserving pain and temperature sensation synapse in the posterior horn. Postsynaptic second-order sensory neurons send their axons through the anterior white commissure to the opposite side, where they form the lateral spinothalamic tract. This tract terminates in many brainstem structures but principally in the thalamus (Fig. 1–5). Sensory nerve fibers subserving crude touch synapse in other layers of the posterior horn. Postsynaptic second-order sensory axons form the contralateral ventral spinothalamic tract, with some fibers remaining ipsilateral. The termination of this tract is also largely in the thalamus. Large myelinated sensory nerve fibers subserving discriminatory sensation, and to some degree vibratory perception, ascend without interposed synapses on the ipsilateral side of the cord to nuclei cuneatus and gracilis in the medulla oblongata (Fig. 1–6). Visceral afferent fibers synapse within one or two segments of entry in the posterior portion of the intermediate cell column and then ascend on the same and opposite sides in close proximity to the gray matter to reach different brainstem structures and the hypothalamus.

The spinocerebellar system is divided into a dorsal and a ventral spinocerebellar tract. Peripheral nerve fibers that form the dorsal spinocerebellar tract synapse with cell bodies located in the ventral and medial portion of the posterior horn. Postsynaptic fibers form the dorsal spinocerebellar tract on the same side, fibers of which reach the cerebellum via the inferior cerebellar peduncle. Fibers that ultimately form the ventral spinocerebellar tract synapse at the level of entry with cell bodies of the posterior horn. Postsynaptic fibers remain on the same side or cross over and enter the cerebellum via the superior cerebellar peduncle. There are, of course, many other ascending and descending paths, but since none of them can presently be adequately evaluated clinically, they will not be discussed. (Fig. 1–7).

The blood supply to the spinal cord is from one anterior spinal artery and two posterior spinal arteries, which are formed by branches of the vertebral arteries. In addition, radicular arteries enter the spinal canal and contribute to spinal cord blood supply at each level; a large radicular artery, entering somewhere between T-6 and T-12 (greater medullar artery), supplies almost all the blood to the spinal cord from this level down. The anterior spinal artery perfuses the anterior two thirds of the spinal cord and the posterior spinal arteries the posterior one

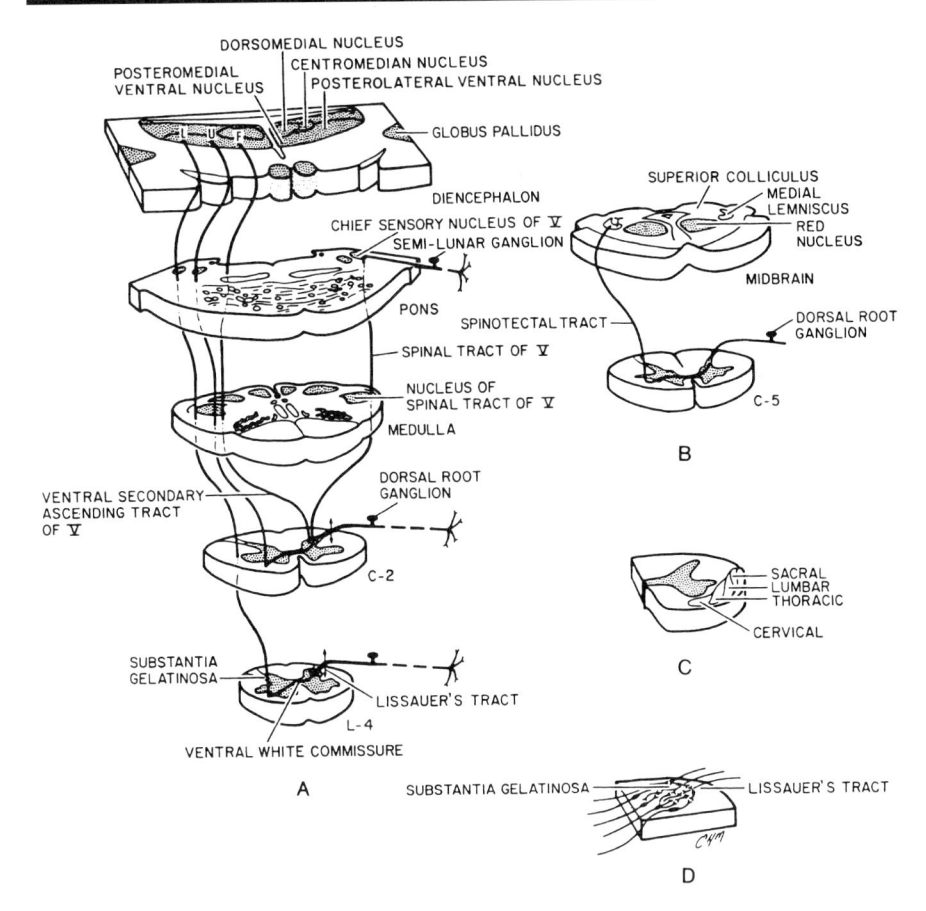

FIGURE 1–5. Diagram of some pathways concerned with transmission of impulses activated by peripheral painful and thermal stimuli. Entering peripheral nerve fibers ascend and descend several segments and then cross over to ascend to the thalamus on the opposite side of entry (A) (L, lower extremity; U, upper extremity; F, face). Many fibers terminate in the mesencephalon (B). Layering of fibers in the lateral spinothalamic tract is shown in C and details of synapses in D. Pain and temperature fibers from the face descend from the midpontine level to the upper cervical levels before postsynaptic fibers synapse and cross to the opposite side.

third. A small rim of the spinal cord is supplied by perforating branches from radicular arteries.

CLINICAL CORRELATION. A complete transection of the spinal cord produces paralysis below the transection, with spasticity, hyperreflexia,

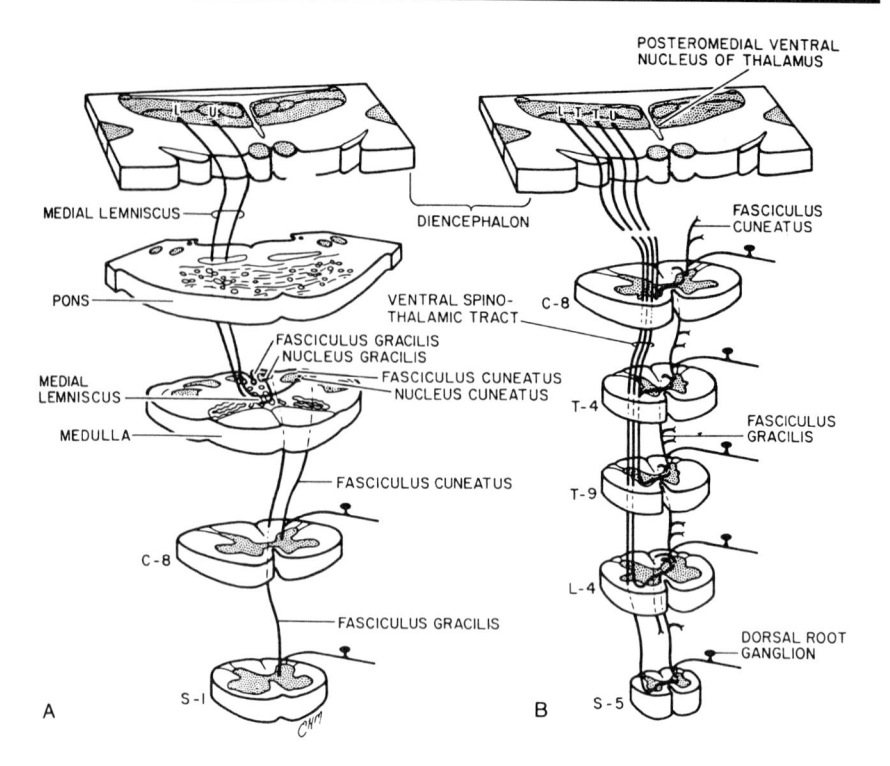

FIGURE 1–6. Diagram of pathways concerned with discriminatory tactile sensibility (A) and crude tactile sensibility (B) (L, lower extremity; U, upper extremity; T, trunk).

and upgoing toes. In addition, all sensation is lost below the level of the lesion. Destruction of the anterior two thirds of the spinal cord, such as is seen with occlusion of the anterior spinal artery, produces loss of pain, temperature, and crude touch sensation on both sides below the level of the lesion. If the lesion extends sufficiently posteriorly, there may also be bilateral spastic paralysis. When the posterior one third of the cord is destroyed acutely, discriminatory sensation and vibratory perception may be lost but considerable recovery usually occurs. In so-called subacute combined degeneration, which is most frequently secondary to vitamin B^{12} deficiency, the posterior columns and the lateral corticospinal tracts are involved. The clinical picture is that of a bilateral spastic paraparesis and loss of discriminatory sensation. Pain and temperature sensation remain essentially intact.

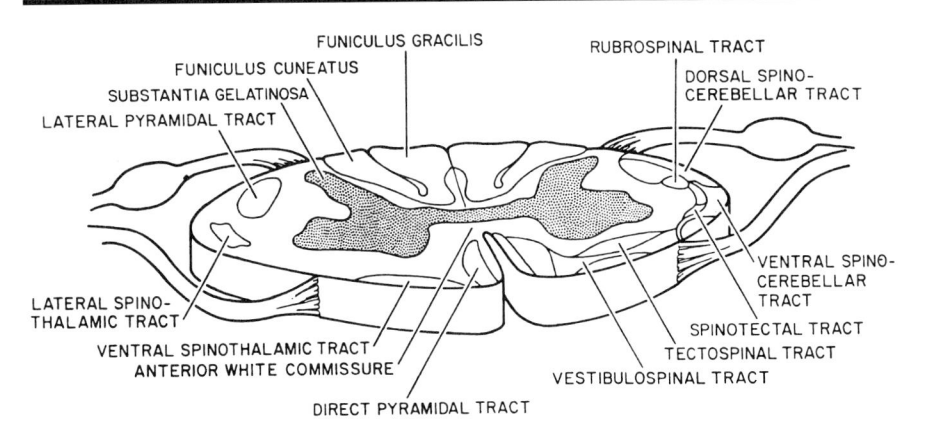

FIGURE 1-7. Diagrammatic cross-section of the spinal cord with major descending and ascending pathways.

BRAINSTEM

Anatomically, the brainstem consists of the hypothalamus, epithalamus, thalamus, basal ganglia, mesencephalon, rhombencephalon, and medulla oblongata. Only the last three structures are referred to as the brainstem in colloquial clinical usage. The organization of brainstem nuclei very much resembles the organization within the gray matter of the spinal cord, except that the orientation is from medial to lateral. In the most medial position are found somatic and branchial efferent nuclei, including nuclei of the third, fourth, sixth, seventh, eleventh, and twelfth nerves. During development, both the seventh-nerve nucleus and the ambiguous nucleus migrate to a slightly more lateral and ventral position. Just lateral to this position are located visceral efferent nuclei. The main representative is the dorsal efferent nucleus of the vagus. Farther lateral are found structures principally concerned with general or special visceral sensory functions. These include the gustatory nuclei and the nucleus of the tractus solitarius. Except for the nucleus gracilis and nucleus cuneatus, which are in a median and paramedian location, other somatosensory nuclei are situated in the lateral field of the brainstem. In midpons these include the fifth-nerve nucleus, with its mesencephalic and spinal extension. The two cochlear and four vestibular nuclei are located in the medulla, pons, and spinal cord. Almost all cranial nerve nuclei are located either directly below or not far from the floor of the fourth ventricle or in close proximity to the aqueduct.

The cerebellum caps the brainstem and is connected with it through three peduncles. The superior is connected to the mesencephalon, the middle to the pons, and the inferior to the medulla. Fibers of passage in the brainstem include motor and sensory tracts, located in ventral and lateral positions. Reticular nuclei are found throughout the brainstem in ventral median and lateral positions.

The blood supply to the brainstem is from the two vertebral arteries that join at the pontomedullary junction to form the basilar artery. At the most rostral mesencephalic level, the basilar artery ends and forms the two posterior cerebral arteries. The perfusion territories of these arteries can be grossly subdivided into a median field supplied by short perforating branches, a paramedian field supplied by short circumferential arteries, and a lateral field supplied by long circumferential arteries that also supply the cerebellum.

Medulla

Several distinct levels of the brainstem can be recognized clinically. The lowermost medullary level is characterized by the twelfth nerve, its nucleus in a median dorsal location, and its axons traveling ventrally to exit between the pyramids (Fig. 1–8). Immediately below this level, the corticospinal tract fibers cross and form the medullospinal junction. At the lower third of the medulla, the gracilis and cuneate nuclei are well developed, and their postsynaptic fibers form the crossed medial lemniscus in a paramedian location. The medial lemniscus ascends, gradually assumes a more horizontal position, and ultimately joins all other sensory tracts in the lateral field of the mesencephalon. The next most rostral level is characterized by nuclei of the ninth and tenth nerves.

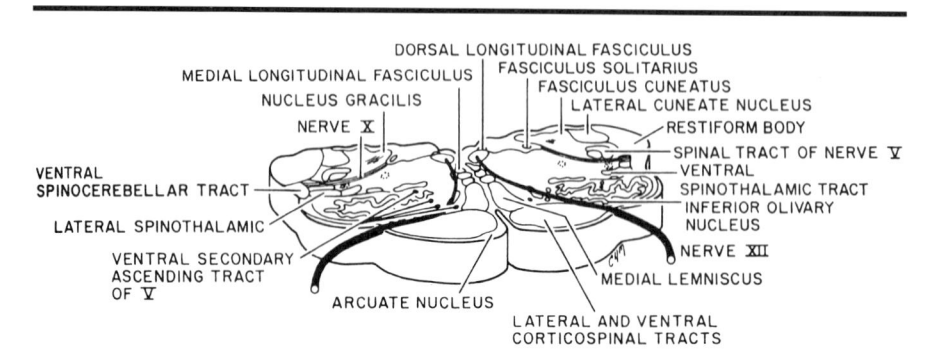

FIGURE 1–8. Diagram of the medulla at the level of cranial nerve XII.

At the uppermost level of the medulla, the vestibular and cochlear nuclei are well developed (Fig. 1–9). Throughout the medulla, the corticospinal tract is in a ventral position. It forms the two pyramids, bordered laterally and somewhat dorsally by the inferior olive. The medial lemniscus is in a median position, whereas the descending tract of the fifth nerve and its nucleus, as well as the ascending fibers of the lateral and ventral spinothalamic tracts, are in the lateral field.

CLINICAL CORRELATION. A ventral, unilateral lesion in the lower medulla above the decussation of the pyramidal tract will produce a contralateral hemiparesis and ipsilateral weakness and atrophy of the tongue, secondary to involvement of the twelfth nerve as it emerges in a ventral position. A laterally placed medullary lesion will produce decreased or absent hearing on the same side due to involvement of the cochlear nuclei. The patient will also be vertiginous and fall to the same side of the lesion because of vestibular nuclei and inferior cerebellar peduncle involvement. The patient will be hoarse because of involvement of the ambiguous nucleus, which produces paralysis of the ipsilateral vocal cord. Impairment of the descending tract of the fifth cranial nerve leads to ipsilateral loss of pain and temperature sensations in the face. Involvement of the lateral spinothalamic tract produces contralateral decreased or absent pain and temperature sensation on the body.

Pons

In the pons, the corticospinal tracts are buried in the large expansion of the basis pontis, which in addition contains scattered pontine nuclei,

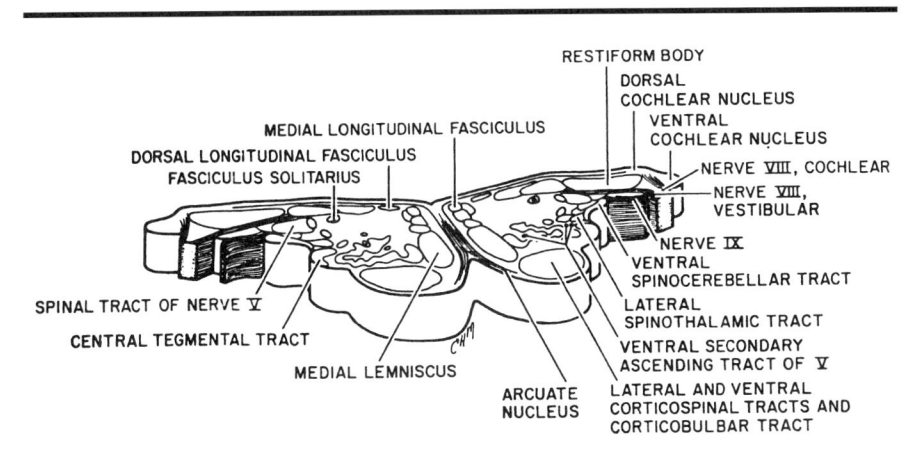

FIGURE 1–9. Diagram of the medulla at the level of cranial nerves VIII and IX.

corticopontine, and pontocerebellar fibers. Corticopontine fibers synapse on the ipsilateral side of the pons and then cross to the other side to reach the cerebellum via the middle cerebellar peduncle. The lower one third of the pons is characterized by the dorsally and medially located sixth-nerve (abducens) nucleus. Around the sixth-nerve nucleus loop axons form the seventh (facial) nucleus. The sixth nerve exits the pons ventrally, whereas the seventh nerve exits laterally. The medial lemniscus assumes a horizontal position at this level and lies between the basis pontis ventrally and the tegmentum pontis dorsally (Fig. 1–10). Other sensory tracts remain in the lateral field. At the midpontine level, the motor nucleus of the fifth nerve, which supplies ipsilateral muscles of mastication, can be identified. Slightly lateral to it is located the main or chief sensory nucleus of the fifth nerve. All sensory fibers of the fifth nerve enter at this level and pursue separate pathways according to their function. Those concerned with pain and temperature (descending tract of V) descend in the lateral field as far as C-2 or even C-4 in the spinal cord. These fibers synapse in the medially located nucleus. Postsynaptic fibers form the ventral secondary ascending tract of the fifth nerve. These ascending fibers reach the lateral field on the opposite side at upper medullary and lower pontine levels to proceed to the thalamus. Axons that convey crude tactile perception synapse in the chief sensory nucleus of the fifth nerve. Postsynaptic fibers cross over as the dorsal secondary ascending tract to reach the opposite lateral field and, ultimately, the thalamus. Those fibers that transmit discriminatory sensory information ascend to the mesencephalon as the mes-

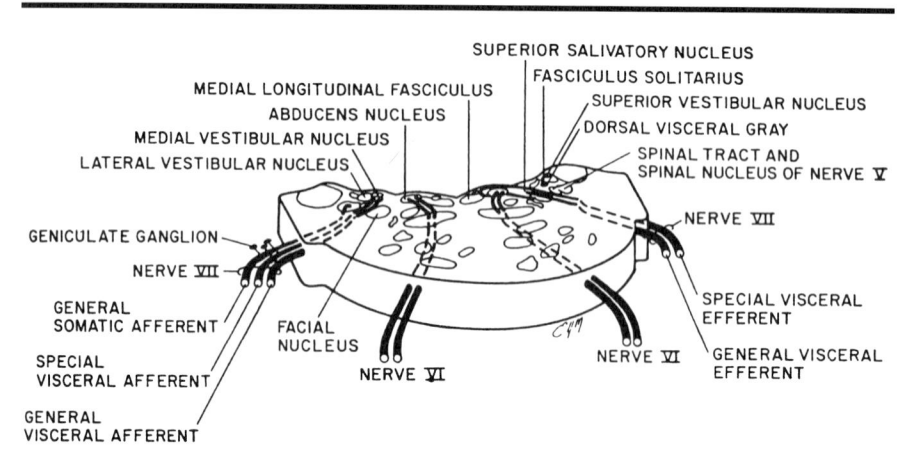

FIGURE 1–10. Diagram of the pons at the level of cranial nerves VI and VII.

encephalic tract of the fifth nerve. Postsynaptic fibers descend to the chief sensory nucleus of the fifth nerve and cross over to form the dorsal secondary ascending tract of the fifth nerve. At the upper third of the pons, there are no cranial nerve nuclei. However, a very important structure, the nucleus of the locus coerulus, is present. This latter structure is intimately involved in the regulation of sleep.

CLINICAL CORRELATION. Unilateral ventral lesions of the pons produce contralateral hemiparesis and apraxia secondary to involvement of both corticospinal tract fibers and corticopontine fibers. If the lesion is caudally located, the sixth nerve will be involved, leading to an ipsilateral sixth-nerve paresis characterized by inability to move the eye laterally.

Lesions in the lateral field will lead to loss of pain and temperature and other sensory modalities on the ipsilateral side of the face, but in addition there may be some decrease of pain and temperature perception in contralateral parts of the face because of involvement of the ventral secondary ascending tract of the fifth nerve, which has crossed at this level and is located in the lateral field. As in a lateral medullary lesion, pain and temperature perception will be decreased or lost on the entire body on the contralateral side. If the motor component of the fifth cranial nerve is involved, the patient will have difficulty chewing on the same side as the lesion.

Mesencephalon

The mesencephalon is in a rostral position and can be divided into an upper and a lower part. The lower part is characterized by the trochlear (fourth) nerve nucleus in a median location, axons of which loop around the central gray matter and exit on the opposite side to reach the superior oblique muscle of the eye. Ventrally, a large white matter structure is seen, which is the decussation of the main cerebellar outflow, the dentatorubrothalamic tract. Farther ventrally, the basis pontis is no longer present but is replaced by the two cerebral peduncles. These structures contain, in the most medial position, the frontopontine fibers, followed by the pyramidal tract, within which face fibers are most medial and leg fibers most lateral. In the most lateral position are parietal corticopontine fibers. Dorsally, one encounters the inferior colliculi, which are part of the auditory system. In the upper portion of the mesencephalon, the superior colliculi are located dorsally, with the pretectal area just in front. Both the pretectal area and the superior colliculi are intimately involved with the visual system. At this level, the central gray matter surrounds the central canal (cerebral aqueduct). Ventral to the gray matter is the oculomotor nuclear complex (cranial nerve III). Axons of the third nerve exit ventrally between the cerebral peduncles. These fibers course through the red nucleus, which is seen on the ventral side of the mesencephalon in a similar location as the decussation of the cerebellar outflow at a more caudad level (Fig. 1–11). All somatosensory tracts are grouped together and are located in the lateral field. Between the red nucleus dorsally and the cerebral peduncle ventrally lies the substantia nigra.

CLINICAL CORRELATION. Unilateral ventral lesions involving the cerebral peduncle and the third nerve produce contralateral hemiparesis with facial involvement and an ipsilateral third-nerve paralysis characterized by lateral deviation of the eye, inability to move the eye up and down and medially, a large nonreactive pupil, and ptosis of the upper eyelid.

Laterally placed lesions, since they involve all sensory pathways, will produce contralateral decrease or loss of all types of sensation, both in the face and the rest of the body.

CEREBELLUM

Dorsal to the brainstem and participating in the formation of the fourth ventricle is the cerebellum. The cerebellum is connected to the brainstem by three cerebellar peduncles. The major input to the cerebellum from the cortex is via the middle cerebellar peduncle; peripheral input is via the inferior cerebellar peduncle and the superior cerebellar peduncle. The main output from the cerebellum, both to the cortex and

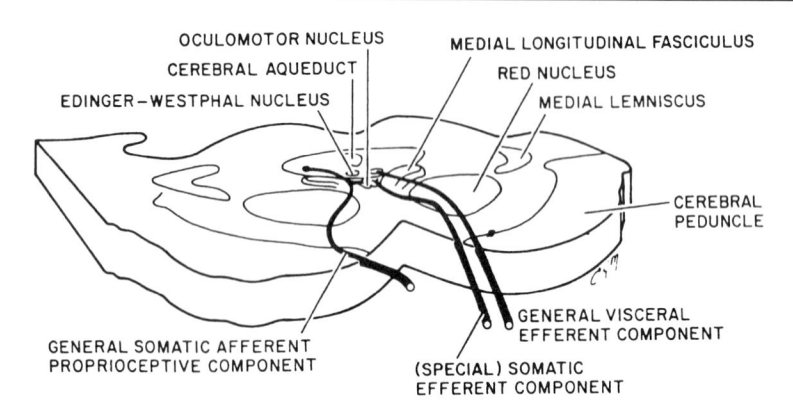

FIGURE 1–11. Diagram of the mesencephalon at the level of cranial nerve III.

brainstem as well as the spinal cord, is through the superior cerebellar peduncle. All peripheral afferent fibers to the cerebellum terminate ipsilaterally. Similarly, cerebellar efferents terminate ipsilaterally in the periphery. It should be noted, however, that most cerebellar afferents and efferents terminate ipsilaterally by crossing and then recrossing. For example, efferent cerebellar fibers cross over in the lower half of the mesencephalon to reach the area of the red nucleus. After synapsing in that location, they immediately recross to descend to the lower brainstem and spinal cord. Fibers to the cortex do not recross. Therefore, for all practical purposes, a so-called cerebellar deficit, due to a lesion in the cerebellum or the afferent and efferent pathways to and from the periphery, will always produce an ipsilateral deficit. The only exception to this is a lesion in the red nucleus and its vicinity.

The cerebellum is subdivided into a medially located vermis and two cerebellar hemispheres. In general, any cerebellar deficit will produce disintegration and irregularity of movements. Truncal stability and gait will be most affected by lesions in the anterior vermis. Cerebellar hemisphere lesions are usually accompanied by disintegration of movement in the upper or lower extremity on the same side.

VISCERAL NERVOUS SYSTEM

The visceral nervous system, including the parasympathetic and sympathetic subsystems, is controlled by the hypothalamus. The parasympathetic outflow is principally via the third, ninth, and tenth cranial nerves. All peripheral structures, including the eye, are innervated by this outflow with the exception of the descending colon, sigmoid, rectum, and bladder, which are innervated by the sacral parasympathetic outflow from S-2 through S-4. All sympathetic fibers exit at spinal levels T-1 through L-2 and reach all structures with their appropriate peripheral nerves.

THALAMUS AND HYPOTHALAMUS

The thalamus is located deep in the paramedian area of the forebrain. The third ventricle is located medially and the internal capsule laterally. Its primary function is to serve as a relay station for sensory information from the spinal cord, brainstem, cerebellum, and basal ganglia. The blood supply to this structure is derived mainly from branches of the posterior cerebral arteries. The anterior nuclear group receives input from the mamillary body and fornix and projects to the cingulate gyrus. The dorsal medial nucleus receives and relays fibers from other thalamic nuclei, receives fibers from the amygdala, and projects to the hypothalamus and prefrontal cortex. The intralaminar nuclei receive input from the globus pallidus, brainstem reticular formation, and spinal cord. Their projection is principally to the caudate and putamen. The lateral nuclear group receives input from and projects to the cortex. The ventral nuclear group, which is the largest subdivision of the thalamus, relays sensory impulses from spinothalamic tracts, medial lemniscus, and fifth nerve. Projections from these nuclei are principally to the sensory cortex. The most posterior area of the thalamus contains two small structures: the medial geniculate body, an auditory relay nucleus that connects with the inferior colliculus and auditory cortex, and the lateral geniculate body, a visual relay nucleus connecting the optic tracts with the visual cortex. The projections from the thalamus to the cortex are principally through the posterior portion of the posterior limb of the internal capsule, with some fibers projecting through the anterior limb of the internal capsule to the cortex.

The hypothalamus, which is located on the ventral and rostral aspect of the forebrain, is concerned with visceral, autonomic, and endocrine functions. Its blood supply is derived from the anterior cerebral artery, anterior communicating artery, and posterior communicating artery. Attached to it, through the pituitary stalk, is the pituitary gland. The supraoptic and paraventricular nuclei project to the posterior pituitary and the tuberal region to the anterior pituitary. The anterior medial hypothalamus is associated with parasympathetic activity, whereas sympathetic activity is related to lateral and posterior hypothalamic areas. There are innumerable connections to the cortex, olfactory regions, hippocampus, amygdala, thalamus, retina, midbrain, medulla, and spinal cord.

BASAL GANGLIA

The basal ganglia, as the name implies, are buried deep in the forebrain and consist of the caudate nucleus, putamen, globus pallidus, subthalamic nucleus, and substantia nigra. The blood supply is derived mainly from the middle cerebral artery via lenticulostriate branches. Input to the caudate and putamen is from the cortex, thalamus, and substantia nigra. Output from these two structures is principally to the globus pallidus and, to a lesser degree, the substantia nigra. The globus pallidus receives its largest input from the caudate and putamen and a smaller input from the subthalamic nucleus and the substantia nigra. Efferent fibers project to the thalamus as the ansa lenticularis, the lenticular fasciculus, and the thalamic fasciculus. Additional efferents project to the subthalamic nucleus and to the tegmental reticular formation. The major connections of the subthalamic nucleus are with the globus pallidus and the mesencephalic reticular formation.

CLINICAL CORRELATION. Lesions in the basal ganglia produce abnormal movements, including chorea, athetosis, hemiballismus, and dystonic posturing. The most commonly encountered disorder is Parkinson's disease.

INTERNAL CAPSULE

The internal capsule is bounded medially and anteriorly by the head of the caudate nucleus and medially and posteriorly by the thalamus. Laterally, it is bounded by the basal ganglia. It forms a V pointing toward the midline, with an anterior and posterior limb and knee. Thalamocortical fibers project through the anterior limb of the internal capsule. Corticobulbar and corticospinal fibers course through the knee and the anterior portion of the posterior limb. Sensory fibers from the thalamus, including visual and auditory raditions, pass through the most posterior part of the posterior limb of the internal capsule (see Fig. 1–4).

PINEAL GLAND

The pineal gland is attached to the most posterior portion of the third ventricle and is situated just above the superior colliculi and the pretectal area.

CEREBRAL HEMISPHERES

The paired cerebral hemispheres are separated by the longitudinal fissure, and they are connected through the corpus callosum and the anterior and posterior commissures. Each hemisphere is subdivided into frontal, temporal, parietal, and occipital lobes. Frontal and parietal lobes are separated by the central sulcus. The lateral fissure separates the frontal and parietal lobes from the temporal lobe below. The major portion of the occipital lobe lies on the medial aspect of the hemisphere and is delineated by a line drawn between the parieto-occipital fissure and the occipital notch on the inferior lateral surface of the temporal lobe. On the medial surface of the hemispheres, frontal and parietal lobes are separated by the medial extension of the central sulcus. The temporal lobe also has a large medial representation. Its most medial inferior aspect is the hippocampal gyrus from which the uncus protrudes. This latter structure lies just above the tentorial notch. The cingulate gyrus lies just above the corpus callosum and extends anteriorly into the frontal lobe to the anterior hypothalamic area. The arterial supply to the forebrain consists of an anterior and a posterior portion. The anterior is derived from the internal carotid artery and comprises most of the lateral hemispheres and the anterior two thirds of the medial portion of the hemispheres. The posterior circulation is derived from the two posterior cerebral arteries, which are the end branches of the basilar artery. The posterior cerebral arteries supply the occipital lobes, the inferior and medial portion of the temporal lobes, and most of the thalamus.

VISUAL SYSTEM

Fibers from each retina form the optic nerve. In the optic chiasm, all optic nerve fibers from the medial retina cross over to the opposite side, whereas those from the lateral retina remain on the same side. The optic tracts are formed by ipsilateral temporal retinal fibers and contralateral medial retinal fibers. They proceed to the lateral geniculate body of the thalamus, from which postsynaptic fibers project to the occipital lobes. Lesions anterior to the optic chiasm will produce unilateral visual loss, whereas lesions behind the chiasm will always produce homonymous field defects—that is, vision will be impaired in both visual fields of each eye in homologous areas. Compression of the optic chiasm frequently will lead to field defects involving both superior temporal fields (Fig. 1–12).

EYE MOVEMENTS

Eye movements are organized in such a fashion that the object to be in focus will project on both foveas. This end is accomplished by moving the eyes conjugately. This means that the eyes move in the same direction at exactly the same speed. The only exception is for near vision. In this situation, when an object is between the near point and the eyes, both eyes will converge with the aim, again, of having the object projected on both foveas. The center of convergence of the eyes is part of the third-nerve nuclei. The center for vertical conjugate movements is located in the pretectal area, with its output to the third and fourth cranial nerves. The two centers for horizontal conjugate eye movements are located on each side of the pons in close proximity to the sixth-nerve nucleus. The output from each center for horizontal conjugate gaze is to the ipsilateral sixth-nerve nucleus and to the opposite third-nerve nucleus via the medial longitudinal fasciculus (Fig. 1–13). Any input from any part of the nervous system, from the cortex to the brainstem to the periphery, that produces either vertical or horizontal conjugate eye movements, or a combination thereof, projects to the appropriate centers in the pretectal area (vertical conjugate movement) and pons (horizontal conjugate movement). Consequently, movement

REVIEW OF CLINICAL NEUROANATOMY 21

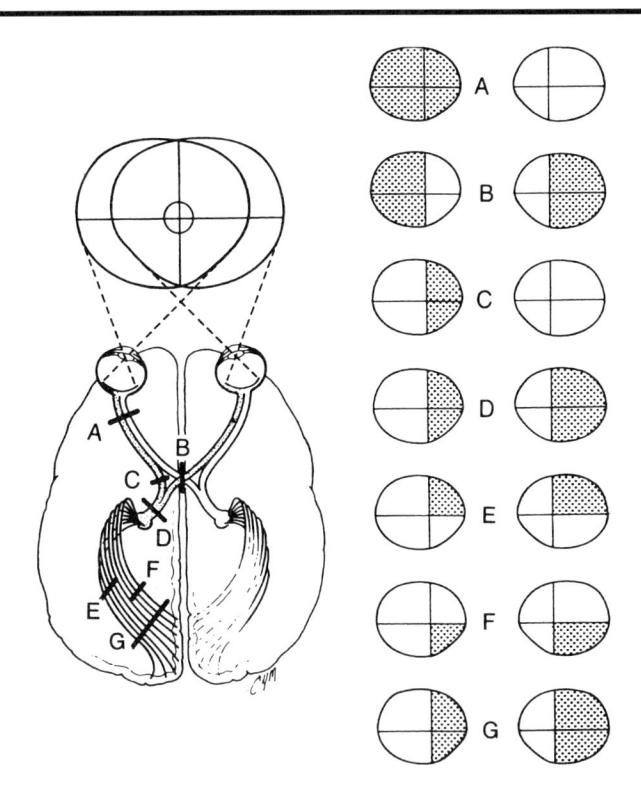

FIGURE 1-12. Diagram of lesions of optic pathways with corresponding field defects. Defects are drawn as if patient were facing the page: (A) left optic nerve (B) optic chiasm, (C) uncrossed temporal retinal fibers of optic nerve, (D) left optic tract, (E) left temporal lobe, (F) left parietal lobe, and (G) occipital lobe.

abnormalities of one eye will be due to lesions in the respective eye muscle nucleus or its nerve. Any lesion involving pathways to the centers for conjugate movements will produce paresis of conjugate movement. Since the eyes are driven by each hemisphere in the direction contralateral to that hemisphere, a cortical lesion that interferes with conjugate movements will produce tonic deviation of the eyes toward the side of the lesion. This deviation arises because of the unopposed input from the healthy hemisphere. In this situation, however, the eyes can move past the midline when other input is used, such as caloric stimulation of the inner ear or rotation of the head. In internuclear ophthalmoplegia, the lesion is in one or both medial longitudinal fasciculi. If the lesion is in the left medial longitudinal fasciculus, on attempted right lateral gaze, the eyes will show the following: the right eye will move laterally in a normal fashion, whereas the left eye either will not

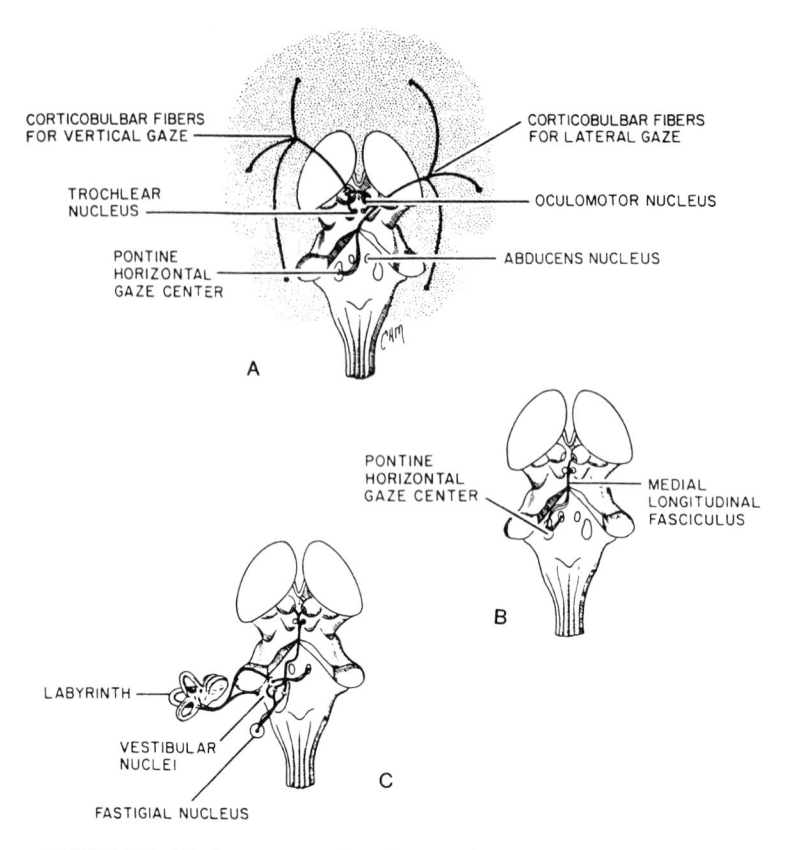

FIGURE 1-13. Some neural pathways for eye movements (A–C).

move nasally at all or will do so only partially, depending on how many fibers in the medial longitudinal fasciculus are nonfunctioning. In order to exclude a peripheral medial rectus paresis of the left eye, the patient is asked to converge the eyes. This action can be performed normally because the center for convergence, which is part of the third-nerve nuclear complex, is not disturbed.

REFERENCES

Daube JR, Sandok, BA: Medical Neurosciences. Boston, Little, Brown, 1978.

Brodel A: Neurological Anatomy in Relation to Clinical Medicine. New York, Oxford University Press, 1981.

Netter FH: Nervous System, part I and II. The Ciba Collection of Medical Illustrations, vol 1. West Caldwell, NJ, Ciba Pharmaceutical Company, 1983.

2

Neurologic History and Examination

History and examination are inseparable. The examination begins the moment the physician is first introduced to the patient. Observations made during the interview are essential and frequently reveal more about the patient's true neurologic deficit than is apparent during the subsequent formal examination. A patient with functional weakness may move all extremities quite appropriately during the history taking but may show profound weakness during the formal examination. Just as the patient is examined through observation during the history, pertinent questions should be asked as one proceeds in an orderly fashion through the examination. At the end of the history taking, the physician should know what the patient has and what the neurologic deficit will be. The formal examination serves to verify this impression and to grade the degree of abnormalities.

Each patient is unique. Although initially the patient should talk about his or her problems spontaneously, sooner or later the physician will have to ask specific questions. Most patients are poor historians because they are not in the habit of recording accurately and precisely their symptoms and signs, nor are they trained to do so. As a matter of fact, as soon as their symptoms or signs have subsided, most patients would rather forget them than dwell on them. The physician needs to recognize that it is the neurotic patient who, preoccupied with his bodily functions, very often gives the best history. In patients who are demented or have altered states of consciousness, observations by relatives, friends, or colleagues are indispensable.

A great obstacle in obtaining valid histories is that patients and physicians do not use the same terminology. The physician, therefore, has to ascertain what patients mean when they use certain terms. Three terms that patients with neurologic problems use rather frequently are "weakness," "dizziness," and "numbness." These words have a variety of different meanings to patients. Only rarely do patients use the term *weakness* to describe loss of strength. What patients most often mean is a general feeling of inertia, lack of energy, or fatigue. Whether or not true lack of strength exists can usually be elicited by asking specific questions, such as, "Can you get up from a chair without using your arms?" "Can you carry and lift objects as easily as you could before?" "When walking up a flight of stairs, do you have to pull yourself up with your hands on the banister?" The term *dizziness* very often describes almost any deviation from feeling normal. It is commonly used to describe vertigo, an ill-defined feeling inside the head, unsteadiness when walking, general fatigue, nervousness, and even depression. A similar multitude of altered sensations may hide behind the term *numbness*. Very often the true nature of a patient's complaint can be ascertained by tactfully asking for a description of symptoms in different terms. If this method does not succeed, the physician should offer different terms and let the patient choose the one that best describes the sensation. Care should be taken not to lead the patient into accepting descriptive terms just to please the physician.

Neurologic disorders may be stable or progressive, but many have superimposed intermittent symptoms or signs, while others are characterized by intermittent symptoms and signs with a normal state between them. An adequate neurologic history, therefore, should include inquiry about the following: onset, character, severity, localization, duration, and frequency of symptoms and signs; associated complaints; precipitating, aggravating, and alleviating factors; progression, remission, and exacerbations; and familial occurrence of similar problems.

While the patient relates the history, the physician should concurrently analyze which part of the nervous system may be involved, what diagnostic possibilities should be considered, and what additional evidence is needed either to confirm or discard preliminary hypotheses.

During the first interview, it is not unusual for patients not to volunteer, or simply not to know, if other members of their family have had similar or other neurologic problems. Consequently, if one suspects that a patient's problem may be hereditary, the patient should again tactfully be asked to inquire more specifically into problems that other members of the family now have or may have had in the past. At times it may even be necessary to interview and examine other family members. Gentle persistence in pursuing the possibility of a hereditary disorder very often will pay off handsomely, thereby avoiding unnecessary expenses and providing the correct diagnosis.

The patient's general behavior, mannerisms, and ability (or lack thereof) to give a coherent history and to respond appropriately to questions will almost invariably reveal whether or not the problem is a psychiatric disorder or a dementing illness. Often, patients with a true memory deficit will not be able to remember that they have a memory problem and therefore will not complain about it. A patient with a memory problem will, however, often display inconsistencies and variability in recounting events, understanding questions, or both. If a patient relates a reasonably consistent history, speaks and understands normally, and responds appropriately to questions, it is unlikely that a disorder of higher cortical functions will subsequently be detected.

Some neurologic disorders manifest themselves in a disturbance of other bodily functions, and the neurologic problem may be only one aspect of a more general illness. Therefore, an inventory of the patient's past medical history is in order. This inventory can be conveniently obtained at the appropriate points in the neurologic history and during the examination. Intimate questions, particularly those related to sexual dysfunction, should probably be asked at the end of the examination, at which time the patient is much more comfortable discussing such problems.

There probably is no best way to conduct a neurologic examination. Very often, the specific situation will dictate how the examination, or some specific tests, are carried out. In most instances the mental status examination follows the history; but in an anxious, insecure patient, it may be better conducted later. There are, on the other hand, certain approaches that make the neurologic examination more logical and more efficient. Regional examination, which includes testing muscle strength, sensation, and muscle stretch reflexes, is much more appropriate than doing each of these examinations separately. For example, a muscle stretch reflex cannot be properly interpreted unless one has completed the motor and sensory examination. Since many neurologic disorders affect only one side of the body, both sides should be examined either simultaneously or in close temporal proximity to provide the best chance of detecting subtle abnormalities. Regardless of which component of the nervous system is tested, the goal is always to establish the least stimulus intensity that will produce a normal response.

Because much of neurologic testing requires the patient's active participation, it cannot be overemphasized how important it is that patients understand what they are being asked to do. In most instances, a simple demonstration of a specific test is understood much more readily than an elaborate verbal description and is thus followed by successful, cooperative performance. Mental status and sensory examinations are unreliable when performed while the patient, the physician, or both are tired or fatigued. Since some of the tools used in the neurologic examination, such as the reflex hammer or a needle, may be frightening, the patient should be informed and reassured before they are used.

In most patients, the following suggested order of examination works well. Mental status examination easily follows the history taking. The patient is then asked to walk; stand tandem; stand on one foot and then the other, with the eyes alternately open and closed; hop on one foot and then the other; squat and get up; and step onto a chair, first with one foot and then with the other. This procedure is followed by examination of the cranial nerves. Next, all the muscles of the upper extremities and sensation are tested, followed by reflex testing. There is little point in doing a formal motor examination of the legs if the patient has performed well on the above tests, because the likelihood of finding an abnormality in this situation is almost zero. If some abnormality is detected, a formal motor examination of the legs is carried out. However, the extensor digitorum brevis should always be examined, because it may be the only muscle involved early in a peripheral neuropathy. Sensory examination and reflex testing of the legs should always be done. At this point, the patient may be asked to undress. Abdominal, cremasteric, and anal reflexes are tested; and a rectal examination and an examination of the heart, lung, and abdomen may be performed. Examination of peripheral blood vessels, including the neck, is done after examination of the cranial nerves and extremities. In this fashion, the general physical examination is readily incorporated into the neurologic examination. During the history taking and the neurologic examination, appropriate observations regarding abnormal movements and physical abnormalities, such as cranial defects and skin lesions, are made.

MENTAL STATUS EXAMINATION

For proper evaluation of a patient's mental status, knowledge of the patient's social, cultural, and educational background is essential. What may be normal for someone with little intellectual endowment may be abnormal for someone with a greater intellectual potential. Although speech is not totally dependent on higher cortical functions, it will be included here. A widely used brief mental status test is the Mini-Mental State Examination (MMSE). The areas of inquiry in a detailed mental status examination are as follows:

1. Level of consciousness
2. Orientation
3. Speech
4. Language
5. Memory
6. General information

7. Calculation
8. Abstraction and judgment
9. Other

Level of Consciousness

Changes in level of consciousness may indicate worsening or improvement of a neurologic condition. The range of altered states of consciousness includes slight drowsiness; obtundation; light coma, in which the patient may be briefly aroused by noxious stimuli; and deep coma, in which even the most noxious stimuli will not produce arousal. Conditions seen in the awake patient include inattention, confusion, delirium, hallucinations, and delusions.

Orientation

A patient is tested for orientation to time, place, and person. Orientation to time is the most tenuous, and it is impaired early in many mild organic brain syndromes. Disorientation to place is seen in moderate disturbances of cerebral function, and impairment of orientation as to person is present with severe cerebral dysfunction.

Speech

Speech is produced by the delicate coordination of respiratory muscles, vocal cords, soft palate, tongue, and lips. Dysfunction in any of these will produce distinctive speech abnormalities. Partial or complete paralysis of one vocal cord produces hoarseness; paralysis of both vocal cords results in aphonia. Dysfunction of the soft palate produces a distinctive, hypernasal speech. The classical pseudobulbar speech, seen in bilateral subcortical lesions, is characterized by hypernasality, slurring of words, and an apparent great effort with reduced output. Patients with multiple sclerosis frequently exhibit "scanning" speech, in which each syllable is pronounced with equal strength and the normal melody of speech (prosody) is lost. In patients with Parkinson's disease, speech becomes very soft and may be barely audible. Most speech abnormalities can easily be detected during conversation with the patient. Lip movements may be tested by asking the patient to say "memememe," tongue movements by "lalalalala" and palatal movements by "gagagaga." In addition, phrases such as "around the rugged rock the ragged rascal ran" may be used. Practically all speech abnormalities except speech apraxia imply peripheral, brainstem, and/or cerebellar dysfunction.

Language

In contrast to speech dysfunction, impairment of the ability to use abstract language symbols implies cortical damage, usually of the dominant hemisphere. Rarely, patients with thalamic lesions will be aphasic. Aphasic patients may have difficulty expressing themselves in speaking or in writing, or they may have difficulty comprehending spoken or written language. Although one of these functions may be prominently impaired, more often than not all four functions are disturbed to some degree. Language comprehension is best tested by asking the patient to follow both spoken and written commands and by determining if the patient comprehends what has been said or written. Language production is tested by asking the patient to talk and write. Eight types of aphasia can usually be recognized. These aphasias and their typical features are listed in Table 2–1.

In patients with Broca's aphasia, the lesion is located in the inferior and posterior portion of the dominant frontal lobe. Patients with this aphasia typically are nonfluent and use substantive words; their speech is slow, produced with great effort, and poorly articulated. There is marked reduction of language output, but comprehension is usually good. The same mistakes are seen when the patient writes. The ability to name objects is also affected frequently. This type of aphasia is usually accompanied by a hemiparesis on the contralateral side that is worse in the arm than in the leg. The patient is aware of the deficit and is frequently frustrated and depressed.

In Wernicke's aphasia, the lesion is located in the posterior and superior portion of the dominant temporal lobe. Language production is fluent, with normal articulation and melody, but is very often empty and studded with errors in word choice or word substitution. The patient's ability to comprehend written and verbal language is impaired. Frequently, writing ability is also impaired, as is the ability to repeat and to name objects. In this type of aphasia, hemiparesis is usually absent. The patient very often does not realize that a deficit exists and, therefore, may appear unconcerned or become paranoid.

In conduction aphasia, the lesion is between Broca's and Wernicke's area. Speech is fluent. The most prominent abnormalities are in repetition and writing. The transcortical aphasias are very similar to Broca's and Wernicke's aphasias, except that repetition is normal. The responsible lesion is adjacent to Broca's area and/or Wernicke's area. Anomic aphasia cannot be localized, but the lesion is often posteriorly located. In global aphasia, all language functions are impaired. The lesion is usually very large, involving frontal, parietal, and temporal areas.

TABLE 2–1. Classification of Common Aphasias

Aphasia	Speech Production	Repetition	Comprehension	Naming	Reading	Writing
Broca's	Impaired	Impaired	Normal	May be impaired	May be impaired	Impaired
Wernicke's	Normal	Impaired	Impaired	Impaired	Impaired	Impaired
Conduction	Normal	Impaired	Normal	May be impaired	Normal	Impaired
Transcortical motor	Impaired	Normal	Normal	May be impaired	May be impaired	Impaired
Transcortical sensory	Normal	Normal	Impaired	Impaired	Impaired	Impaired
Transcortical mixed	Impaired	Normal	Impaired	Impaired	Impaired	Impaired
Anomic	Normal	Normal	May be impaired	May be impaired	Impaired	May be impaired
Global	Impaired	Impaired	Impaired	Impaired	Impaired	Impaired

Memory

Memory is conveniently divided into a hold function, recent memory, and remote memory. The hold function is tested by asking the patient to repeat six to seven digits forward and three to four digits backward. Retention of this information normally is only a few seconds. Recent memory is tested by asking the patient to remember a name and an address, or a short story consisting of no more than four or five sentences, or a set of simple words such as "house, orange, car, love, river." It is important to ask the patient to repeat what is to be remembered to make sure that the information has been properly understood and held. After a few minutes, the patient is asked to repeat what he or she was asked to remember. If the patient cannot remember spontaneously, several choices should be given, including those items that should have been remembered. Many anxious patients who do not remember anything spontaneously will then be able to remember. Remote memory is tested by asking questions about significant national and international events in the past and about significant events in the patient's life. Nonverbal memory is tested by showing the patient several simple geometric figures and later asking the patient to identify them again. The hold function is impaired when a primary sensory receiving area is affected. Impairment of recent memory usually implies bilateral medial temporal lobe dysfunction, whereas impairment of remote memory implies rather widespread and severe brain dysfunction.

General Information

General information should be commensurate with the patient's educational background and interests. This information, once accumulated, is not lost until there is severe loss of brain substance or severe impairment of function. Except for occasional patients who have been totally deprived socially and educationally for a long time, most should be able to name five cities, five rivers, and five animals. Inquiry into the patient's knowledge of his or her specific job may sometimes reveal an early dementia. The main purpose of testing knowledge is to determine if patients have an adequate fund of knowledge in keeping with their stated profession or job and their educational background.

Calculation

The ability to calculate varies rather widely in normal people. Simple additions, subtractions, and multiplications should be avoided, because these are usually overlearned responses that do not test the ability to calculate. Subtractions are more difficult than additions, and divisions are more difficult than multiplications. For most patients, questions have to be simple, such as 4×12, $100 - 7$, $50 \div 2$, or 2×28. More difficult questions would be $3 \times 11\frac{1}{2}$ or $90 \div 18$. Another good test question is to ask the patient how much change will be returned after tendering a $10 bill for three bottles of a soft drink at $.60 each. It should be kept in mind that a significant number of normal persons will not be able to answer this question accurately. Impairment of calculation implies dominant parietal lobe damage.

Abstraction and Judgment

Abstraction and judgment, the ability to project into the future and draw on experience, require intact frontal lobe function. The patient is presented with a proverb, such as, "A stitch in time saves nine," and is asked to interpret it. An appropriate response would be that taking care of a problem as it arises saves a greater effort later. A concrete and abnormal interpretation is that a tear in a garment should be repaired. The patient is then asked to describe in which way apples are different from oranges and in which way they are similar. Another question might be, "What would you do if you found a stamped, addressed letter on the sidewalk?" An appropriate response would be to put it into the next mailbox; an inappropriate response would be to deliver it to the address written on it.

Other Skills

A number of tasks, not covered under any of the previous headings, are useful in demonstrating cognitive, perceptive, and praxis deficits. Ask the patient to demonstrate how to use a comb or pencil. Have the patient pretend to hold a toothbrush and to brush his or her teeth. Ask the patient to follow three-part commands, for example, "Pick up the pen, close your eyes, and then open your mouth." If the patient cannot follow three-step commands, proceed to two-step commands. Have the patient copy simple geometric figures and draw the face of a clock showing 3:45. Ask the patient to identify his or her right ear, left foot, and so on and to point to the examiner's right arm.

A wide range of formal neuropsychological evaluation procedures is available. Two basic approaches to evaluate altered brain functions are utilized. One uses a tailored approach to fit an individual patient's needs; the other uses a battery of standardized neuropsychological tests. The latter approach is more widely used, because abilities are tested systematically and the testing can be done by a trained technician. Patients who are not clearly demented or in whom detailed documentation is needed for sequential observations or treatment purposes should be referred to a behavioral neurologist or neuropsychologist.

EXAMINATION OF HEAD AND NECK

The head and neck are inspected and palpated for abnormalities. The external ear canal and eardrum should always be examined. Bruits are detected by applying a bell-shaped stethoscope lightly at the level of the larynx anterior to the sternomastoid muscle to listen for carotid bruits, at about the same level behind the sternomastoid to listen for vertebral artery bruits, in the supraclavicular fossa to listen for subclavian bruits, and over each eye to listen for bruits originating from stenotic lesions in the internal carotid artery distal to the common carotid bifurcation. When the patient describes abnormal noises, it is advisable to listen over several parts of the head in order to detect bruits from intracranial arteriovenous malformations. A carotid bruit can usually be distinguished from a transmitted cardiac murmur by the fact that it is loudest at the level of the carotid bifurcation and is transmitted distally but not proximally. A great number of noninvasive vascular tests—including tests for Doppler effect, recording of bruits, and ocular plethysmography—are available. These tests are helpful in the evaluation of extracranial vascular disease in the neck. After listening for bruits, the neck may be examined for tender areas in patients with neck complaints; limitations of motion are detected by rotating, flexing, and extending the head in all directions. This part of the examination should be done with great caution or not at all when the possibility of an acute neck injury exists.

CRANIAL NERVES

FIRST CRANIAL NERVE (OLFACTION). One nostril is occluded by the examiner's finger, and the patient is asked to sniff a substance held directly under the other nostril. The substances used may be camphor, ground coffee, or mint. Testing should then be repeated on the other side. The most common reason for a patient's inability to smell is obstruction of the nasal passages, which may have to be opened with a nasal decongestant prior to testing.

CRANIAL NERVES II, III, IV, V, AND VI (VISION, EYE MOVEMENTS, PUPILS). Visual acuity should be tested with a standard visual chart, and a patient who normally wears glasses should wear them during the test. Each eye should be tested separately. The presence of normal visual acuity implies normal central vision. To test peripheral vision, the examiner stands with abducted arms approximately 1 m away from the patient and then asks the patient to cover one eye and look at the examiner's forehead. The examiner then randomly moves a finger on one or both hands in the upper and lower parts of the patient's visual field. The patient is asked to indicate which finger(s) is (are) moving. This procedure is then repeated for the other eye. Lesions of the eye and optic tract will produce visual defects in the visual field of one eye only. Lesions in the optic chiasm in general will produce bilateral but nonhomonymous defects. Any lesion behind the chiasm will produce homonymous defects in both fields of vision.

Pupils should be approximately equal in size and round. Slight asymmetries are normal. When a bright light is flashed into one eye, both pupils should briskly constrict. Pupillary constriction on near vision is tested by asking the patient to look first at a distant object and then at a close object. Eye movements should always be smooth. Both eyes should move in the same direction and at the same speed, except for convergence, where both eyes will move medially. Smooth pursuit movements are tested by having the patient follow the examiner's finger to the extreme left and right in the horizontal plane, as well as up and down in two planes about 30–40 degrees medially and laterally to the primary axis of vision. Saccadic eye movements are tested by asking the patient to look to the extreme right and extreme left, and up and down. When patients complain of double vision, or when abnormalities of eye movements are detected, even though the patient may not complain of double vision, examination and definition of abnormalities are greatly facilitated by using a Maddox rod. This is a red glass that rotates light and produces a red streak. When a normal subject looks at a white light with one eye covered by the red glass, the red streak should always go through the white light in all eye positions. When an eye movement abnormality exists, the relationship will be different. Except during conversion, the image (white or red) that is farthest in the direction of the eye movement is always the abnormal one. For example, if the patient looks to the right with the red glass in front of the left eye and the red streak is to the right of the white light, the left eye is the abnormal one. In this situation, the medial rectus muscle on the left is not functioning properly. The Maddox rod can be conveniently rotated so that the streak will be vertical for testing of horizontal movements and horizontal for testing of vertical movements. Movements of the eyes to the right in the horizontal plane test the right lateral rectus and the left medial rectus. Movements to the left test the left lateral rectus and the right medial rectus. Convergence tests both medial rectus muscles. Movements up and down and to the right test the right superior rectus, right inferior rectus, and left superior and inferior obliques. Movements of the eyes up and down to the left test the left superior and inferior rectus, and the right superior and inferior oblique muscles (see Fig. 2–1).

```
        Right Eye                    Left Eye
   SR           IO              IO           SR


LR  ←————————→ MR  ←————————→ LR


   IR           SO              SO           IR
```

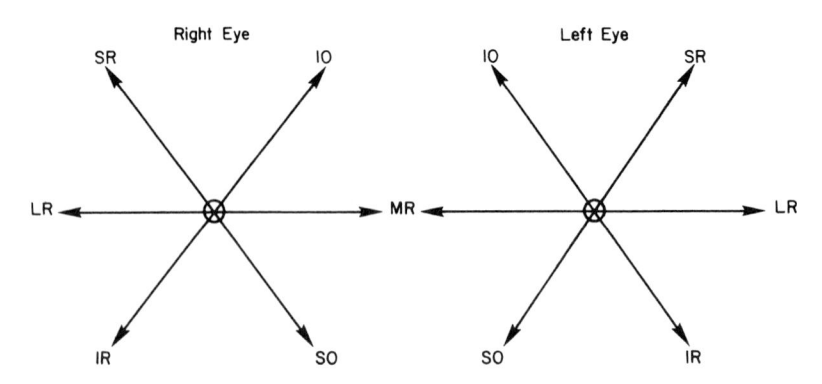

FIGURE 2-1. Cardinal positions of gaze, looking at the subject. Impairment in movement of one or both eyes in the directions indicated suggests weakness of the corresponding muscles. Muscles innervated by the oculomotor or third nerve: MR, medial rectus; SR, superior rectus; IR, inferior rectus; and IO, inferior oblique. Muscle innervated by trochlear or fourth nerve: SO, superior oblique. Muscle innervated by abducens or sixth nerve: LR, lateral rectus.

The corneal reflex is tested by placing a wisp of cotton just in front of the center of the cornea and then gently touching the cornea. The appropriate response is a bilateral blink. Care should be taken in each eye always to place the wisp of cotton on the center of the cornea, because more distal parts of the cornea are less sensitive.

Finally, the patient's fundus is examined. The patient is instructed to look at a distant object with the eye not being examined and is asked to indicate when the examiner's hair or head obstructs vision. If the patient is unable to fixate on a distant object, the eyes will move, and the examination will become unduly difficult. Of particular interest in neurologic diagnosis is the optic disc. The normal optic disc should have a pink color and, in most instances, a physiological cup that varies in size considerably. The temporal disc margins are usually quite sharply outlined, whereas the nasal disc margins, even in normal persons, are often somewhat less distinct. The presence of venous pulsation for all practical purposes excludes papilledema; absence does not necessarily indicate papilledema. In early papilledema, the physiological cup may not be obliterated, but the optic disc margins are blurred and the disc is elevated. Disappearance of blood vessels as they cross the disc margin, followed by their reemergence distally, is a reliable sign of papilledema. Splinter hemorrhages in close proximity to the optic disc frequently accompany papilledema. In optic atrophy, disc margins are unusually sharp, the disc appears pale, and the number of arterioles crossing the disc margin is reduced. Usually three to four small arterioles cross the disc margin between the superior and inferior temporal retinal arteries. Disc pallor is best appreciated by directing the light just slightly away from the disc and then observing the disc.

Ptosis, i.e., drooping of the upper eyelid, indicates third-nerve impairment, whereas narrowing of the palpebral fissure, i.e., lowering of the upper lid and raising of the lower lid, suggests Horner's syndrome, which is accompanied by a small but reactive pupil.

FIFTH CRANIAL NERVE (FACIAL SENSATION AND MASTICATION). Sensation to the face and to the nasal and oral cavities is mediated via the fifth cranial nerve. This nerve has three distinct divisions: ophthalmic, maxillary, and mandibular. Each division is tested separately for appreciation of a lightly applied tactile stimulus and painful stimulus, and the left and right sides are compared. Testing the corneal reflexes as described in the preceding section also tests the fifth nerve. Muscles of mastication are also innervated by the fifth nerve. They are tested by palpation of masseter and temporalis muscles and by asking the patient to keep the mouth closed while the examiner tries to open it.

SEVENTH CRANIAL NERVE (FACIAL MOVEMENTS). All facial muscles are innervated by the seventh nerve and are tested by having the patient show his or her teeth, blow out the cheeks against resistance, close the eyes, and wrinkle the forehead.

EIGHTH CRANIAL NERVE (HEARING AND VESTIBULAR FUNCTION). After examination of the external canal and tympanic membrane, hearing is tested. The examiner produces a high-frequency sound by gently rubbing fingers and notes the distance from the ear at which the patient hears the sound. This type of hearing is frequently reduced in elderly patients and in those exposed to a noisy environment. Low-frequency hearing is tested by placing a large tuning fork on the mastoid process and asking the patient to say when the sound is no longer audible. The tuning fork is then removed and held directly in front of the patient's ear. A normal person should then still hear the sound from the tuning fork for 10 to 15 seconds. Small tuning forks are inappropriate for this test because their decay time is too rapid. When obstruction of the external ear canal is present, the patient will not hear the tuning fork when it is removed from the mastoid process and placed in front of the ear. Vestibular function can be tested by the following method: In the recumbent position, the patient's head is slightly flexed, and each ear is separately irrigated with approximately 5 ml of ice water after inspection of the external ear canal and tympanic membrane. In the awake patient, the normal response is nystagmus with the fast component away from the irrigated ear and the slow component toward the irrigated ear. More precise testing of vestibular function requires specially equipped laboratories.

CRANIAL NERVES IX AND X. These nerves are essential for swallowing and phonation. They are tested by listening for hoarseness as the patient talks and by having the patient swallow a few sips of water. The pharynx and the soft palate are inspected directly; they should contract when a tongue blade is pushed gently against the posterior pharynx on each side separately (gag reflex).

ELEVENTH CRANIAL NERVE. This nerve supplies the ipsilateral sternomastoid and upper trapezius muscles. The patient is asked to rotate the head to one side and to resist the examiner's effort to turn it in the opposite direction. This procedure tests the sternomastoid muscle in the opposite direction of the head movement.

TWELFTH CRANIAL NERVE (TONGUE MOVEMENTS). The patient is asked to stick out his or her tongue and wiggle it from left to right and in and out of the mouth. Atrophy and fasciculations may be observed as the patient rests the tongue in the mouth. In addition, the patient is asked to put his or her tongue into the cheek, while the examiner then attempts to push the tongue back into the mouth.

MOTOR SYSTEM

Any motor act requires the proper function of a multitude of central and peripheral nervous system components. These include the pyramidal and extrapyramidal systems, cerebellum, peripheral nerves (both motor and sensory), neuromuscular junction, and contractile apparatus of the muscle. When examining abnormalities of the motor system, therefore, it is necessary to determine which of these systems is impaired. Dysfunction of the muscle itself will produce weakness and atrophy identical to that seen with anterior horn or peripheral motor nerve lesions. Impaired peripheral or central sensory input and processing produce incoordination of movements. Lesions in the corticospinal and extrapyramidal motor system will produce weakness but little or no atrophy, and very often changes in muscle tone—including spasticity, rigidity, and hypotonia. In addition, extrapyramidal motor system involvement may produce abnormal movements such as chorea, athetosis, hemiballismus, and dystonic posturing. Spasticity is characterized by increasing resistance to the examiner's passive movement of a limb, followed by complete and sudden relaxation of the muscle tested. In rigidity, resistance is about equal throughout the entire range of motion. Lesions in afferent and efferent cerebellar pathways, as well as the cerebellum, will produce irregular movements. Cortical lesions, usually in the parietal lobes, may produce deficits of skilled movements in the presence of well-preserved strength (apraxia).

During the history taking, it will become abundantly clear if skilled motor acts are impaired, because normal people continually move their face, arms, and hands. They shift from one side to the other, and they talk. On formal testing of strength and movements, best results are obtained when the patient is asked to resist the examiner's effort to displace a limb or parts of a limb. Subtle abnormalities in skilled motor acts are detected by asking the patient to tap fingers rapidly, to rotate the hand rapidly, and to touch his or her nose or the examiner's finger.

Testing strength of the upper extremities can be rapidly and accurately done by testing both upper limbs at the same time. With this technique, subtle differences between left and right will readily be detected. The patient is asked to grasp the examiner's finger tightly (finger flexors). Subsequently, the patient is requested to extend his or her fingers and hands to resist the examiner's effort to push fingers and hands down (finger and wrist extensors), push the fists up (wrist flexors), internally rotate the hands (external rotators of the hand or supinators), and externally rotate the hands (internal rotators of the hand or pronators). Next, the patient is asked to resist the examiner's attempt to push the fists downward and outward (arm flexors, internal rotators, and adductors at the shoulder). Finally, the patient resists the examiner's effort to push both fists upward and inward (arm extensor, abductors, and external rotators at the shoulder). Examining the upper extremities in this fashion tests practically all muscles and can be completed in a little more than a minute.

Lower extremity functions can best be assessed by having the patient stand, walk, and hop. When more detailed examination on the basis of an observed abnormality is required, the patient is asked to lift each leg individually and to resist the following movements: downward pressure (hip flexors), pulling the knees apart (thigh adductors), pushing the knees together (thigh abductors), flexion of the leg (leg extensors), straightening of the flexed leg (leg flexors), pushing down the dorsiflexed foot (dorsiflexors), and pulling apart the inverted feet (invertors). Since the gastrocnemius-soleus muscle is very powerful, even significant weakness can rarely be adequately detected by pushing against the patient's plantar-flexed foot. The appropriate test to detect moderate and small degrees of weakness is to have the patient walk on tiptoe. Like the upper extremit muscles, most muscles of the lower extremity can be tested simultaneously, which facilitates detection of a subtle weakness.

Lower Motor Neuron

The lower motor neuron is defined as the anterior horn cell, or the appropriate cranial nerve nucleus, with its motor axons, the neuromuscular junction, and the muscle. A lesion anywhere in the lower motor neuron will produce weakness, atrophy, and fasciculations.

Upper Motor Neuron

The upper motor neuron consists of those pathways that impinge on cranial nerve nuclei and anterior horn cells. Abnormalities in this system will produce minimal to severe weakness, minimal or no atrophy, no fasciculations, frequently increased tone, increased muscle stretch reflexes, and upgoing toes on plantar stimulation.

SENSORY SYSTEM

Light touch, pain, vibration, and position sense are tested in every patient. It is impossible to test every square centimeter of the skin. Usually the face, both the radial and ulnar aspect of the hand, and the feet are tested. For testing light touch, the examiner's finger is an appropriate instrument because the degree of pressure, as well as the area contacted, can be easily controlled. A piece of cotton serves just as well. The lightest stimulus the patient can perceive is determined, and this is compared to normal on the examiner or the patient's normal side. For assessing pain, a sharp pin should be used. Safety pins are inadequate, because they are almost always too dull. Care should be taken not to penetrate the patient's skin. The examiner determines with a pin the lightest pressure that can produce a painful stimulus. All pins need to be discarded after use on one patient. For vibratory perception, a large tuning fork with a long decay time is appropriate, because left and right can readily be tested without too much decay of the tuning fork. When comparing left and right or abnormal and normal areas, great care must always be taken to ensure that the stimulus intensities are identical. The tuning fork is placed on the fingers, toes, ankles, and knees; and differences between normal and abnormal and left and right are observed. In many patients over the age of 60, vibratory perception is significantly diminished in the feet.

When testing position sense, the examiner must make sure that the patient understands precisely how to respond. To accomplish this task best, the examiner holds a finger or toe laterally with the patient looking at it, moves the finger or toe in very tiny steps in an irregular fashion up or down, and then asks the patient to tell whether the toe is being moved up or down. Practically every patient examined in this way will quickly learn how to respond appropriately. At this point, the patient is asked to indicate—with eyes closed—whether the movement is up or down or, if uncertain, to say, "I don't know." If small movements are not properly perceived, the amplitude of the movement should be increased to the point at which the patient's responses are correct.

MUSCLE STRETCH REFLEXES

Muscle stretch reflexes should always be tested after motor and sensory examinations have been completed. In order to obtain maximal information from this testing, the examiner's finger is first placed across the tendon of the muscle to be tested and then hit repeatedly with the reflex hammer to determine the least intensity of the blow that can produce a barely perceptible contraction. The advantage of this method is that it allows the examiner at all times to feel the tension of the muscle, monitor the intensity of the blow, and detect the least degree of contraction—including contractions that may not even be visible. Furthermore, this method does not subject patients to a direct blow from the hammer. Since muscle stretch reflexes have little to do with the tendon, it is unnecessary always to try to hit the tendon. For example, to test the gastrocnemius-soleus reflex in a bedridden patient, the examiner places a hand over the ball of the patient's foot and then strikes the hand with the reflex hammer. This action produces an appropriate stretch of the muscle. Rather than testing all reflexes in one extremity and then moving to the other, it is best to test one reflex repeatedly and then test the homologous reflex in the other extremity. This method greatly facilitates detection of subtle differences. An outline of muscle stretch reflexes and their segmental and peripheral innervation is provided in Table 2–2.

TABLE 2–2. Muscle Stretch Reflexes and Their Segmental and Peripheral Innervation

Muscle	Nerve Root(s)	Peripheral Nerve
Biceps	C5, C6	Musculocutaneous
Brachioradialis	C5, C6	Radial
Triceps	C7, C8	Radial
Quadriceps	L3, L4	Femoral
Medial hamstrings	L5	Sciatic
Lateral hamstrings	S1	Sciatic
Gastrocnemius-soleus	S1, S2	Sciatic (tibial)

OTHER REFLEXES

GLABELLAR REFLEX. The forehead is lightly tapped with the finger, and the patient is observed for blinking of the eyelids. In a normal person, blinking occurs once or twice but then stops, even though the examiner continues to tap the forehead.

POUTING REFLEX. The examiner lightly taps the upper lip in the center. An abnormal response is pouting of the lips.

SUCKING REFLEX. Lips are gently stroked laterally. An abnormal response is a sucking movement of the lips. The sucking, pouting, and glabellar reflexes are not frontal release signs and are seen in many normal elderly subjects. However, they are commonly found in patients with extrapyramidal disorders and other forebrain diseases and suggest emergence of primitive brainstem reflexes.

ABDOMINAL REFLEXES. The patient's abdominal wall is lightly stroked from central to lateral with a tongue blade or a pin. A normal response is contraction of the abdominal muscles, with movement of the umbilicus to the side that was stroked. This reflex is frequently absent in obese persons and in women who have had multiple pregnancies. The reflex is often diminished or absent in upper motor neuron lesions.

CREMASTERIC REFLEX. The inner aspect of the upper thigh is briskly stroked. The normal response is a rapid elevation of the testicle.

ANAL REFLEX. With the patient lying on one side, the buttocks are pulled apart and the perianal area is briskly stroked with a pin. The normal response is a quick contraction of the external anal sphincter.

PLANTAR REFLEX. The patient's foot is firmly stroked from the heel to the ball of the foot laterally. The normal response in subjects older than 1 year is plantar flexion of the toes. The abnormal response consists of dorsiflexion of the big toe, often accompanied by fanning and dorsiflexion of the remaining toes. This abnormal response (Babinski sign) is normally seen in infants up to 8 to 12 months of age. If this maneuver does not produce a response, the lateral dorsal part of the foot may be stroked.

EXAMINATION OF THE COMATOSE PATIENT

The comatose patient should be examined in an organized, efficient manner to determine whether or not he or she is most likely in toxic metabolic coma or in coma secondary to a structural lesion of the CNS. First, the patient's respiration is observed and abnormal patterns noted. If any abnormalities are present, ready accessibility to a mechanical respirator needs to be assured. While the patient's respiration is observed, a needle should be placed in a vein through which blood is withdrawn for appropriate studies. Then 100–200 ml of 10% glucose in water is given to cover the possibility that the patient is hypoglycemic. It is always advisable to simultaneously give 100 mg thiamine. The intravenous needle is kept open with a slow drip of 5% glucose in one-quarter strength saline. Depth of coma is established by applying noxious stimuli and observing if the patient responds. The patient is then examined for evidence of head trauma, which requires palpation of the head and examination of the external ear canals, nose, and pharynx for evidence of bleeding. If the possibility of neck injury exists, care should be taken not to move the patient's head. Next, the patient's eyes are examined; particular emphasis should be placed on position of eyes, size and shape of pupils, pupillary reactions, and corneal responses followed by ophthalmoscopy. If the patient's eyes do not move spontaneously and if neck injury can be absolutely excluded, the patient's head is quickly rotated from one side to the other to observe normal eye movements in the opposite direction of head movement. The patient's head is then flexed and extended and, again, normal eye movements in the opposite direction of head movement are observed. If the eyes do not move with these maneuvers, each ear in turn is irrigated with 5 ml of ice water. In coma the normal response is tonic deviation of both eyes toward the ear stimulated. Facial movements and possible sensory deficits in the distribution of the fifth nerve are checked by applying noxious stimuli to the face and observing presence or absence of appropriate facial movements. The patient's head and extremities are moved to detect increased tone, and then noxious stimuli are applied to determine if these are followed by movements. Next, muscle stretch reflexes and plantar responses are tested. This examination should take no more than 5 to 10 minutes. If no abnormalities are detected, it is extremely unlikely that the patient's coma is due to a structural lesion of the CNS. Only profound endogenous or exogenous intoxication will produce abnormalities on the neurologic examination.

REFERENCES

Folstein MF, Folstein SE, McHugh PR: "Mini-Mental State": A practical method for grading the cognitive state of patients for the clinician. Pychiatr Res 1975; 12:189–198.

Sections of Neurology, Mayo Clinic and Mayo Foundation: Clinical Examinations in Neurology, 4th ed. Philadelphia, WB Saunders, 1976.

DeJong RN: The Neurologic Examination. Hagerstown, MD, Harper, 1979.

Plum F, Posner JB: The Diagnosis of Stupor and Coma, 3rd ed. Philadelphia, FA Davis, 1980.

3

Ancillary Methods of Study

LUMBAR PUNCTURE

Lumbar puncture (LP) was first performed by Quincke in 1891 and has been a mainstay of neurologic diagnosis since. Even today it is the most important tool to diagnose infections of the brain. A computed tomography (CT) scan or magnetic resonance imaging (MRI) of the brain should be performed in most situations prior to LP, except in those cases where the delay of a diagnosis of meningitis would unduly delay institution of appropriate antibiotic treatment.

Meningitis and encephalitis are the major indications for LP. If focal neurologic signs are present, a brain scan should be done expeditiously prior to an LP. When a patient is suspected of having a subarachnoid hemorrhage, a brain scan has to be done first. If the scan is negative for bleeding, an LP is indicated because a small percentage of patients will have blood in the cerebrospinal fluid (CSF). If the scan shows clear evidence of a bleed, an LP is not necessary; in massive bleeds it is contraindicated. Other indications for an LP include multiple sclerosis, pseudotumor cerebri, Guillain-Barré syndrome and other peripheral neuropathies, neurosyphilis, fungal infections, and meningeal carcinomatosis. An LP is also used to inject contrast material and therapeutic agents.

Contraindications include infection at the site of the LP, an intracranial mass lesion, suspected spinal cord compression, papilledema, and bleeding disorders. Platelet counts of less than 15,000 and prothrombin time greater than 15 seconds are relative contraindications and should be corrected prior to LP.

Informed consent must be obtained prior to an LP. A platelet count, prothrombin time (PT), and partial thromboplastin time (PTT) should be obtained prior to all elective LPs. Complications of LP include postspinal headache, bleeding, arachnoiditis, exacerbation of spinal cord compression, cerebral herniation, spinal cord or root injury, infection, and epidermoid tumor. Except for headaches, which occur in about 10% of patients, the other complications are exceedingly rare, and most can be avoided by using proper technique.

Proper positioning of the patient is the single most important aspect of performing a successful LP. The patient is positioned on the side on a firm surface with the back perpendicular to the examination table. The knees are pulled up as far as possible and the head is flexed. Lumbar lordosis must be overcome to open the space between spinous processes; otherwise the needle cannot be inserted in the subarachnoid space. After proper cleansing of the puncture site, a small area between the L4 and L5 spinous processes is anesthetized with 1–2 cc of lidocaine. There is no need to inject lidocaine in the subcutaneous tissue or muscle. An LP should not be attempted above the L3–L4 interspace in adults and L4–L5 in children. The 20 or 22 gauge spinal needle is then inserted, with the stylet in place and the bevel facing up. The needle should be at a right angle to the back and aimed slightly toward the navel. When the needle is advanced 4–5 cm a slight give is often felt when it penetrates the dura mater. The stylet is withdrawn, and if no spinal fluid appears, the stylet is reinserted and the needle is advanced in small steps until spinal fluid is obtained. Sometimes the needle will touch a root in the subarachnoid space, producing pain that may radiate into a leg or the back. Such an occurrence does not indicate failure of the procedure but is sometimes unavoidable. The pain is usually present only momentarily. When firm resistance is encountered, the needle should not be forced. If no spinal fluid can be obtained, the needle should be completely withdrawn and repositioned for another attempt. If three attempts are unsuccessful, it is prudent to ask someone for help. When CSF appears, the patient can relax and straighten the head and legs. The manometer is then attached to the needle and the opening pressure measured. Normal pressure is between 50 and 200 mm CSF. If the pressure is very high, about 2 cc of CSF (sufficient for cell count, glucose, and protein) is obtained and the procedure terminated. Following the procedure, the patient should lie on his or her stomach for about 15 minutes. Maintaining this position for longer periods does not appear to reduce the likelihood of postspinal headache. Postspinal headache is relieved by lying down. If an LP is unsuccessful in the lateral position, it can be tried in the sitting position with the patient bent forward as far as possible. Once the needle is in the subarachnoid, the stylet is replaced and the patient should lie down on his or her side.

Normal CSF is clear and colorless. There is no reliable method of differentiating subarachnoid hemorrhage from bleeding induced by the spinal needle. If there is frank blood in the first CSF sample and subsequent clearing, the bleeding is most likely due to needle trauma. Since practically no LP is ever totally nontraumatic, usually a few red blood cells are found in the CSF. If an individual with normal hemoglobin and red cells has an overtly bloody LP, one can expect 1 white blood cell per 700 red blood cells and 1 mg% protein per 700 red blood cells. Normal CSF contains less than 5 lymphocytes and no polymorphonuclear neutrophils. At steady state, CSF glucose is two thirds of blood glucose. Glucose values of 40 mg or lower are almost always abnormal. Normal CSF protein is greater than 10 mg and less than 50 mg.

In premature and neonatal infants the normal CSF is clear but may be slightly xanthochromic and contains less than 40 white blood cells. In addition, red cells are frequently found, the protein varies between 20 and 150 mg, and the CSF glucose is about equal to plasma levels.

Causes of increased intracranial pressure include tumor, abscess, hemorrhage, head trauma, infection, stroke, hydrocephalus, hypertensive encephalopathy, pseudotumor cerebri, and miscellaneous causes, e.g., congestive heart failure and chronic pulmonary obstructive disease. The presence of polymorphonuclear neutrophils suggests bacterial infections. Increased lymphocytes suggest viral, fungal, parasitic, and tuberculous infections or chronic inflammatory processes. A few white blood cells may also be seen in subarachnoid hemorrhage, stroke, tumor, and demyelinating diseases. Atypical lymphocytes suggest meningeal carcinomatosis or lymphoma, and a cytological examination is indicated. Glucose in the CSF may be decreased in meningitis, subarachnoid hemorrhage, meningeal carcinomatosis, chemical meningitis, sarcoidosis, and systemic hypoglycemia. The CSF protein is elevated in brain and spinal cord tumors, meningitis, encephalitis, arachnoiditis, abscess, spinal subarachnoid block, subarachnoid and intracerebral hemorrhage, neuropathies, neurosyphilis, multiple sclerosis, CNS degenerative disorders, and systemic diseases—e.g., uremia, connective tissue diseases, or myxedema. CSF gamma globulin is increased in multiple sclerosis, neurosyphilis, subacute sclerosing panencephalitis (SSPE), progressive rubella panencephalitis (PRPE), multiple myeloma, monoclonal gammopathies, sarcoidosis, carcinomatous meningitis, and paraneoplastic syndromes. It is occasionally elevated in viral, parasitic, and fungal infections and in collagen vascular diseases involving the CNS.

Tumor cells may be identified on cytological examination. Stains and cultures are requested whenever a CNS infection is suspected. Antigen and antibody titers are helpful in diagnosing fungal and viral infections.

NERVE CONDUCTION STUDIES AND ELECTROMYOGRAPHY

Nerve conduction studies and electromyography (EMG) are useful in the diagnosis of muscle disease and diseases of the neuromuscular junction—e.g. myasthenia gravis, peripheral neuropathies—including radiculopathies—and anterior horn cell disease. These techniques are of limited value in spinal cord diseases. Often these electrical tests provide objective evidence of a lesion. There are few contraindications except local skin infections, and some patients cannot tolerate the discomfort associated with electrical stimulation and needle examination of muscles. Complications, e.g., hematoma and infection, are exceedingly rare.

Nerve conduction studies are used to assess motor and sensory latencies, conduction velocities, and certain other parameters—e.g., H reflex and F wave. Slowing of conduction velocities and increased latencies are seen with demyelinating disorders. When the primary pathology is loss of axons, conduction velocities and latencies do not change; but the summated action potential, sensory or motor, is decreased in amplitude. In proximal disorders, e.g., plexopathies and radiculopathies, the H reflex and the F-wave latencies and velocities may be decreased. Repetitive stimulation studies are useful in evaluation of disorders of neuromuscular transmission.

In EMG a small needle is inserted in muscles and insertional, resting, and voluntary electrical activity of the muscle is studied. Some insertional activity is normally present due to direct irritation of muscle fibers. Prolonged insertional activity is observed in denervated muscle, and decreased or absent activity is seen in severe muscle atrophy where muscle tissue is replaced by connective tissue and fat. Normal spontaneous activity, when the needle is not moved and the muscle is relaxed, is seen when the tip of the needle is near neuromuscular junctions. Fibrillation potentials and positive sharp waves are seen in the resting muscle when the muscle is denervated and also in primary muscle disorders. These potentials first appear 14 to 20 days after anterior horn cell damage or proximal nerve injury and 7 to 14 days after facial nerve injury. Abnormal high-frequency discharges are most commonly seen in patients with myotonic muscular dystrophy but may also occur in certain lower motor neuron disorders. Fasciculation potentials are spontaneous discharges of motor units and are most often seen in anterior horn cell disease. Fasciculations are frequently visible through the skin as small muscle twitches. Patients with anterior horn cell disease almost always do not feel these twitches. So-called benign fasciculations, commonly seen in athletes and people who have recently increased their physical activities, are always felt by the individual. The electrical activity of muscle fibers of a single motor unit, which lie within the recording range of the needle electrode, represent the motor unit potential. With increasing volitional effort, more and more motor units are recruited. A weak effort by the patient or an upper motor lesion produces few, slowly firing motor unit potentials. Decreased numbers of motor unit potentials, firing rapidly, are seen in certain peripheral neuropathies and anterior horn cell disease. Individual motor unit potentials are polyphasic and of small amplitude and short duration in primary muscle disorders. In contrast, in chronic motor neuropathies individual potentials are polyphasic and of large amplitude and long duration.

ELECTROENCEPHALOGRAPHY

Electroencephalography has been used in clinical practice for over 50 years. Introduction of new techniques has changed its place in the evaluation of clinical problems. Yet even today, it is an indispensable tool because it is one of the few tests that reflects ongoing activity of the brain rather than static anatomical changes. Unlike the electrocardiogram (ECG), which records the electrical activity of a rather uniform muscle and a simple conduction system, the electroencephalogram (EEG) reflects the ongoing activity of many billion brain cells. In light of this, it is surprising how much specific information the EEG can provide when appropriately applied, although one might expect little useful information because of the complexity of the multitude of generators within the brain. Electroencephalographic activity largely reflects summated postsynaptic potentials rather than axonally conducted spike discharges. Electrical activity as generated in the brain is severely attenuated by the skull and scalp and has to be amplified approximately 1 million times in order to visualize potentials in the 20–60 uV range. Surface scalp electrodes can only record electrical activity that is no more than a few centimeters underneath the skull. Therefore, large portions of the brain buried in its sulci, deep brain nuclei, or brainstem are not accessible for surface recording. In abnormal states, however, disturbances in these deep structures may secondarily affect more superficially located cortex activity that can be recorded from the scalp. Different parts of the brain produce different patterns of electrical activity and, consequently, recording has to be made from many surface locations. Electroencephalographic patterns change profoundly during development and do not approach the adult pattern until the late teenage years or early twenties. Interpretation of EEG, therefore, takes into account the changing patterns related to age; the different locations of different electrical activity; and the changing patterns associated with alertness, drowsiness, and sleep.

Since many EEG abnormalities occur transiently, a certain minimum recording period is essential. For practical purposes, it is approximately 0.5–1 hour, because the yield of detecting transient abnormalities beyond this amount of time is rather small and is required only in certain special situations, such as monitoring epileptiform abnormalities. The EEG is very much prone to the intrusion of noncerebral activity, including electrical field changes generated by the heart and body, tongue, and eyes. Resultant electrical activity recorded from the surface of the scalp is so overwhelming at times that the recognition of brain waves is impossible; at other times, noncerebral artifacts are subtle and may be mistaken for abnormal brain waves. It is for this reason that a highly trained EEG technologist is indispensable not only to assure the technical adequacy of an EEG but also to monitor patients' behavior and movements during the recording session. Electroencephalographic reports emanating from laboratories that do not employ highly trained technologists are, therefore, of dubious value.

In the adult, the typical brain rhythm of the normal EEG during relaxed wakefulness is the alpha rhythm, which has a frequency of approximately 8–12 cps and is usually maximal in amplitude over the posterior portions of the head. There is very little asymmetry between recording from the left and the right side. Some minimal activity in the frequency range of 0.5–3 cps (delta waves), in the frequency range of 7 cps (theta waves), and in the frequency range of 13–30 cps (fast activity) is seen in most normal people. During drowsiness and sleep, the normal alpha activity first attenuates, then disappears, and is finally replaced by specific wave patterns characteristic of different depths of sleep. During sleep, the brain goes through a sequence of different stages that are repeated 4 to 6 times every night. In routine electroencephalography, short sleep studies are helpful in detecting transient epileptiform abnormalities that may not be seen during the alert wakeful stage. Periods of hyperventilation and photic stimulation are used for the same purpose. Prolonged EEG monitoring in certain epileptic patients and for detection of sleep apnea is done only in specialized laboratories.

In the interpretation of EEG, the most important question to be answered is, "Is the abnormality generalized or focal?" When a generalized abnormality is persistent, it may show an abundance of theta waves compatible with a variety of early toxic metabolic disturbances of brain function. In more severe conditions of this nature, the generalized abnormality usually consists of delta waves or an intermixture of theta and delta waves. Generalized delta waves may also suggest rather widespread cortical destruction, usually secondary to ischemic or anoxic necrosis. Some generalized abnormalities, such as triphasic waves, suggest hepatic coma or, at times, uremic encephalopathy. Persistent generalized epileptiform activity (spike and waves and multispike and wave discharges) are compatible with status epilepticus and may also be seen as an ominous sign in patients with severe postanoxic encephalopathy. Intermittent generalized abnormalities that consist of spikes and waves and multispikes and waves suggest an underlying epileptiform disorder. Intermittent generalized rhythmic delta waves, which frequently are more prominent over the anterior than the posterior head regions, are compatible with dysfunction of deep subcortical structure, including the brainstem. Focal abnormalities may consist of persistent or intermittent theta waves, delta waves, or more specific discharges such as spikes or spikes and waves. A persistent focal increase in theta waves is suggestive of an underlying destructive process that is still rather small in size; but it may also be seen in late EEG recordings after a focal infarct or, in some patients, is suggestive of an epileptogenic focus. Persistent focal delta waves are almost always associated with an underlying destructive process, such as a tumor or an infarct. It should be noted that such a focal abnormality in a patient with a stroke will be apparent immediately after the stroke has occurred, whereas a focal lesion on the CT or MRI scan may not be visualized until 24 to 48 hours after the acute event. Persistent focal epileptiform activity is usually associated clinically with focal status epilepticus. Persistent, rather widespread, but almost always strictly unilateral epileptiform activity and delta waves are often seen in patients with acute stokes or relatively large underlying tumors. Intermittent focal abnormalities, such as spikes, spike and wave discharges, multispike and wave discharges, and rhythmic intermittent delta waves strongly suggest the existence of an underlying epileptogenic focus.

The principal value of the EEG is in detecting functional abnormalities. Its value is vastly enhanced when the electroencephalographer is provided with good clinical information and is asked specific questions that the EEG may be able to answer. Historically, the EEG is most often used in the evaluation of patients with epilepsy. It is still extremely useful in this situation and may strengthen or corroborate clinical information; detect whether a patient has a focal or a generalized seizure disorder; and, on occasion, when an abundance of electroencephalographic seizures are present in the EEG, serve as a guide in therapy. The EEG should be ordered in all situations in which there is a transient change in a patient's behavior, even though it may be very subtle. The EEG is an invaluable tool in assessing children with behavior disorders, because children may not be able to give an accurate history. Because the EEG is only a very short sample (usually 0.5 hour) a normal EEG does not exclude a seizure disorder, because neither seizures nor spike discharges on the EEG occur all the time. In special situations, it may be worthwhile either to obtain a prolonged EEG recording or a repeat EEG or to use activation procedures such as hyperventilation, photic stimulation, and recording during sleep. Another setting in which the EEG may provide valuable clinical information, but in which it is unfortunately totally underused, is in the evaluation of patients in coma. In this situation, the EEG very often may give a clue as to whether or not the coma is due to a toxic-metabolic disturbance of brain functionor secondary to a destructive process. Furthermore, in some situations the EEG abnormality may clearly indicate that a patient is suffering from a rather specific encephalopathy, such as that observed secondary to liver or renal failure. The EEG can also be used to determine whether a patient is in the postictal state following a series of seizures. The presence of an abundance of fast activity in the EEG usually suggests an overdose of one of the barbiturates. In coma secondary to overdose with other drugs, the EEG usually shows nonspecific, generalized abnormalities. Since therapeutic paralysis of patients to aid in proper ventilation is quite common in adults, children, and infants, the EEG may be the only tool for monitoring brain function. In this situation, particularly in children, nonrecognized epileptiform abnormalities may be readily seen. In some situations, the level of coma may be monitored with the help of the EEG. Another area in which the EEG is increasingly important is in the evaluation of elderly patients with impairment of higher cortical function. In this particular setting, it is a good tool to screen patients for toxic-metabolic disturbances secondary to endogenous problems or exogenous intoxications, including iatrogenic drug overdose. In this situation the EEG will frequently suggest the possibility of structural brain lesions, including tumors. Although CT and MRI scans are indispensable in the evaluation of patients with acute head trauma, the EEG nevertheless has a place here too. It is helpful in detecting posttraumatic epilepsy and may be used when a patient is comatose to monitor the level of coma. Total absence of any cerebral electric activity in a profoundly comatose patient who has no brainstem reflexes and is not intoxicated is compatible with brain death if the findings persist for a period of 24 hours.

In general, the EEG is of little help in the evaluation of patients with headaches that have been present for decades. If the EEG is used primarily for the purpose of detecting functional abnormalities, then it is extremely helpful in providing the clinician with specific information that cannot be obtained with any other test.

In the last decade, brain mapping, because of easily available technology, has become rather popular. Without a doubt it can be a valuable adjunct to routine EEG in the hands of electroencephalographers trained in this new area. Its value in day-to-day practice, however, has not yet been established.

EVOKED POTENTIALS

Sensory stimulation (electrical, acoustic, visual) produces evoked electrical potentials in the peripheral and central nervous system. These potentials, when recorded from skin overlying the spinal cord or brain, are of such low amplitude that they can be recorded only by averaging the response to a large number of stimuli. Sensory stimuli sequentially activate rostral sensory pathways, each producing a distinct potential, which frequently allows precise anatomical localization of a lesion. The most common clinical application is in patients with suspected multiple sclerosis, in which these tests may indicate sublinical lesions. In addition to diagnostic purposes, evoked potentials are used in intraoperative monitoring. In common use are somatosensory evoked potentials (SSEP), brainstem auditory evoked potentials (BAEP), and visual evoked potentials (VEP).

NEURORADIOLOGY

Neuroradiology is a specialty with an array of sophisticated and efficient procedures that permit visualization of almost all gross anatomical abnormalities of the CNS and many physiological and dynamic disturbances. Plain skull films are rarely used today but may yield important information about fracture lines, abnormalities of sutures, congenital malformations, and abnormalities of the bone matrix.

Noninvasive Ultrasonography

Ultrasound examination of the carotid arteries in the neck is now a common procedure. Most commonly, pulsed Doppler technique, together with frequency analysis, is used for examination of the carotid arteries in the neck. Frequency analysis of the reflected sound results in a good assessment of blood flow rate in the examined segment of the artery. When blood traverses a stenosed segment of an artery, blood flow rate is markedly increased. When B-mode ultrasound scanning and the Doppler flow examination are combined into "duplex scanning," a very good estimate of the anatomical integrity and the patency of the lumen can be obtained. There are several sources of error and shortcomings inherent in all ultrasound examinations of the carotid arteries, e.g., short and thick neck, inability to distinguish between complete occlusion and severe stenosis of carotid arteries, and inability to assess the vertebrobasilar vasculature. Transcranial Doppler studies are technically feasible and are becoming more reliable in estimating intracranial blood flow. Transcranial Doppler B-mode ultrasound scanning is very reliable in the diagnosis of intracerebral hemorrhages in newborns and infants.

Cerebral Angiography

Cerebral angiography accurately shows the vascular anatomy of the brain. Vessels with a diameter as small as 0.1–0.2 mm can be made visible. Angiography clearly demonstrates almost all vascular abnormalities, such as displacement, stretching and deformation of arteries and veins, abnormal vasculature in malignant tumors or arteriovenous malformations, and intracranial aneurysms and accompanying arterial spasm. Interventional angiography is successfully used for patients with arteriovenous malformations and fistulae. Intravascular catheters are used to selectively perfuse certain brain tumors with chemotherapeutic agents. In addition, angioplastic procedures are being developed to dilate stenosed carotid arteries in the neck. Cerebral angiography is an invasive technique and thus carries a certain risk. Morbidity is 1–3%; this rate includes reactions to the contrast medium, hematomas in the groin, and strokes, most of which are fortunately minor and usually reverse. The use of digital subtraction angiography can reduce the amount of contrast injected by about 60% to 75%, make catheter placement much less critical, and thus shorten the examination time. All these factors reduce complications, make the examination more comfortable for the patient, and allow it to be performed on an outpatient basis. Digital subtraction angiography is suitable for visualization of the carotid arteries in the neck and for overviews of the intracranial circulation. Full-scale angiography is needed for precise visualization of the carotid bifurcation and intracranial vasculature.

Computed Tomography

Computed tomography (CT) enables the examiner to distinguish very small differences in density between various tissues and fluids. In head trauma, CT will show extracerebral and intracerebral hematomas, cerebral edema, and herniation of the brain. It is also an excellent technique to visualize nontraumatic intracerebral hematomas. Approximately 80% of cerebral infarcts can be detected, but they are usually not visualized until 2 to 3 days after the clinical event. Arterial aneurysms can be detected, provided their diameter is greater than 4–5 mm. Curvilinear calcifications and dilated vascular spaces suggest the presence of arteriovenous malformations. Localized inflammatory processes are shown with a high degree of accuracy. The detection rate of primary and secondary brain tumors is about 90%. About 5% of all brain tumors are low-grade astrocytomas, which have a density similar to that of the surrounding brain, do not enhance following contrast injection, exert no mass effect, and are thus missed by CT. Similarly, small aneurysms and small tumors in the posterior fossa and pituitary tumors may be missed because of their location adjacent to the dense skull base.

Magnetic Resonance Imaging

Magnetic resonance imaging (MRI) uses magnetic properties of protons to create images of biological tissues. No biological hazards from MRI have been recorded to date, and the patients are not exposed to any form of ionizing radiation. MRI determines proton density, i.e. hydrogen density, and proton relaxation time factors known as T1 and T2. These factors are primarily responsible for tissue characterization in the images. MRI also detects and determines the rate of flow of fluids, such as blood and CSF. Soft tissue distinction is much better on MRI than on CT. Different tissue types render signals of widely varying strength. On T1 weighted images, fat, brain tissue, and old hematomas deliver relatively strong signals; on the other hand, CSF, cartilage, calcifications, and bone give off weaker signals. Signal intensities can be modified by adjustment of the radiofrequency pulse sequence. Since bony structures give off almost no signal, there is no disturbing influence on the images, in contrast with CT. MRI is the most versatile and powerful technique for imaging the brain.

Intracranial neoplasms down to about 5 mm are almost always well visualized. Tumors of the brainstem and the cerebellum are particularly well seen. Ischemic cerebral infarcts usually show within 6 to 12 hours of the clinical event. Acute hemorrhages are sometimes difficult to delineate because the signal intensity of hemoglobin is similar to that of brain tissue. MR scans readily shown inflammatory lesions but give poor images of healed, calcified inflammatory foci.

MRI is excellent in showing abnormalities of the white matter, e.g., in multiple sclerosis. Small, numerous white matter lesions are commonly seen in older persons. Some of these lesions are due to intracerebral small vessel disease, and others represent foci of demyelination of uncertain etiology. MR angiography is becoming more refined and presently is an excellent tool for screening for vascular disease in the neck and head. Limitations of MRI are mainly due to its relative inability to detect acute hematomas and calcifications. Contraindications to MR examination are patients with surgically implanted metallic devices such as pacemakers. Further, severely ill patients attached to monitors and other equipment with ferromagnetic components cannot be examined.

Plain film radiography of the spine still has its place in the neuroradiological armamentarium. Plain films demonstrate bony structures and soft tissue calcifications, and they permit excellent visualization of all major abnormalities of the spine, e.g., scoliosis, kyphosis, congenital malformations, and degenerative diseases. Radioisotope bone scans are more reliable than plain films for detection of areas of bone destruction.

Plain radiographic myelography is still used occasionally, but most often in conjunction with CT scanning. With CT, critical bony and soft tissue features of many spinal disorders can be visualized. In lumbar intervertebral disc disease, CT will show both the herniated disc and the compression of the thecal sac or the nerve roots. In metastatic disease to the spine, CT is able to demonstrate areas of bone destruction and extension of the lesion into the spinal canal. CT is indispensable in spinal trauma. Fractures of vertebral bodies and neural arches are accurately shown, as are bony fragments and foreign bodies within the spinal canal. CT of the spine will not show intrinsic spinal cord abnormalities. Furthermore, it is not possible to distinguish postoperative scars from recurrent disc herniation or other soft tissue masses. MRI of the spine, with contrast material, allows differentiation between scar tissue and other soft tissues. In addition, the quality of the intervertebral discs can be assessed. Healthy discs have a high water content and consequently produce a high MRI signal on T2 weighted images. In contrast, aging, degenerated discs become desiccated and lose their signal intensity. Furthermore, MRI allows direct visualization of the spinal cord.

NEUROPSYCHOLOGICAL TESTING

The field of neuropsychological testing is complex. No agreement exists on which method of testing the behavioral correlates of brain function is optimal. At one extreme is the tailored approach, which suits the needs of the individual patient. At the other extreme is the psychometric approach, in which an assortment of established tests is administered to all patients. Most neuropsychological testing will include the Minnesota Multiphasic Personality Inventory (MMPI) to assess the potential influence of psychopathology on test performance. Each approach has advantages and disadvantages. Regardless of approach, neuropsychological testing can provide a reliable inventory of the behavioral manifestations of brain disorders and thus is useful in neurologic diagnosis, in treatment planning, and in monitoring treatment and illness outcome. If neuropsychological testing appears indicated, the optimal choice is to refer the patient to a neurologist with special expertise in the field of behavioral neurology.

REFERENCES

Kooi KA: Fundamentals of Electroencephalography. New York, Harper, 1971.

Epstein BS: The Spine: A Radiological Text and Atlas, 4th ed. Philadelphia, Lea and Fiegiger, 1976.

Aminoff MJ: Electromyography in Clinical Practice. Menlo Park, CA, Addison-Wesley, 1979.

Fishman RA: Cerebrospinal Fluid in Diseases of the Nervous System. Philadelphia, WB Saunders, 1980.

Johnson ML, Rumack CM: Ultrasonic evaluation of the neonatal brain. Radiol Clin North Am 1980; 18(1):117–31.

Kiloh LG, McComas AJ, Osselton JW, Upton, ARM: Clinical Electroencephalography, 4th ed. London, UK, Butterworth, 1981.

Halliday AM (ed): Evoked Potentials in Clinical Testing. Edinburgh, UK, Churchill Livingstone, 1982.

Chiappa KH: Evoked Potentials in Clinical Medicine. New York, Raven Press, 1983.

Goodgold J, Eberstein A: Electrodiagnosis of Neuromuscular Diseases, 3rd ed. Baltimore, Williams and Wilkins, 1983.

Kimura J: Electrodiagnosis in Diseases of Nerve and Muscle: Principles and Practice. Philadelphia, FA Davis, 1983.

Kramer DM: Principles of magnetic resonance imaging. Radiol Clin North Am 1984; 22(4):765–78.

Stockard JJ, Iragui VJ: Clinically useful applications of evoked potentials in adult neurology. J Clin Neurophysiol 1984; 1:159–202.

Adams, JP, Kassell NF, Torner JC: Usefulness of computed tomography in predicting outcome after aneurysmal subarachnoid hemorrhage: A preliminary report of the cooperative aneurysm study. Neurology 1985; 35:1263–7.

Bradley WG, Adey WR, Hasso AN: Magnetic Resonance Imaging of the Brain, Head and Neck. Rockville, MD, Aspen Publishing Co, 1985.

Foley WD, Milde MJ: Intra-arterial digital subtraction. Radiol Clin North Am 1985; 23(2):293–319.

Grant EG: Duplex ultrasonography: Its expanding role in non-invasive vascular diagnosis. Radiol Clin North Am 1985; 23(3):563–582.

Latchaw RE: Computed Tomography of the Head, Neck and Spine. Chicago, Year Book Medical Publishers, 1985.

Spehlmann R: Evoked Potential Primer. Boston, Butterworth, 1985.

Cracco RG, Bodis-Woller I (eds): Evoked Potentials. New York, Alan Liss Inc., 1986.

Modic MT, Masaryk TJ, Paushter DM: Magnetic resonance imaging of the spine. Radiol Clin North Am 1986; 24(2):229–245.

4
Headache

Headache is one of the most common symptoms for which patients consult physicians. It has a marked emotional component, and its significance for the patient is greatly increased because of the fear that it may be caused by a brain tumor. Even though 90% of all headaches are not due to serious illness, a small percentage are of sinister nature with potentially disastrous consequences. Therefore, many physicians are ill at ease dealing with patients suffering from headaches. Much of this anxiety can be relieved by taking a careful history followed by examination, at times laboratory studies, and prudent management. The single most important feature of the evaluation of a patient with headaches is the history.

The vast majority of patients with headaches from serious intracranial disease do not complain of headache alone but almost invariably have other symptoms and neurologic signs that suggest the correct diagnosis. More often than not, the character of the headache is nonspecific. Headache of sudden onset and brief duration, of exceptional severity, accompanied by neurologic abnormalities, an organic mental syndrome, altered state of consciousness, or following trauma or convulsions, often suggests intracranial disease. Headache of recent onset superimposed on a long history of another type of headache is indicative of intra- or extracranial pathology.

HISTORY

Since headaches are often an expression of systemic or local diseases, a general health history is essential. In addition, inquiry should be made into (1) type of pain; (2) location of pain; (3) aggravating and alleviating factors; (4) onset, progression, and duration; (5) age of onset; (6) family history; and (7) current medications, substances, alcohol, cigarettes, and caffeine.

The type of pain may be pressurelike, pulsating, stabbing, burning, lancinating, or bandlike. Throbbing headaches are usually vascular in origin, but cluster headaches are almost always nonthrobbing. A number of drugs can precipitate throbbing, pounding headaches; these include nitrites, hydralazine, alphaadrenergic agonists, nicotine, caffeine, histamine, MAO inhibitors, alcohol, quinidine, and potentially any drug that can affect the cerebral vasculature. Tension-type headaches are frequently described as pressurelike or bandlike pains. Brief lancinating pains occur in trigeminal neuralgia. Burning-type pain often occurs in the setting of cranial neuralgias or thalamic lesions. The acute pain accompanying subarachnoid hemorrhage is often described by patients as the worst headache of their life. Although none of the different types of pain is highly specific, knowledge of them often provides clues to their etiologies. Sharply localized pain often occurs in the setting of diseases of the eyes, ears, teeth, or sinuses. An exception to that is cluster headaches, in which the pain is usually most intense in one eye and is often accompanied by lacrimation and stuffiness of the nose. Migraine-type headaches are often unilateral, while tension-type headaches are usually bilateral but may be predominantly frontal, occipital, or temporal. In migraine headaches the pain is often perceived as much worse when exposed to bright lights or loud noises, and patients have a tendency to retire to a quiet and dark room. Acute sinus headaches may be worse when lying down and may be aggravated by blowing the nose. Headache from meningeal irritation is aggravated by neck flexion. Chewing worsens the pain of temporomandibular joint disease. Trigeminal neuralgia pain is often brought on by chewing or any contact with lips or cheek. In some patients with temporal arteritis, chewing may lead to bilateral jaw pain (claudication). A whole host of environmental factors—including certain foods, drugs, organic solvents, gases, and other toxins—may aggravate or produce headaches. Stress at times may exacerbate tension and migraine headaches, but both of these types occur without any overt stress. The type of headache that awakens the patient from a sound sleep is most commonly a cluster or migraine headache. The onset of the headache associated with subarachnoid hemorrhage is abrupt, while migraine headaches usually progress to their peak within 0.5 to 1 hour; tension-type headaches have an insidious onset and then fluctuate in intensity from day to day and from week to week. Knowing under what circumstances the headache started may provide a clue to the etiology. Migraine headaches usually last for a day or two, while tension headaches frequently last weeks or are present all the time with varying intensity. Age of onset of headaches is important to know; migraine headaches frequently start in the second or third decade of life, although they may start during the first decade or even as late as the sixth decade. Even though headaches that have their onset after the age of 50 may still be migraine or tension-type, one should be much more concerned in this age group about temporal arteritis, stroke, transient ischemic attacks (TIAs), cerebral hemorrhage, subarachnoid hemorrhage, brain tumor, and glaucoma. Tension headaches often make their appearance late in teenage years. A positive family history is found in the majority of patients with migraine. Because migraine headaches fluctuate widely in their frequency, patients sometimes are not aware of the fact that their parents suffered from these headaches. Cluster-type headaches have a very strong family history and are almost invariably seen in men. In many patients with tension-type headaches, a positive family history can also be obtained. Inquiry into use of drugs is important because the extremely wide use of prescription, nonprescription, and recreational drugs may produce headaches, either through use or withdrawal from them.

EXAMINATION

Besides a general medical examination, which may detect systemic illnesses, examination of all cranial structures, including cranial nerves, is of great importance. Even though palpation of the skull rarely provides any clues to the etiology of headaches, it should be done routinely; more often than not, patients will spontaneously say, "You are the first doctor who ever put your finger on where my problem really is." Pressure on the external ear canal may aggravate the pain associated with otitis media, and tapping with a finger on the frontal and maxillary sinuses often aggravates acute pain from sinusitis. Touching a patient's tongue, lips, or face may precipitate the pain of trigeminal neuralgia. Unfortunately, in many patients with proven temporal arteritis one cannot palpate a tender nodular temporal artery. If one suspects that a patient's head pain may be related to root canal disease, tapping of the teeth with a metal tool will aggravate the pain associated with that condition. Funduscopy is helpful in detecting subarachnoid hemorrhage, pseudotumor cerebri, acute papillitis, optic neuritis, and other intracranial processes leading to headaches. Detailed neurologic examination of all cranial nerves, including smell, may point to central or peripheral nervous system etiologies. Granted, in the majority of patients with headaches no abnormalities will be found; nevertheless, a normal neurologic and general examination of the head is helpful in narrowing the etiological possibilities. Head pain primarily caused by disease of the cervical spine is not common, but a routine examination in a patient with headaches should include testing for range of motion of head and neck.

Work-up of Patients with Headaches

There is no standard work-up for patients with headaches; the procedure has to be individualized. The vast majority of patients with headaches will have migraine and/or tension-type headaches, requiring no further work-up. Patients with headaches and neurologic symptoms and signs or patients with obvious local pathology require further work-up. Headache that is steadily worsening or is changing in character should be considered for further work-up. CT and MRI are helpful in detecting brain tumors, hydrocephalus, abscesses, infarctions, hemorrhages, sinusitis, and other focal abnormalities. Plain x-rays of the skull and neck are of limited usefulness but can be helpful in patients with platybasia, basilar impression, sinusitis, and cervical spine disease. The EEG is useful only in patients suspected of having encephalopathies or seizures. An LP is mandatory if one suspects a CNS infection. An LP is also important in patients with pseudotumor cerebri and in normal pressure hydrocephalus. Other laboratory tests are indicated only if a specific etiology is suspected that may reveal its nature by such tests. Consultations with other specialists and dentists are often helpful in ruling out certain specific diseases and should be freely used.

CLASSIFICATION

Even though the specific etiology and pathogenesis of most headaches are unknown, it is helpful in the management of patients with headaches to use some classification. The classification provided here (see Table 4–1) may appear overwhelming but it has the advantage of being rather inclusive and may serve as a guideline for diagnosing rare but possibly treatable conditions. Many patients suffer from more than one type of headache, the most frequent combination being migraine and tension-type headache.

TREATMENT

General Considerations

Headache is a common affliction often ignored or belittled by both the family and the treating physician. The most commonly encountered types of headaches are chronic and intermittent in nature and should be dealt with like any other chronic medical condition. Both the physician and the patient with headaches have to accept that most headaches cannot be cured but that the pain can often be aborted, lessened, or prevented. Since many patients are fearful that their headache is caused by a brain tumor, each patient needs to be reassured that this is not the case. The history, examination, and—if necessary—further work-up will lead to a diagnosis, on the basis of which a rational treatment plan should be designed. Realistic treatment goals have to be established and communicated to the patient. In patients with obvious disease, e.g., otitis media or root canal disease, the medical or surgical treatment required is straightforward and the pain need be treated with analgesics only. Patients with headache disorders should be seen and reexamined at regular intervals, the frequency of which should be specific to the patient's needs. The first goal of treatment is to eliminate or minimize factors that precipitate or aggravate headaches. For example, in patients with migraine who smoke, abstinence from any form of nicotine often leads to a dramatic reduction in the frequency and severity of headaches. The second goal is to treat the pain symptomatically. In patients with infrequent headaches this may be all that is required. On the other hand, in patients with frequent and disabling headaches prophylactic treatment should be attempted. Early symptomatic treatment of headaches is often as important as the specific therapy used. Most patients will already have experience with taking different analgesics but may not have taken enough or have taken them too late. Often, two or three aspirins or acetaminophen tablets at the beginning of a headache are more beneficial than a handful when the headache has been present for hours and has become intolerable. The first drug to be used should always be a simple analgesic, which, if taken early, may be all that is required. More potent analgesics can always be added later. Oral narcotics should be avoided in outpatients, because patients become rapidly tolerant and require larger and larger doses. Abortive or prophylactic drug therapy is used in patients with migraine, cluster headaches, paroxysmal hemicrania, postherpetic neuralgia, glossopharyngeal neuralgia, and trigeminal neuralgia. Patients who experience nausea and/or vomiting with their headaches are helped with the addition of antiemetics. Patients who are extremely anxious or depressed will benefit from anxiolytic agents and antidepressants. It will become clear from the following discussion that there is no single approach or drug that is invariably effective in the management of patients with headaches. Because there are no specific markers for any of the common headache types, diagnostic accuracy is not great, and it is not surprising that specificity of drug treatment is low.

SPECIFIC HEADACHES

Migraine

CLINICAL PRESENTATION. Migraine headaches are periodic. They occur daily, weekly, monthly, or every few years. Not all migraine headaches

TABLE 4–1. Classification of Headaches

1. MIGRAINE

Migraine without aura
Migraine with aura
  Migraine with typical aura
  Migraine with prolonged aura
  Familial hemiplegic migraine
  Basilar migraine
  Migraine aura without headache
  Migraine with acute onset aura
Ophthalmoplegic migraine
Retinal migraine
Childhood periodic syndromes that may be precursors of or associated with migraine
  Benign paroxysmal vertigo of childhood
  Alternating hemiplegia of childhood
Complications of migraine
  Status migrainosus
  Migrainous infarction
Migrainous disorder not fulfilling above criteria

2. TENSION-TYPE HEADACHE

Episodic tension-type headache
  Episodic tension-type headache associated with disorder of pericranial muscles
  Episodic tension-type headache unassociated with disorder of pericranial muscles
Chronic tension-type headache
  Chronic tension-type headache associated with disorder of pericranial muscles
  Chronic tension-type headache unassociated with disorder of pericranial muscles
Headache of the tension-type not fulfilling above criteria

3. CLUSTER HEADACHE AND CHRONIC PAROXYSMAL HEMICRANIA

Cluster headache
  Cluster headache, periodicity undetermined
  Episodic
  Chronic
    Unremitting from onset
    Evolved from episodic
Chronic paroxysmal hemicrania
Cluster headache–type disorder not fulfilling above criteria

4. MISCELLANEOUS HEADACHES UNASSOCIATED WITH STRUCTURAL LESION

Idiopathic stabbing headache: "ice-pick pains"
External compression headache: "swim-goggle headache"
Cold stimulus headache
  External application of a cold stimulus
  Ingestion of a cold stimulus: "ice cream headache"
Benign cough headache
Benign exertional headache
Headaches associated with sexual activity: "benign sex headache" (coital cephalgia)
  Dull type
  Explosive type
  Postural type

5. HEADACHE ASSOCIATED WITH HEAD TRAUMA

Acute posttraumatic headache
  With significant head trauma and/or confirmatory signs
Chronic posttraumatic headache
  With significant head trauma and/or confirmatory signs
  With minor head trauma and no confirmatory signs

TABLE 4–1. Classification of Headaches *(Continued)*

6. HEADACHE ASSOCIATED WITH VASCULAR DISORDERS

Acute ischemic cerebrovascular disease
  TIAs
  Thromboembolic stroke
Intracranial hematoma
  Parenchymal hematoma
  Subdural hematoma
  Epidural hematoma
Subarachnoid hemorrhage
Unruptured vascular malformation
  Arteriovenous malformation
  Saccular aneurysm
Arteritis
  Giant cell arteritis
  Other systemic arteritides
  Primary intracranial arteritis
Carotid or vertebral artery pain
  Carotid or vertebral dissection
  Carotidynia (idiopathic)
  Postendarterectomy headache
Venous thrombosis
Arterial hypertension
  Acute pressor response to exogenous agent
  Pheochromocytoma
  Malignant (accelerated) hypertension
  Preeclampsia and eclampsia
Headache associated with other vascular disorder

7. HEADACHE ASSOCIATED WITH NONVASCULAR INTRACRANIAL DISORDERS

High CSF pressure
  Benign intracranial hypertension
  High pressure hydrocephalus
Low CSF pressure
  Post–lumbar puncture headache
  CSF fistula headache
Intracranial infection
Intracranial sarcoidosis and other noninfectious inflammatory diseases
Headache related to intrathecal injections
  Direct effect
  Due to chemical meningitis
Intracranial neoplasm
Headache associated with other intracranial disorder

8. HEADACHE ASSOCIATED WITH SUBSTANCES OR THEIR WITHDRAWAL

Headache induced by acute substance use or exposure
  Nitrate/nitrite-induced headache
  Monosodium glutamate–induced headache
  Carbon monoxide–induced headache
  Alcohol-induced headache
  Other substances
Headache induced by chronic substance use or exposure
  Ergotamine-induced headache
  Analgesic-induced headache
  Other substances
Headache from substance withdrawal (acute use)

Table continued on following page

TABLE 4–1. Classification of Headaches *(Continued)*

Headache from substance withdrawal (chronic use)
    Ergotamine-withdrawal headache
    Caffeine-withdrawal headache
    Narcotics abstinence headache
    Other substances
Headache associated with substances but with uncertain mechanism
    Birth control pills or estrogens
    Other substances

9. HEADACHE ASSOCIATED WITH NONCEPHALIC INFECTION

Viral infection
    Focal noncephalic
    Systemic
Bacterial infection
    Focal noncephalic
    Systemic (septicemia)
Headache related to other infection

10. HEADACHE ASSOCIATED WITH METABOLIC DISORDERS

Hypoxia
    High-altitude headache
    Hypoxic headache (low-pressure environment, pulmonary diseases causing hypoxia)
    Sleep apnea headache
Hypercapnia
Mixed hypoxia and hypercapnia
Hypoglycemia
Dialysis
Headache related to other metabolic abnormality

11. HEADACHE OR FACIAL PAIN ASSOCIATED WITH DISORDER OF CRANIUM, NECK, EYES, EARS, NOSE, SINUSES, TEETH, MOUTH, OR OTHER FACIAL CRANIAL STRUCTURES

Cranial bone
Neck
    Cervical spine
    Retropharyngeal tendinitis
Eyes
    Acute glaucoma
    Refractive errors
    Heterophoria or heterotropia
Ears
Nose and sinuses
    Acute sinus headache
    Other diseases of nose or sinuses
Teeth, jaws, and related sources
Temporomandibular joint disease (functional disorders are coded to group 2)

12. CRANIAL NEURALGIAS, NERVE TRUNK PAIN, AND DEAFFERENTATION PAIN

Persistent (in contrast to ticlike) pain of cranial nerve origin
    Compression or distortion of cranial nerves and second or third cervical roots
    Demyelination of cranial nerves
        Optic neuritis (retrobulbar neuritis)
    Infarction of cranial nerves
        Diabetic neuritis
    Inflammation of cranial nerves
        Herpes zoster
    Tolosa-Hunt syndrome

TABLE 4-1. Classification of Headaches *(Continued)*

Neck-tongue syndrome
Other causes of persistent pain of cranial nerve origin
Trigeminal neuralgia (tic douloureux)
  Idiopathic trigeminal neuralgia
  Symptomatic trigeminal neuralgia
    Compression of trigeminal root or ganglion
    Central lesions
Glossopharyngeal neuralgia
  Idiopathic
  Symptomatic
Nervus intermedius neuralgia
Superior laryngeal neuralgia
Occipital neuralgia
Central causes of facial pain other than tic douloureux
  Anesthesia dolorosa
  Thalamic pain
Facial pain not fulfilling criteria in groups 11 and 12

13. HEADACHE NOT CLASSIFIABLE

are throbbing in nature, but many are. The typical headache lasts less than 24 hours, but it is not unusual for one to go on for several days.

Migraine without an aura is the most common type of migraine headache encountered. It often begins at a young age, but may begin at any age. Some patients will have a prodrome prior to a headache, which may consist of vague abdominal discomfort, mild head pain, stuffiness of nose or head, or other nonspecific complaints. The headache may be unilateral or bilateral and progressively increases in severity. The patient may have nausea and, less often, vomiting during the headache. Patients often have photophobia and must lie down during the headache. "Sick headaches" are usually migraine headaches. Headaches may occur during the day or night and can wake the patient from sleep.

Headaches occur in discrete attacks lasting from 1 to 24 hours, the average being 3 to 4 hours. Various factors trigger migraine, including menarche, menstruation, and menopause. Headaches may be worse or better during pregnancy. Birth control pills can precipitate migraine. Because birth control pills are believed to increase the risk of stroke in patients with migraine, they are contraindicated for such patients. Foods that precipitate migraine in some patients include alcohol, cheese, chocolate, hot dogs, monosodium glutamate, and ice cream. Emotion and tension may precipitate migraine. Weather and changes of barometric pressure are well-known triggers of migraine in some patients. Many patients have a history of motion sickness. There is family history of migraine in well over 50% of patients. Migraine patients have a slightly increased risk for stroke and seizures. The neurologic examination is normal, except that some patients may develop a transient or persistent Horner's syndrome. Laboratory tests are invariably normal.

Migraine with aura affects approximately 10% of all migraine patients. The aura typically lasts for 10 to 30 minutes. The most common aura consists of visual manifestations. These may involve part of or all of the visual field. Some patients have circular or lightning-bolt flashes of light that begin in the center and progress to the periphery, or vice versa. The flashing lights may be large or small, multiple or single, and they may be colored. Visual distortions occur, as well as expanding figures with scintillating edges that often leave behind areas of blindness for up to 30 minutes. Tunnel vision due to bilateral occipital lobe ischemia occurs as a migraine aura. Uncommonly, a migraine aura leaves permanent cortical blindness or a hemianopic field defect. Scintillating scotomata that occur in both homologous visual fields are almost diagnostic of migraine. After the visual aura, the headache occurs. Headaches are pounding, unilateral or bilateral, often associated with nausea and vomiting, and last for hours. Otherwise the headache, family history, and other aspects of the disorder are very similar to that seen in other forms of migraine. Episodic visual disturbances without headaches are not uncommon, and some patients rarely have headaches. In some sporadic and familial cases, the headache is preceded by hemiplegia. Rarely, the neurologic deficit may come on or persist during a headache.

In basilar migraine, patients may have diplopia, visual blurring, blindness, tinnitus, vertigo, dysarthria, hemiparesis, quadriparesis, or bilateral sensory symptoms. Occasionally there may be loss of consciousness associated with other basilar artery symptoms.

Patients with ophthalmoplegic migraine usually have a long history of classic migraine or a family history of migraine. The ocular motor paresis often occurs when a headache is resolving but may also precede it. The third cranial nerve is most frequently affected, the fourth and sixth rarely so. Repeated attacks may lead to permanent paralysis of the affected cranial nerve. One should always be on the lookout for a posterior communicating aneurysm, the Tolosa Hunt syndrome, or other parasellar processes that may mimic the ophthalmoplegic migraine syndrome. In retinal migraine, patients develop visual field defects in one eye, which are transient and may or may not be followed by a headache, usually ipsilateral to the affected eye.

Children develop typical migraine syndromes, which sometimes are preceded by episodes of benign paroxysmal vertigo of childhood or alternating hemiplegia of childhood. Periodic abdominal pain with vomiting and confusional states without a headache and without another explanation have also been thought to be precursors of migraine. There is often a family history of migraine, which may help in the diagnosis.

The diagnosis often becomes clear in retrospect after the patient has established typical migraine.

A small percentage of migraine sufferers at times develop *status migrainosus*, which is defined as a migrainous attack that lasts longer than 72 hours. Because of vomiting, many of these patients become severely dehydrated and may require hospitalization.

DIFFERENTIAL DIAGNOSIS. One of the most common headache disorders seen by physicians is migraine without aura. It ordinarily varies in severity over the patient's lifetime and is usually exacerbated at times of significant stress. If the headaches are typical of a long history of similar headaches, further work-up is usually not indicated. Patients who have experienced new onset headaches, changes in the character of their headaches, or focal neurologic symptoms or signs associated with the headache may require further work-up, including CT or MR brain scans. In patients with transient focal neurologic symptoms during their headaches, the following differential diagnosis should be kept in mind: (1) migraine; (2) seizures; (3) TIAs; (4) mass lesions; (5) symptomatic migraine (new medication, drug withdrawal, head trauma, stress, etc.); (6) demyelinating disease; (7) infectious disease.

The visual symptoms that occur during migraine typically involve homologous portions of both visual fields simultaneously. Positive visual phenomena can occur in several other disease states, however, including occipital and temporal lobe seizures, TIAs, strokes, and retinal or vitreous tears and detachments. Hemiplegic, ophthalmoplegic, and basilar artery symptoms that occur in some migraine patients must be differentiated from other causes, including stroke and TIAs.

TREATMENT. The pharmacologic treatment of migraine can be divided into three classes: (1) abortive drugs, (2) prophylactic drugs, and (3) analgesic drugs. Abortive therapy is excellent for migraine headaches that occur once per week or less frequently. The ergotamin drugs are most frequently used, and typical preparations, doses, and side effects are listed in Table 4–2. Any abortive therapy should be given as early in a headache or aura as possible and in a large enough dose to abort the headache completely. Patients should carry the abortive medication with them at all times. Side effects from ergot compounds are frequent, particularly on initiation of therapy. The oral, sublingual, and rectal routes have fewer side effects and are best tolerated by patients. Intramuscular ergots are the most effective but have frequent side effects and generally cannot be self-administered. An exception is the recently introduced drug sumatriptan succinate, which is given subcutaneously and can be self-administered. It should not be prescribed for patients with basilar and hemiplegic migraine. Aspirin, acetaminophen, and

TABLE 4–2. Abortive Therapy for Migraine*

Drug	Dose	Route
Ergotamine preparations		
Ergotamine and caffeine	2 tablets, repeat in 1 h; max 4 per day	Oral
Ergotamine and caffeine	1 suppository, repeat in 1 h; max 2 per day	Rectal
Ergotaminel	1 tablet, repeat in 1 h; max 2 per day	Sublingual
Serotonin-receptor agonists		
Dihydroergotamine	0.5–1 ml	Intramuscular Subcutaneous Intravenous
5-HT1 receptor agonist		
Sumatriptan	6 mg, may repeat after 1 h, max 2 per day	Subcutaneous
Sympathomimetics	(with or without barbiturates or codeine)	
Isometheptene	2 capsules, repeat in 1 h, max 2 per day	Oral
Acetaminophen	2 capsules, repeat in 1 h, max 2 per day	Oral
Dichloralphenazone	2 capsules, repeat in 1 h, max 2 per day	Oral
Nonsteroidal anti-inflammatory drugs		
Naproxen	550–750 mg, repeat in 1 h; max 3 times per week	Oral
Meclofenamate	100–200 mg, repeat in 1 h; max 3 times per week	Oral
Flurbiprofen	50–100 mg, repeat in 1 h; max 3 times per week	Oral
Ibuprofen	200–300 mg, repeat in 1 h; max 3 times per week	Oral
Antiemetics		
Promethazine	50–125 mg	Oral Intramuscular
Prochlorperazine	1–25 mg 2.5–25 mg (suppository) 5–10 mg	Oral Rectal Intramuscular
Chlorpromazine	10–25 mg 50–100 mg (suppository) Up to 35 mg	Oral Rectal Intravenous
Trimetobenzamide	250 mg 200 mg	Oral Rectal
Metoclopramide	5–10 mg 10 mg 5–10 mg	Oral Intramuscular Intravenous
Dimenhydrinate	50 mg	Oral

*The manufacturer's drug insert should be consulted for side effects and contraindications prior to prescribing any of these drugs.

HEADACHE

propoxyphene may abort migraine if taken in adequate doses at the very onset of headaches.

In the treatment of acute migraine headaches it is as important to treat the nausea and vomiting as it is to treat the headache. Vomiting per se may increase the severity of the headache. The gastrointestinal disturbances that accompany migraine probably impair absorption of medications. Therefore, either metaclopramide (10–50 mg orally), compazine (10–25 mg rectally), or phenergan (50 mg intramuscularly) should be given prior to giving pain medication. Once nausea and vomiting are controlled, an analgesic should be given orally, rectally, or intramuscularly. Aspirin (5–20 grains), acetaminophen (5–20 grains), propoxyphene (50–150 mg), Fiorinal (1–2 tablets), or various codeine preparations (aspirin or acetaminophen with codeine) can be used orally and are often effective if nausea is first controlled.

Most patients in status migrainosus require hospitalization and parenteral medication and intravenous fluid replacement to control dehydration and electrolyte imbalance. Methylprednisolone (40–80 mg) or dexamethasone, (12–16 mg) intramuscularly often can abort an attack. Dihydroergotamine (DHE-45) (1 mg intravenously, after an initial test dose of 0.5 mg) is also an effective agent. A major advantage is that it appears to be effective even if the headache has been present for hours or days and may be used repeatedly. Along with DHE-45, metoclopramide (10 mg) can be used to control nausea and vomiting. Most patients will benefit from the addition of a sedative. Severe headaches following acute ergotamine withdrawal in habituated patients is treated in a similar fashion.

If abortive therapy is ineffective, side effects are limiting, migraine headaches occur more than once per week, or it is desirable to minimize the number of headaches, then prophylactic migraine therapy is used. The prophylactic medications, their dosages, and their side effects are listed in Table 4–3. The prophylactic medications are initiated at a low dose, and the dose is increased until either the headaches are reduced to an acceptable frequency or until unacceptable side effects occur. Many patients fail with prophylactic medication because the drug dosage was not adjusted properly. If a prophylactic is ineffective or has unpleasant or dangerous side effects, another drug is chosen. A given prophylactic only has a 40% to 80% success rate. Amitriptyline probably has the highest success rate. Recently, valproic acid has been used with some success. The starting dose is 600 mg twice a day and should be gradually increased to optimal plasma levels of 700 µmol/p. Side effects are weight gain and drowsiness, and liver functions should be monitored to avoid hepatotoxicity.

Most migraine headache disorders are reasonably controlled with abortive or prophylactic therapy. Patients may not be completely

TABLE 4-3. Prophylactic Therapy for Migraine*

Drug	Oral dosage per day
β-Blockers	
Propranolol	40–240 mg
Nadolol	20–80 mg
Atenolol	50–150 mg
Timolol	20–60 mg
Metropolol	50–300 mg
Calcium channel blockers	
Verapamil	120–240 mg
Diltiazem	90–180 mg
Nifedipine	30–120 mg
Serotonin antagonists and agonists	
Cyproheptadine	4–8 mg
Methysergide	4–8 mg
Methylergonovine	0.2 mg tid or qid
Tricyclic antidepressants	
Amitriptyline	10–200 mg
Nortriptyline	10–150 mg
Doxepin	10–200 mg
Imipramin	10–200 mg
MAO inhibitors	
Phenelezine	30–90 mg
Serotonin reuptake inhibitors	
Fluoxetine	10–30 mg
Trazodone	50–300 mg
Anticonvulsants	
Phenytoin	300–500 mg
Carbamazepine	200–1200 mg
Divalproex sodium	250–1500 mg
Nonsteroidal anti-inflammatory drugs	
Naproxen	550–1100 mg
Meclofenamate	100–400 mg
Flurbiprofen	50–200 mg
Ibuprofen	300–1200 mg
α-Adrenergic blockers	
Clonidine	0.1 mg bid or tid

*The manufacturer's drug insert should be consulted for side effects and contraindications prior to prescribing any of these drugs.

headache-free but are usually significantly improved. Psychiatric consultation, biofeedback, and acupuncture may be helpful in some patients.

Tension-type Headache

Tension-type headache is extremely common but is poorly defined. Other names attached to this disorder include muscle contraction headache, psychogenic headache, and stress headache. Tension headaches are sometimes associated with adverse reactions to life stresses. There is no prodrome, and they are almost always bilateral. The areas of major discomfort are the back of the head and neck and frontal areas. The headaches are described as covering the head, like a cap or a headband; are nonpulsatile; and produce discomfort described as tight, squeezing, pressing, crawling, or viselike. Many patients also complain that their scalp is overly sensitive. These headaches are not periodic, though they may occur daily toward the end of the day. They may wake patients out of sleep. They are frequently continuous but wax and wane from day to day. Neurologic examination is normal. Occasionally, the examination will reveal tenderness and stiffness of the neck muscles. Probably some of these headaches are related to osteoarthritis or bony abnormalities of the neck.

There is no single good therapy for tension headaches. Some patients will do well with the use of aspirin or other minor analgesics. Narcotics should be avoided, since patients who suffer from tension headaches tend to have them for many years and decades, and such headaches often become refractory to any medication. Muscle relaxants, anti-anxiety agents, and antidepressants are helpful in some patients. Psychiatric, social, and psychological evaluation may be useful. Massage and biofeedback benefit some patients. The continued support and encouragement of the physician is very important over the long run; but excessive testing, doctoring, and medicating should be avoided.

Cluster Headaches

CLINICAL PRESENTATION. Cluster headaches are periodic headaches of severe intensity. They occur in clusters that last weeks or months, frequently waking the patient at night with a severe, piercing or knifelike pain. Such pain is usually associated with a Horner's syndrome, nasal stuffiness, lacrimation, and conjunctival injection on the side of the pain. The pain is almost always most intense behind the eye or in the orbitotemporal region and generally lasts 20 to 60 minutes.

Headaches frequently occur at the same time every day. Headaches often occur at night and wake patients from sleep. There is no prodrome and no associated nausea or vomiting. Men are affected 5 to 10 times as frequently as women, and one can usually obtain a strong family history of similar headaches. Alcohol, nitrites, and other vasodilators may precipitate these headaches during clusters.

The pathogenesis of cluster headaches is probably different from migraine. Increases in whole blood histamine have been demonstrated at the onset of a cluster. Injection of histamine may precipitate a cluster headache. Occasional patients have typical migraine and cluster headaches, and at times it may be difficult to distinguish clearly between them. Retro-orbital processes may produce severe eye pain, but it is generally not of the character and periodicity of cluster headaches. Chronic paroxysmal hemicrania (see below) is a disorder very similar to cluster headaches but has a slightly different history and different therapy.

TREATMENT. Cluster headaches are treated primarily with prophylactic medications as outlined in Table 4–4. Analgesic drugs are of little use because of the short duration of the headache. Lithium, (300 mg by mouth 3 times per day) is useful, particularly if there are multiple headaches every day. Blood levels and side effects should be carefully monitored. Sansert is very effective and is the drug of choice in patients with short clusters. Occasionally, attacks may be aborted with sublingual Ergomar or by inhalation of 100% oxygen. Prednisone is sometimes used (starting with 100 mg and tapering to 0 mg over a period of 7 days). Usually, a prophylactic must be used with prednisone, because headaches often resume once prednisone is stopped. Thorazine is used as the last resort because of the frequency and severity of side effects that occur with high doses of this medication. Once patients are headache-free on a particular prophylactic, it is continued for another 6 to 8 weeks. The prophylactic is then tapered over 4 weeks. If headaches do not recur, no further treatment is necessary until the next cluster begins.

Chronic Paroxysmal Hemicrania

CLINICAL PRESENTATION. Chronic paroxysmal hemicrania resembles cluster headaches in a number of respects. The headache is unilateral and remains so in subsequent occurrences. Symptoms are periodic. Headaches have an abrupt onset; last 20 to 30 minutes, sometimes an

TABLE 4–4. Treatment for Cluster Headaches*

Drug	Dose
Sansert	2 mg po, bid to 5 times per day
Ergotamine tartrate (Ergomar)	2 mg po at bedtime or per attack
Lithium	300 mg po, bid to qid
Prednisone	100 mg/day; taper to zero over 1–2 weeks
Thorazine	25 mg po at bedtime to 50 po, qid
Oxygen	100% per attack

*The manufacturer's drug insert should be consulted for side effects and contraindications prior to prescribing any of these drugs.

hour; and then subside. Pain begins and is most severe behind the eye or in the temporal region, but it may spread to involve the orbit, jaw, neck, maxilla, and occasionally the shoulder. A Horner's syndrome, rhinorrhea, and lacrimation often accompany the headache. Patients usually do not have nausea and vomiting with these headaches. Chronic paroxysmal hemicrania can be distinguished from cluster headache by the history. Unlike cluster headaches, the headache occurs every day of the patient's life. In chronic paroxysmal hemicrania, there are 5 to 20 headaches per day that occur throughout the day and night, and they show no evidence of nocturnal preponderance, as in cluster.

TREATMENT. Aspirin is partially effective in alleviating this headache, and indomethacin is often curative. Because both indomethacin and aspirin inhibit prostaglandin biosynthesis, prostaglandins may be involved in the pathogenesis of this headache. Naproxen may also be useful.

Miscellaneous Headaches Unassociated with Structural Lesion

The idiopathic stabbing headache or "ice-pick pain" is very severe and frightening to the patient, but it is of a benign nature and often seen in patients with migraine. Other benign headaches in this group can be easily diagnosed by a careful history.

Headaches Associated with Head Trauma

Fractures of the temporal bone, often with hematympanon, produce localized head pain. Fractures through the cribriform plate or temporal bone can result in CSF leakage with resulting headaches similar to post-LP headaches. CSF leakage should be suspected if a headache is aggravated by standing and relieved by lying down. If bed rest, fluids, and time do not stop the CSF leak, surgical intervention may be necessary. The most serious potential complication of any CSF leak is meningitis. Acute, and in some patients a chronic, subdural hematoma can give rise to unilateral headaches. Tenderness to percussion of the skull on the affected side may be present.

Headaches following even trivial head trauma are common and occur with equal frequency in patients with or without a prior history of headaches. Their clinical presentation is indistinguishable from migraine and tension-type headaches. Treatment is the same as for those headaches. They may last for weeks, months, or years. In about 70% of patients, headaches will subside within 1 year following head trauma. The older the patient, the poorer the prognosis.

Headache Associated with Vascular Disorders

Headaches may be caused by thrombosis of, or occlusion by, emboli of neck and intracranial arteries and veins; venous thrombosis; subdural, epidural, and parenchymal hematomas; arteriovenous malformations and aneurysms; and arteritis. None of these headaches is specific, but they are often localized, and the presence of neurologic deficits allows correct diagnosis in most instances.

Subarachnoid Hemorrhage

Subarachnoid hemorrhage headache is characterized by the sudden onset of what the patient may dub the "worst headache of my life." The headache is of severe intensity. Drowsiness, nausea, and vomiting are frequent accompanying symptoms. Some patients immediately lapse into coma after a subarachnoid hemorrhage without a preceding headache. The headache of subarachnoid hemorrhage usually persists at a very high intensity for a few days to a week and slowly subsides thereafter. A few hours after the initial headache, patients develop a stiff neck, fever, and hypertension. The neurologic examination is usually nonfocal, unless there has been bleeding into the cerebral parenchyma. If a subarachnoid hemorrhage is suspected, a CT brain scan should be performed immediately. A CT scan will detect subarachnoid blood in over 70% of cases and will also demonstrate intraparenchymal blood. If a CT scan does not show blood in the subarachnoid space, an LP will increase the likelihood of detecting blood by a few percentage points. In most instances of subarachnoid hemorrhage, angiography will be needed to detect aneurysms and arteriovenous malformations.

GIANT CELL ARTERITIS. The new onset of a headache in any patient over the age of 50 should raise the possibility of temporal arteritis. The headache associated with it can be a vague tensionlike headache or a pounding headache localized to the temporal areas. Some patients cannot sleep on one side of the head because of localized temporal pain. There can be occipital pain and localized neck tenderness as well. A number of patients with temporal arteritis also have polymyalgia rheumatica. This syndrome consists of malaise, occasional anorexia, low-grade fever, and moderate to severe muscle pains. The syndrome can be short-lived or protracted. Giant cell arteritis is discussed in more detail in Chapter 5.

CAROTIDYNIA. Carotidynia is an episodic, occasionally throbbing, pain in the neck. The pain is probably due to swelling and tenderness of the wall of the carotid artery. Slight pressure on the carotid causes pain, but firm pressure may completely relieve the symptoms. Carotidynia is related to migraine and occurs in patients who have otherwise typical migraine headaches but in addition have a tender carotid during he headache. Patients may also have a tender carotid in the interval between headaches. Occasionally, tender carotid arteries are the patient's only manifestation of a migrainelike syndrome. These patients respond to migraine medication.

Headache Associated with Nonvascular Intracranial Disorders

HIGH CEREBROSPINAL PRESSURE. The headache associated with brain tumor and increased intracranial pressure is often nondescript. Headaches that tend to occur on waking and are aggravated by bending or coughing may be associated with increased intracranial pressure. However, all of these features also occur in migraine and, occasionally, in tension headache. One aspect of headaches associated with increased intracranial pressure is that over a period of time—days, weeks, or months—they often become progressively more severe. Seeing many patients with headache, one soon becomes impressed with the fact that very few have increased intracranial pressure. Conversely, patients who actually have cerebral tumors often have headaches that are not severe. Patients with extremely severe headaches usually have migraine.

Pseudotumor cerebri is an important, though uncommon, cause of increased intracranial pressure. Patients may present with headache, diplopia, menstrual irregularities, visual complaints, and usually obesity. Examination is normal except for papilledema and, occasionally, a sixth-nerve palsy. LP should be normal except for increased intracranial pressure and occasional abnormalities of protein. CT brain scan, MRI, EEG, and arteriogram are normal. Pseudotumor may be idiopathic or associated with obesity, menstrual irregularities, empty sella syndrome, pregnancy, menarche, vitamin A intoxication, tetracyclines, steroid withdrawal, hypoparathyroidism, systemic lupus erythematosus, increased right heart pressure, and cerebral venous occlusion. Blindness from prolonged papilledema is a complication of pseudotumor. Treatment is aimed at maintaining normal intracranial pressure. Frequent LPs often relieve the headache but are insufficient for long-term treatment. Diamox (250 mg by mouth 4 times per day) is first administered. If the CSF pressure is not near normal within 2 to 3 weeks, or if vision is failing, then prednisone (60 mg per day in divided doses) is added. Medical treatment is continued until CSF pressure remains normal. If vision begins to fail, lumboperitoneal shunting, or subtemporal or orbital decompression, can be performed to try to save vision.

LOW CEREBROSPINAL PRESSURE. Post-LP headache occurs in about 1 out of 10 patients. Using a small needle, keeping attempts at LP to a minimum, and having the patient lie on the abdomen for 15 minutes after the puncture reduces the frequency of such headaches. The headache may appear immediately after the procedure or a few hours to several days later. The headache is precipitated by standing or sitting and is relieved by lying down. It is usually a dull, deep ache but may be throbbing. It is often bifrontal and occasionally occipital. Shaking the head, coughing, or straining makes the headache worse. There may be moderate neck stiffness associated with the headache. The mechanism is believed to be due to persistent leakage of CSF from a hole in the dura created by the LP needle. The headache lasts for days to weeks; on rare occasions, it lasts for months. Treatment of LP headache includes bed rest, oral fluids, minor analgesics, and time. The headache is usually resistant to all types of treatment except bed rest, but almost all cases resolve spontaneously. If the headache persists for several weeks, placement of an epidural blood patch to close the dural hole may be beneficial; but this procedure is not without potential complications, e.g. injury of nerve roots.

INTRACRANIAL INFECTION. Inflammation of the meninges causes headaches. Bacterial, fungal, viral, tuberculous, and parasitic meningitis all cause headaches. Irritation of the meninges from blood, air, and other foreign substances in the subarachnoid space also cause headaches. These headaches are associated with signs of meningismus and pain on head flexion but not rotation. In small children, headaches may be absent even in the presence of overwhelming bacterial meningitis.

Headache Associated with Substances or Their Withdrawal

Nitrates and nitrites, monosodium glutamate, carbon monoxide, and alcohol all may acutely induce headaches. Chronic use of analgesics and ergotamines may be the cause of headaches. Birth control pills may cause or exacerbate preexisting headaches. Caffeine withdrawal and narcotic abstinence are frequently accompanied by headaches. Ergotamine withdrawal may produce severe headaches and may require inpatient management.

Headache Associated with Noncephalic Infection

Many viral syndromes and sepsis are associated with rather nonspecific headaches.

Headache Associated with Metabolic Disorders

Many metabolic disorders may cause headaches. High-altitude sickness, almost always associated with headaches, can be partially prevented by pretreatment with diamox and/or short-acting steroids. Once severe headaches are present, rapid descent to lower altitudes is not only beneficial but may be lifesaving.

Severe, uncontrolled idiopathic hypertension, pheochromocytoma, and carcinoid syndrome may be associated with headaches. Organic chemicals, solvents, and many gases in high concentration may precipitate headaches.

Headache or Facial Pain Associated with Disease Affecting Cranial and Facial Structures

A detailed history and examination of cranial and facial structures will usually lead to the identification of the source of the pain. Once identified, further work-up and specialty referral are usually indicated.

Costen's is the syndrome of pain due to temporomandibular joint disease. It is characterized by pain over or around the temporomandibular joint, which is usually unilateral but occasionally bilateral. Causes include trauma, bruxism, rheumatoid arthritis, osteoarthritis, and congenital jaw malformations. Patients complain of pain while chewing, yawning, singing, or overextending the jaw. On examination, there is local tenderness or crepitus over the temporomandibular joint involved. X-rays may show degenerative changes of the joint. Treatment is variable. Simple analgesics may help. The condition may be relieved by prosthetic devices that prevent overbite. These devices can be provided by an orthodontist. In severe cases, bite correction surgery may be required if there is a severe overbite or underbite or severe pain due to degenerative changes. Face and head pains should not be attributed to temporomandibular joint disease unless it is the obvious cause of the complaint or is verified as such by a dentist with specialized expertise in this condition.

Cranial Neuralgias, Nerve Trunk Pain, and Deafferentation Pain

A variety of diseases of cranial nerves and intracranial structure lead to head and face pains. Some of the more common ones are postherpetic neuralgia and trigeminal neuralgia.

POSTHERPETIC NEURALGIA. Postherpetic neuralgia rarely poses a diagnostic problem. The herpetic infection is usually obvious. However, at the onset of herpes zoster, in the 3 to 5 days between the onset of the initial pain and the eruption of vesicles, there may be a considerable diagnostic dilemma. Ophthalmic division herpes zoster in the elderly may mimic temporal arteritis. However, the sedimentation rate is usually normal. The neuralgia itself may occur prior to the onset of vesicles, during the onset of vesicles, or afterwards. When postherpetic neuralgia develops, as it does in about 10% of patients, the pain changes to a continual burning sensation exacerbated by touching the affected skin. The scars themselves are usually insensitive to pain, and it is the normal-looking skin between the scars that is extremely sensitive. The pain itself may be continuous and contribute to a severe disability. The pain may last days, weeks, months, and sometimes years. Those patients with persistent pain present a distressing and formidable problem. Minor analgesics are usually ineffective, and even narcotics often do not control the pain. Treatment modalities include the following: (1) Tegretol (from 200 mg by mouth twice a day to 200 mg 6 times a day), (2) Dilantin (300–400 mg by mouth at bedtime), (3) antidepressants, including Elavil (25–300 mg by mouth at bedtime), (4) combinations of a phenothiazine and tricyclic antidepressants. The latter combination has been reported to be very effective in the control of pain from postherpetic neuralgia. The therapeutic regimen is Triavil 2–25; (one tablet by mouth 3 times a day for 7 days increasing to 2 tablets 3 times a day for 7 days); if there is still no response, the daily dosage is increased by one tablet per week. Early treatment of herpes zoster with acyclovir may decrease the likelihood of developing the neuralgia.

TRIGEMINAL NEURALGIA (TIC DOULOUREUX). The pain of tic douloureux is characteristic. Shooting or stabbing, electrical, hot needle, or searing-type pains occur in the affected zone. Each pain lasts but a few seconds but may recur many times. Typically, the patient is pain-free between attacks, and the attacks vary from every few seconds to every week or month. Pains shoot along the distribution of one branch of the fifth cranial nerve on one side. The mandibular (jaw) and maxillary (cheek) branches are most commonly involved. The pains need not occur in the entire distribution of the mandibular or maxillary branches. At the height of the pain, many patients have difficulty locating it accurately. Many patients with trigeminal neuralgia have trigger zones with attacks precipitated by chewing, smiling, yawning, drinking hot or cold fluids, or touching particular areas of the face. Neurologic examination of patients with trigeminal neuralgia is usually normal, but areas of hypesthesia may be found. Trigeminal neuralgia may be a manifestation of multiple sclerosis, and in some patients it is due to compression of the fifth cranial nerve by a tortuous posterior fossa artery. Treatment of trigeminal neuralgia should begin with drug therapy. The most effective drug is Tegretol (200 mg by mouth 2 to 6 times per day). Dosage should be increased slowly in elderly patients, because early side effects of confusion and ataxia may lead to rejection of an effective treatment. Dilantin (300–500 mg by mouth at bedtime) is sometimes effective. Occasionally, patients respond to Dilantin plus Tegretol. Narcotic analgesics are usually ineffective. Various surgical procedures are used for the treatment of trigeminal neuralgia if drug therapy fails or is not tolerated. These include alcohol injection, phenol injection, radiofrequency lesions of the involved branch(es) of the fifth nerve, and a posterior fossa operation to place a sponge between the affected branch of the fifth cranial nerve and a tortuous artery compressing it.

GLOSSOPHARYNGEAL NEURALGIA. Glossopharyngeal neuralgia is similar to trigeminal neuralgia. Short bouts of throat, neck, or ear pain are precipitated by swallowing. It is also treatable with Tegretol and/or Dilantin.

ATYPICAL FACE PAIN. This poorly characterized pain syndrome occurs in adults, is usually localized to one side of the face or cheek, is continuous, and is often present for months to years. Patients complain of unbearable pain but often have an inappropriately flat affect. Many of these patients are depressed and respond to mild analgesics and antidepressants (Elavil 25 mg by mouth at bedtime, increasing to 150 mg). Occasional patients have underlying pharyngeal tumors. In about 25% of patients, the etiology is dental disease, infections, or other organic pathology; and such etiologies should be carefully excluded.

REFERENCES

Friedman AP: Atypical facial pain. Headache 1969; 9:27–30.

Kudrow L: Lithium prophylaxis for chronic cluster headache. Headache 1977; 17:15–18.

Markley HG, Cheronis JCD, Piepho RW: Verapamil in prophylactic therapy of migraine. Neurology 1984; 34:973–976.

Welch KMA, Ellis DJ, Keenan PA: Successful migraine prophylaxis with naproxen sodium. Neurology 1985; 35:1304–1310.

Fogan L: Treatment of cluster headache. Arch Neurol 1985; 42:362–363.

Ziegler DK, Hurwitz A, Hassanein RS et al: Migraine prophylaxis. A comparison of propranolol and amitriptyline. Arch Neurol 1987; 44:486–489.

Raskin JH: Headache, 2nd ed. New York, Churchill Livingstone, 1988.

Headache classification committee of the international headache society. Classification and diagnostic criteria for headache disorders, cranial neuralgias and facial pain. Cephalgia 1988; 8(suppl 7):1–96.

Diamond S: Migraine headaches. Med Clin North Am 1991; 75:545–566.

Lance JW: The Mechanism and Management of Headache, 5th ed. London, UK, Butterworth, 1993.

Baumel B: Migraine: a pharmacologic review with newer options and delivery modalities. Neurology 1994; 44(Supp3):S13–S17.

5
Cerebrovascular Disease

Cerebrovascular disease continues to represent one of the major causes of disability and death, particularly in the aged. It is the third most frequent cause of death in the United States, heart disease and cancer being the first and second. Patients with cerebrovascular disease therefore represent the largest proportion of patients with neurologic disorders seen by primary care physicians. Even though recent epidemiological evidence suggests that the incidence of both thrombotic and hemorrhagic stroke is decreasing, approximately one-half million patients per year in the United States are expected to suffer from strokes of all etiologies. Of these patients, 10% will die during the acute illness, and another 20%–40% will die during the months immediately following the acute stroke. Of those patients who survive stroke, 10% will be disabled, requiring permanent institutional care; 40% will require some special care; 40% will have a persistent, mild neurologic deficit; and only 10% will be normal. The major risk factor is hypertension. Even mild elevation of systolic pressures is followed by an increased risk for cerebrovascular disease. Since hypertension is in most instances a treatable condition, and since long-term reduction of hypertension decreases the risk of subsequent strokes, the single most important measure in preventing strokes is detection and treatment of hypertension. Evidence of arteriosclerosis in other parts of the body, rheumatic heart disease, diabetes, certain types of lipid abnormalities, smoking, and the use of birth control pills are all associated with higher risk of cerebrovascular disease. The younger the patient with TIA or stroke, the more intense should be the search for causes other than arteriosclerotic disease. In a patient with head trauma, the development of TIAs or a stroke suggests the possibility of carotid or vertebral artery dissection. In a number of cases, though, the condition is idiopathic, with medical cystic necrosis present in some.

TABLE 5-1. Causes of Ischemic Cerebrovascular Disease

Vascular disorders
  Large-vessel atherothrombotic disease
  Lacunar disease
  Arterial-to-arterial embolization
  Carotid or vertebral artery dissection
  Fibromuscular dysplasia
  Migraine
  Venous thrombosis
  Radiation
  Complications of arteriography
  Multiple, progressive intracranial arterial occlusions
  Inflammatory disorders
    Giant cell arteritis
    Polyarteritis nodosa
    Systemic lupus erythematosus
    Granulomatous angiitis
    Takayasu's disease
    Arteritis associated with amphetamine, cocaine, or phenylpropanolamine
    Syphilis, mucormycosis
    Sjögren syndrome
    Behçet syndrome
Cardiac disorders
  Rheumatic heart disease
  Mural thrombus
  Arrhythmias
  Mitral valve prolapse
  Prosthetic heart valve
  Endocarditis
  Myxoma
  Paradoxical embolus
Hematologic disorders
  Thrombotic thrombocytopenic purpura
  Sickle cell disease
  Hypercoagulable states
  Polycythemia
  Thrombocytosis
  Leukocytosis
  Lupus anticoagulant

Proportions of different causes of ischemic strokes reported in the literature vary widely. In most recent studies the cause was reported as large-vessel atherothrombotic disease in 10%–50%, lacunar disease in 15%–30%, embolic in 10%–25%, and unknown in 2%–50%. Some of this variation may be due to selection bias, but some may reflect true differences in populations. Some of the more and less common causes of ischemic cerebrovascular disease are listed in Table 5-1.

The conditions included in this chapter are cerebral infarction (nonhemorrhagic and hemorrhagic), TIA, progressing stroke, reversible ischemic neurologic deficit (RIND), intracranial hemorrhage secondary to ruptured aneurysm or arteriovenous malformation, arteritis, and venous sinus thrombosis.

Regardless of the underlying etiology, in the development of a stroke a certain part of the brain does not receive an adequate blood supply for a period of time. If brain tissue is thus deprived of blood supply for 10 to 20 minutes, infarction will occur. Occlusion of a given artery does not necessarily imply infarction of brain tissue in the perfusion territory of the blood vessel, because adequate collateral circulation may exist. Since collateral circulation may be excellent in some patients and extremely poor in others, occlusion of a major artery may be followed by no neurologic deficit at all or by a devastating neurologic deficit secondary to infarction in the entire perfusion territory of the occluded artery. If adequate blood supply is restored to the brain within the 10- to 20-minute time limit, there will be total resolution of the neurologic deficit. Furthermore, the more peripheral portions of ischemic brain tissue may receive sufficient blood through collateral circulation to allow brain tissue to remain viable, leading to ultimate recovery, even though it may be temporarily nonfunctioning. This situation accounts for the rather common early partial or complete recovery of many patients with strokes. In some instances, the total volume of brain tissue that is infarcted and does not recover may be too small to produce a residual neurologic deficit. Therefore, such a patient will clinically recover completely, in spite of having suffered a small infarct. Such small infarcts, which by themselves may be asymptomatic clinically, may nevertheless, when other small infarcts are added over time, produce neurologic deficits that are sometimes rather unexpected. From that, it follows that the most critical time for intervention in stroke is the first 10 to 20 minutes, during which complete resolution may occur, and the next 24 to 48 hours, during which collateral circulation hopefully will improve and reduce the permanent damage to a minimum.

In patients with tight stenosis of an artery that still permits adequate perfusion, systemic hypotension may sufficiently reduce flow across the stenotic lesion, rendering the poststenotic perfusion territory ischemic; if hypotension persists for longer than 10 to 20 minutes, it will result in infarction even though the artery never became occluded. This situation is not uncommonly encountered in patients who are taking antihypertensive medication, which may be accompanied by orthostatic hypotension. A stenotic lesion may ultimately become so narrow that no significant blood flow across the lesion occurs. In addition, an artery may become occluded by local thrombus formation, which most commonly takes place at a stenotic site. Emboli, either from an arterial ulcerating lesion or from the heart, may occlude arteries and usually lodge at bifurcations. Cerebral infarction secondary to embolic occlusion is more commonly of the hemorrhagic type, because when the embolus breaks up and/or is dissolved, the arterial wall distal to the occlusion is fragile during the first week or so following the insult. Blood leakage of minor or major proportions may occur. Hypertensive intracerebral hemorrhage occurs as a primary event from rupture of arterioles damaged by the hypertensive process. Unfortunately, no reliable clinical signs exist that would allow the clinician to readily separate strokes secondary to ischemic infarction from those due to primary intracerebral hemorrhage. This distinction can only be made through the use of CT or MR scans. The one exception, however, is in patients who develop a focal neurologic deficit that is followed within hours by evidence of cerebral herniation and coma. This condition is almost invariably due to a primary intracerebral hemorrhage. Stroke secondary to arteritic processes may be ischemic or hemorrhagic. Occlusion of the major intracerebral venous sinuses may produce neurologic deficits secondary to infarction of brain tissue in the drainage territory of these sinuses. Such infarcts may be nonhemorrhagic but are very often hemorrhagic. Bleeding from intracranial aneurysms and arteriovenous malformations may be followed by no focal neurologic deficit if the bleeding is primarily into the subarachnoid space. If bleeding occurs into the brain substance, or if there is secondary compression of cranial nerves, focal neurologic deficits will develop.

Terms commonly used in cerebrovascular disease are TIA, progressing stroke, RIND, and completed stroke. Definition of these terms is purely clinical. A TIA is a transient neurologic deficit that persists for less than 24 hours and is followed by complete clinical recovery. Most TIAs do not last longer than 10 to 20 minutes. In progressing stroke, a neurologic deficit may progress continuously or in a stepwise fashion, usually over a period of 24 hours. Strokes secondary to a lesion in the posterior circulation may progress for up to 72 hours. When a neurologic deficit persists for more than 24 hours but less than 3 weeks, the term reversible ischemic neurologic deficit is frequently applied. This condition is rare, and patients who have it recover with no residual abnormalities. A persistent neurologic deficit secondary to cerebrovascular disease that lasts longer than 24 hours and is followed by a persistent residual deficit is called completed stroke. In most instances, the distinction between these different clinical categories can readily be made. Unfortunately, there are situations in which only time will tell; therefore, in the acute management of patients with cerebrovascular disease, it is always wise to assume that the patient can recover. In approximately 10% of patients with completed stroke, a minor or moderate neurologic deficit progresses rapidly to a much more profound deficit within the first 24 hours. At present, there are no clinical or laboratory methods to predict which patients will follow this unfortunate course.

TRANSIENT ISCHEMIC ATTACKS

A patient who has a TIA requires a complete medical and neurologic work-up. The former is done to detect risk factors and noncerebrovascular causes, such as atrial fibrillation, that may be responsible for the patient's symptoms. It is important to determine if the patient's TIA was in the distribution of the internal carotid artery (anterior circulation) or in the distribution of the vertebral and/or basilar arteries (posterior circulation). Symptoms and signs that can be taken as almost absolute evidence for a problem in the anterior circulation include transient monocular blindness (amaurosis fugax) and aphasia. Less reliable signs include hemiparesis, monoparesis, and hemihypesthesia. Symptoms and signs indicative of a posterior circulation problem include diplopia, homonymous hemianopsias, dysarthria, dysphagia, ataxia, vertigo, cranial nerve palsies, weakness of one or more extremities, and drop attacks. Repeated TIAs that occur both in the anterior and posterior circulation, as well as on the right and left side, should always raise the question of emboli originating in the heart. During the examination, particular emphasis should be placed on auscultation of the neck and head. Palpation of the carotid arteries does not yield any useful clinical information and may be dangerous to a patient with an ulcerating lesion at the carotid bifurcation because the procedure may dislodge a clot. Unfortunately, a very tight stenosis or a shallow ulcerating plaque may not produce a bruit. Ocular fundi should also be carefully examined, with the pupils dilated, to look for cholesterol crystals and fibrin and platelet emboli in the retinal arterioles. In most instances, TIAs are probably secondary to embolization of a platelet thrombus originating on an ulcerating arteriosclerotic plaque in one of the major extracranial arteries. Some TIAs may be secondary to arterial spasm.

A number of noninvasive tests are available in this clinical setting. Unfortunately, none of them singly or in combination provides enough information to obviate the need for angiography. Patients with TIAs in the anterior circulation who may be surgical candidates do require angiography as the definitive study. Patients with posterior circulation TIAs do not require angiography because lesions responsible for these symptoms and signs are surgically not correctable. Death as a consequence of angiography occurs in approximately 0.3% of patients, and a permanent and significant neurologic deficit occurs in about 1%. The question of whether or not patients with one TIA in the anterior circulation should be subjected to angiography is not settled. A significant number of these patients never have another attack; moreover, many patients do not have a surgically correctable lesion. The patient who has a clear-cut anterior circulation TIA and a carotid bruit on the appropriate side should have noninvasive carotid studies followed by angiography if a surgically correctable lesion appears to be present. The same procedure applies to the patient who has no bruit but similar symptoms and emboli in the retinal arterioles. Any patient with multiple anterior circulation TIAs occurring within days to weeks should probably be subjected to angiography, regardless of the presence or absence of carotid bruits. Patients with TIAs in the distribution of the anterior circulation and a moderate to severe stenotic lesion at the bifurcation of the carotid artery on the appropriate side, as well as those with large irregular ulcerating but nonstenotic lesions in the same location, should be subjected to carotid endarterectomy. In the hands of the surgeons who will perform the carotid endarterectomy, morbidity should be 5% or less, and mortality 1% or less. This consideration is very important, because if mortality and morbidity were much higher, the risk of undergoing surgery could become equal to or greater than the risk of doing nothing. In patients chosen for good reasons to undergo carotid endarterectomy, and in whom surgery is done by a competent surgeon, the risk of subsequent strokes is substantially reduced over a period of 5 years following the TIA from about 25%–40% to about 10% or less. The addition of aspirin (10 grains bid) after carotid endarterectomy may further reduce the risk of subsequent strokes. This leaves a significant number of patients with posterior circulation TIAs and anterior circulation TIAs who do not have a surgically correctable lesion. What constitutes optimal therapy for these patients is unfortunately an unsettled question. Aspirin (10 grains bid) reduces the risk of stroke or death by 48% in male patients but is of less benefit in women. If aspirin fails, the patient should be treated with ticlopidine (250 mg twice a day). If aspirin and ticlopidine fail, chronic anticoagulation has its advocates, but the evidence to support its efficacy is at best tenuous. Some physicians advocate treating nonsurgical patients who do not respond to aspirin and ticlopidine with chronic anticoagulation for 6 months to 1 year—the period during which the risk of stroke is highest. In cooperative and reliable patients, the risk of intracranial hemorrhage secondary to anticoagulation therapy is least during the first year but increases substantially beyond that time. Undoubtedly, some patients should, and do, respond very well to this form of therapy, but the identification of these individuals remains enigmatic. Patients in whom recurrent TIAs are secondary to emboli originating in the heart should be on chronic anticoagulant therapy. Another unsettled issue concerns patients with an asymptomatic carotid bruit. Recently, the investigators of the Asymptomatic Carotid Atherosclerosis Study (ACAS) reported its interim results. The conclusion is that carotid endarterectomy, performed in medical centers with documented combined perioperative morbidity and mortality for asymptomatic endarterectomy of less than 3% on carefully selected patients who continue to have aggressive modifiable risk factor management, is beneficial for patients who meet eligibility criteria of asymptomatic carotid stenosis exceeding 60% diameter reduction confirmed by arteriography. In recent years, extracranial-intracranial anastomoses have become very popular for patients with occluded extracranial arteries. Although in experienced surgical hands, patency of these anastomoses can be assured in most patients and cerebral perfusion is improved, there is no evidence that these procedures prevent subsequent strokes.

COMPLETED STROKE

The patient with a completed stroke has a fixed neurologic deficit that may have developed abruptly or over a period of time. Infarction may be secondary to occlusion of an artery, secondary to thrombosis in situ, secondary to occlusion by an embolus from a different source, or secondary to hemorrhage. If the infarction is in the cortex, the EEG is likely to show a focal abnormality acutely. The CT or MRI scan may be normal or abnormal, and often does not develop a focal abnormality until 12 to 36 hours after the acute infarction. Since clinically the distinction between a hemorrhage and an ischemic infarct cannot be made, a CT scan in the acute phase is helpful in detecting a hemorrhage. Furthermore, since the completed stroke may change to a stroke in progress requiring anticoagulation, it is advisable to obtain a CT scan acutely to rule out, for all practical purposes, intracerebral hemorrhage. If the CT scan acutely is normal, or shows evidence of nonhemorrhagic infarction, an LP can be done if indicated. Bloody spinal fluid at this time will suggest the possibility of hemorrhage from an aneurysm or arteriovenous malformation. On the other hand, if a patient is suspected of having bled from an aneurysm or arteriovenous malformation with a focal neurologic deficit, LP is contraindicated because of the possibility of herniation. In this situation one should proceed from CT scan to cerebral angiography to rule out vascular abnormalities.

A general medical work-up with particular emphasis on the heart is important. Patients with acute myocardial infarction, rheumatic heart disease, atrial fibrillation, or mitral valve prolapse may have further emboli. Another rare condition is subacute bacterial endocarditis, which secondarily may produce not only cerebral embolization but also formation of intracranial mycotic aneurysms. Atrial or ventricular myxoma must also be considered as a source of emboli. In patients with chronic atrial fibrillation, long-term anticoagulation in addition to other appropriate measures is the treatment of choice. The safest time to start anticoagulation is approximately 7 to 10 days after an acute infarct. Unfortunately, patients with cerebral infarct secondary to emboli originating in the heart may have multiple strokes over a relatively short period of time. Therefore, early anticoagulation—preferably no earlier than 72 hours after the last cerebral event—may have to be instituted even though the risk of significant intracerebral bleeding in a mildly hemorrhagic infarct does exist. This risk, however, is probably less than the risk of subsequent cerebral infarction with more profound neurologic deficits. Patients with bacterial endocarditis and intracranial mycotic aneurysms should be vigorously treated with appropriate antibiotics.

Other vascular work-up of patients with a completed stroke will depend on the rapidity and degree of recovery of the patient's deficit. If within 2 weeks the patient has made a striking, almost complete recovery, a work-up similar to that described for TIAs is probably indicated. Unfortunately, the patient with a residual neurologic deficit, even though it may be of only moderate degree, is not an optimal candidate for carotid endarterectomy, even though all other indications may be excellent.

Coexisting medical problems such as myocardial infarction, congestive heart failure, or gastrointestinal bleeding should be treated appropriately. Many patients who present with completed strokes will have various degrees of hypertension. In the patient who presents with hypertensive encephalopathy—which consists of headaches, seizures, various neurologic deficits, obtundation, dramatically elevated blood pressure, papilledema, severe hypertensive retinopathy, and evidence of renal failure—rapid and drastic reduction of blood pressure is mandatory. Other types of hypertension are best left alone acutely, because with bed rest, the blood pressure will frequently come down spontaneously and long-term antihypertensive management can, and should, be established at a later time. There is evidence to suggest that acutely increasing mean arterial blood pressure to between 100–130 mm Hg may increase perfusion pressure in the ischemic area and provide a better chance for patients to recover more than they otherwise would. The evidence, however, is not sufficiently impressive to recommend this form of therapy routinely. Nevertheless, precipitously lowering blood pressure in patients with acute completed strokes is contraindicated. On the other hand, the patient who presents with hypertensive encephalopathy represents a medical emergency and should be treated promptly with the aim of lowering the diastolic blood pressure below 100 and the systolic pressure below 160 mm Hg. This goal is best achieved with the intravenous administration of trimethaphan or sodium nitroprusside in an intensive care unit under the supervision of a physician experienced in dealing with such a medical emergency. Since cerebral autoregulation is severely impaired in the patient with an acute stroke, even minor degrees of orthostatic hypotension may have a deleterious effect on the patient's neurologic deficit. Bed rest is indicated during the first 48 hours, and the patient's head should not be elevated with more than one pillow. Whether or not hyperosmolar agents such as mannitol or glycerol have any effect beyond transient improvement is not established. There is also no convincing evidence that the routine administration of adrenal corticosteroids is of any benefit. Vasodilators are of no benefit. Deep barbiturate coma appears to be effective in limiting permanent neurologic deficits in some animal models, but this procedure has not been shown to be of benefit in humans. In summary, then, except for bed rest, maintenance of blood pressure, and general medical care, there is no proven effective therapy for patients with acute completed strokes. Early treatment with thrombolytic agents is still in the investigational stage. After 48 hours, patients should begin to ambulate, and an acute physiotherapy program should be instituted. Many patients with completed strokes will show substantial, spontaneous improvement over the next 3 to 4 weeks. Therefore, an assessment for long-term prognosis should be postponed until about 1 month following the acute episode. The earlier the improvement occurs, the better the long-term prognosis. There is no evidence to suggest that long-term anticoagulation in patients with completed stroke is of any benefit. After the acute phase of the completed stroke, long-term antihypertensive medication should be instituted, because it has been shown that, even though the incidence of subsequent strokes may not be reduced, mortality from subsequent cardiac failure is significantly lowered. Proper rehabilitation of the stroke patient requires a concerted effort by the patient's physician, family, physiotherapist, speech therapist, and social worker and at times requires psychiatric counseling for both the patient and the family. Patients who at the end of 3 to 4 weeks still have a profound neurologic deficit cannot be expected to improve much more, but frequently these patients can be helped significantly by being taught to use functions that are still intact to greater advantage. Patients with intracerebral hemorrhage without evidence of an aneurysm or an arteriovenous malformation are treated essentially the same as patients with nonhemorrhagic infarcts. If there is evidence of cerebral herniation secondary to a large intracerebral hematoma and/or cerebral edema, steroids such as prednisone or decadron should be used acutely, and surgical evacuation of the hematoma should be contemplated. The prognosis for patients with deep basal ganglia hematomas is extremely poor, with or without surgery. Candidates for possible surgical intervention are those patients who have large superficial intracerebral hematomas in one of the cerebral lobes and who do not improve substantially during the first 24 hours.

STROKE IN PROGRESS

A patient with a progressing stroke presents initially with a minimal to moderate neurologic deficit that over a period of hours progresses either smoothly or in a stepwise fashion. It is assumed that in some patients with this condition, a thrombus in situ extends, and ultimately occludes, distal branch vessels. The latter reduces collateral blood flow, leading to a larger infarction and, clinically, to a more profound neurologic deficit. In some patients, however, an expanding intracerebral hematoma may produce the same clinical picture. Therefore, the initial work-up of patients with progressing stroke is similar to that described for completed stroke. Because the rate of progression is unpredictable, there is probably greater urgency for a complete work-up in patients with progressing stroke than in patients with completed strokes. If a hemorrhage has been excluded, continuous heparin therapy (approximately 1000 units per hour intravenously) has been advocated, but no definitive studies exist documenting the effectiveness of this treatment. The aim is to maintain plasma recalcification time at approximately 2.5 times normal. If a patient has remained stable or has improved significantly 72 hours after institution of heparin therapy, this therapy may be terminated and the patient treated in the same way as that described for completed stroke.

REVERSIBLE ISCHEMIC NEUROLOGIC DEFICIT

Since this diagnosis is made after the fact and cannot be recognized during the acute period, patients with RIND are essentially treated in the same way as patients with completed stroke.

VENOUS THROMBOSIS

Thrombosis of veins or intracranial venous sinuses leading to infarction is rare but often produces severe neurologic deficits. The infarct is often hemorrhagic, and severe edema may develop. This condition occurs in trauma, cachexia, marasmus, severe dehydration, hyperviscosity states, leukemia, pregnancy, and during the first postpartum week. Anticoagulation with heparin and Coumadin is recommended, but efficacy of this approach has not been established.

SUBARACHNOID HEMORRHAGE

Rupture of a congenital aneurysm, which most often is located at the bifurcation of major intracranial arteries, is the most common cause of subarachnoid hemorrhage. Common sites are the origin of the posterior communicating artery, the anterior communicating artery, and the trifurcation of the middle cerebral artery. Rupture of an aneurysm is exceedingly rare prior to age 20, and the primary consideration during the first two decades of life if subarachnoid hemorrhage occurs should be an arteriovenous malformation. Patients usually describe the sudden onset of a severe headache that, in those who suffer from chronic headaches, is generally distinctly different from their habitual pain. A stiff neck, particularly in children, is not present in all patients, even in those with significant subarachnoid bleeding. Therefore, the absence of a stiff neck does not exclude the possibility of a subarachnoid hemorrhage. If bleeding occurs into the brain substance at the same time, this will produce a mass lesion with a neurologic deficit appropriate to the site of hematoma.

The prognosis and surgical risk are best for patients who initially are alert, have no focal neurologic deficit, and may or may not have a headache. The prognosis is worse in patients who are obtunded, stuporous, or comatose and who have a major neurologic deficit. On initial evaluation, the detection of subhyaloid hemorrhages in the eye is diagnostically extremely helpful, because it is compatible with the presence of subarachnoid blood. As distinct from primary retinal hemorrhages, subhyaloid hemorrhages have a fluid level. Patients with such subhyaloid hemorrhages also may acutely have papilledema. Patients in whom a subarachnoid hemorrhage is expected should immediately be subjected to CT scanning. In some instances, particularly when contrast enhancement is used, aneurysms and arteriovenous malformations may be demonstrated. Furthermore, an intracerebral bleed can be detected by CT scanning. If an intracerebral bleed is present, an LP is contraindicated. In patients with significant intracerebral hematomas, an early angiogram is indicated, and acute evacuation and clipping of the aneurysm—if the aneurysm is in a readily accessible location—is beneficial. In those patients in whom the aneurysm is not readily accessible, evacuation of the blood clot may still be lifesaving, and the aneurysm can be operated on at a later time when the patient's condition has stabilized. The patient in whom a subarachnoid hemorrhage is suspected and in whom a CT scan does not show subarachnoid and intracerebral blood should have an LP to demonstrate the presence or absence of blood in the subarachnoid space. Great care should be taken to do an atraumatic LP, because bleeding secondary to a traumatic procedure cannot be readily distinguished from a primary hemorrhage. It is advantageous to collect CSF in three tubes and to do a count of the red blood cells (RBCs) in each of the tubes. A significant decrease in RBCs from the first to the third tube usually suggests a traumatic LP, but this is not absolute proof. CSF should be centrifuged immediately to determine if the supernatant is xanthochromic (yellow). Any delay will produce xanthochromia of the supernatant fluid, even though the blood was introduced through local trauma.

Once the diagnosis of subarachnoid hemorrhage has been established, patients should be treated with bed rest and sedation. Many neurosurgeons will routinely put patients on anticonvulsant medication. Contrary to standard teaching, the acute lowering of blood pressure during the acute phase is contraindicated, because it increases the likelihood that a neurologic deficit will develop secondary to acute arterial spasm. Whether or not acute moderate elevation of blood pressure is beneficial is unknown. The use of ethylaminocaproic acid (Amicar) to promote thrombosis in the aneurysm is probably not indicated, because it appears to increase the risk of complications. Nimodipine (60 mg by mouth every 4 hours for 21 days) improves outcome and probably reduces the frequency of associated cerebral infarction. The drug should be started within the first 4 days of the bleed. Because rebleeding most commonly occurs during the second week after the initial bleed, patients should have angiography at least by the end of the first week. About 30%–40% of patients die from the first bleed, and an additional 50% die as a consequence of the rebleed. The best time for clipping the aneurysm at its base is probably at the beginning of the second week in a patient who is stable and has no neurologic deficit. A significant number of patients develop delayed arterial spasm with significant morbidity and mortality. This delayed spasm is directly related to the presence of blood in the subarachnoid space; therefore, some surgeons now advocate early aneurysm surgery with removal of blood from the subarachnoid space. Another complication that is usually delayed is the development of hydrocephalus. Such hydrocephalus is best monitored with serial CT scans and may necessitate appropriate shunting procedures.

Patients with arteriovenous malformations may have had preexisting neurologic symptoms or signs before their first bleed. These may consist of focal neurologic deficits and, not uncommonly, focal seizures. When bleeding does occur from these vascular malformations, the degree of bleeding is usually less than that seen in patients with aneurysm. The likelihood of a reasonable clinical recovery is much better. Currently, two methods of treatment appear promising. One is embolization of feeding blood vessels when the malformation can be approached with a catheter. The other method is complete surgical excision, which has become much more feasible and more successful since the introduction of the surgical microscope. With this latter technique, even malformations that were previously considered inoperable and not in a location suitable for embolization can be successfully removed. Both of these procedures, however, are risky and should be performed only by highly skilled and experienced radiologists and neurosurgeons in major medical centers.

ARTERITIS

Many different types of intracranial and extracranial arteritis have been identified. These include systemic lupus erythematosus, polyarteritis nodosa, Takayasu's arteritis, and temporal arteritis. The one that is most commonly encountered and usually lacks obvious systemic symptoms and signs is temporal arteritis, which is frequently associated with polymyalgia rheumatica. The condition occurs almost exclusively in patients above the age of 50 and is more prevalent in men than in women. Many patients will have a period of general malaise, aching, loss of appetite, and weight loss. After a variable duration of these nonspecific symptoms, patients may develop headaches located over the temporal area or may have a more diffuse distribution. Although the headache is persistent in many patients, it may also be intermittent and may mimic migraine headaches. The most common neurologic complication is unilateral or, at times, bilateral blindness secondary to ischemic optic neuritis. A smaller percentage of patients may show other focal neurologic deficits secondary to involvement of intracranial arteries. The disorder is an inflammatory, granulomatous giant cell arteritis that in many patients predominantly involves the extracranial arteries, particularly the temporal artery, but may also involve intracranial arteries, either exclusively or in conjunction with involvement of extracranial arteries.

In some patients, the temporal artery is tender when examined, and in rare cases the physician may be able to palpate the granulomata. Proper and early diagnosis requires a high degree of suspicion, because none of the symptoms or signs is invariably present. In a patient suspected of having temporal arteritis, a sedimentation rate should be obtained, because in the vast majority of patients it is strikingly elevated. As soon as blood has been withdrawn, the patient should be started on prednisone (80–100 mg per day in divided doses) because the risk of visual loss is ever present, and once it has occurred the chance of recovery is at best minimal. Patients should then have a temporal artery biopsy, which may show the typical lesion. Multiple sections need to be taken, because the artery may be perfectly normal a short distance from a granulomatous lesion. Angiography is sometimes helpful in demonstrating lesions of extracranial and/or intracranial arteries. If the sedimentation rate is elevated, this can be used as a guide to continuing therapy. Since patients with chronic fungal meningitis may at times present with a clinical picture similar to that of patients with temporal arteritis, a spinal tap is almost always indicated to rule out the possibility of fungal meningitis if the temporal artery biopsy is normal. Even though the diagnosis of temporal arteritis may turn out to be erroneous, it is always best to start steroid therapy immediately, because early treatment will minimize the risk of visual loss and will have no significant deleterious effect even if chronic fungal meningitis ultimately proves to be the correct diagnosis. Patients with temporal arteritis usually respond rather dramatically to steroid therapy, except that visual loss—if it has already occurred—generally does not improve. Some physicians advocate acute anticoagulant therapy in patients with visual loss, but the value of this therapy is debatable. Since temporal arteritis runs a self-limited course, anywhere from 6 months to 1 year or longer, patients should be treated with steroids for at least 1 year. The long-term dosage is adjusted according to the patient's symptoms and sedimentation rate. Many patients can be adequately controlled by alternate-day steroid therapy after the initial daily therapy, which probably should last from 2 to 4 weeks, depending on the patient's response.

REFERENCES

Hollenhorst RW, Brown JR, Wagener HP, Schick RM: Neurologic aspects of temporal arteritis. Neurology 1960; 10:490–498.

Sundt TM, Whisnant JP: Subarachnoid hemorrhage from intracranial aneurysms: surgical management and natural history of disease. N Engl J Med 1978; 199:116–122.

The Canadian cooperative study group: a randomized trial of aspirin and sulfinpyrazone in threatened stroke. N Engl J Med 1978; 189:53–59.

Siekert RG (ed): Cerebrovascular survey report for joint council subcommittee on cerebrovascular disease. National Institute of Neurological and Communicative Disorders and Stroke and National Heart, Lung, and Blood Institute (revised), January 1980.

Harrison MJG, Dyken ML: Cerebral Vascular Disease. London, UK, Butterworth, 1983.

Barnett HJML: The EC/I bypass study group. Failure of extracranial-intracranial arterial bypass to reduce the risk of ischemic stroke. Results of an international randomized trial. N Engl J Med 1985; 313:1191–1200.

Rothrock JF, Lyden PD, Brody ML, Taft-Alvarez B, Kelly N, Mayer J, Wiederholt WC: An analysis of ischemic stroke in an urban Southern California population. Arch Intern Med 1993; 153:619–624.

Nadeau SE: Decision analysis and carotid endarterectomy. J Stroke Cerebrovasc Dis 1993; 3:244–255.

Haynes RB, Taylor DW, Sackett DL, Math KT, Ferguson GG, Barnett HJM: for the North American Symptomatic Carotid Endarterectomy Trial Collaborators. Prevention of functional impairment by endarterectomy for symptomatic high-grade carotid stenosis. JAMA 1994; 271:1256–1259.

Goldstein LB, Matchar DB: Clinical assessment of stroke. JAMA 1994; 271: 1114–1120.

6
Dementias

DEFINITION OF DEMENTIA

Dementia is a syndrome characterized by progressive intellectual decline that eventually leads to deterioration of occupational, social, and interpersonal functions. Onset is usually insidious with disturbances of memory, frequently attributed to the normal aging process. Sooner or later other areas of cognition become impaired—orientation, language, perceptions, praxis, ability to learn new skills, calculation, abstraction, and judgment. Consciousness is preserved until terminal stages, and other neurologic signs usually do not develop until the syndrome is well established.

EPIDEMIOLOGY

The percentage of people above the age of 60 is gradually increasing. At present, approximately 20 million Americans, or 11% of the total population, are older than 65 years of age. By the year 2000, this number will grow to approximately 32 million. Even though dementia may occur at all ages, the risk for most dementias, including Alzheimer's disease, increases substantially with increasing age. For example, at age 70, the probability of becoming demented is approximately 1.2%, whereas at age 80 the probability is 5.2%. It is estimated that as many as 10% of all elderly persons and 40%–50% of those over the age of 84 probably have Alzheimer's disease. Consequently, as more and more people live 80 to 100 years, the number of demented patients will increase substantially, and practically every physician will have to deal with demented elderly citizens. Of all patients with chronic dementing illnesses, the largest group (approximately 60%) will have Alzheimer's disease; 20% will have some form of vascular dementia; 10% will have a combination of vascular dementia and Alzheimer's disease; and the remaining 10% will have a great number of different illnesses, some of which are treatable.

OLD AGE VERSUS DEMENTIA

Contrary to common medical "wisdom," senescence is not equal to dementia. In old age, mental processes do become slowed, but the healthy older person still retains a firm grasp on reality, is oriented, can reason, has good judgment, and can continue to lead an active and self-supporting life. Many elderly "cantankerous" individuals are too readily labeled demented, when in fact they are simply reacting to the arrogant "know everything" behavior of the younger generation. Like all other organs and biologic systems, the brain ultimately will fail in old age. Severe disturbances of higher cortical functions, except for some slowness, do not occur until weeks to months prior to death. Most aged individuals will show less endurance and a decrease in speed of performance on mental tasks, similar to their decreased endurance and ability to attain peak performance in purely physical tasks. Material already learned is usually well retained, but learning new material becomes more difficult and takes longer. Vocabulary remains well preserved. At a primitive level, the primary senses become somewhat less sharp but are still adequate. Speech may become a bit slow, there may be some awkwardness in skilled movements, and a slight intention tremor may develop. Gait becomes more deliberate, and general stability may be impaired partly secondary to vestibular dysfunction, impaired vision, and loss of peripheral sensory receptors. A patient with dementing illness should be worked up and managed like any other patient with a medical problem. Even though only a small percentage of patients with dementia will have a treatable condition, all should have a complete work-up before a diagnostic label is applied. The primary care physician is ideally situated to make the appropriate diagnosis, supervise the work-up, and manage the patient with the help of neurologists, psychiatrists, social workers, and others.

MANIFESTATIONS OF DEMENTIA

In early stages of dementia, patients very often complain of diminished energy and enthusiasm, show less interest in subjects they previously cherished, and may display lability of affect and heightened anxiety level secondary to the awareness of failing mental functions. It is harder for these patients to recover their mental equilibrium, and defense mechanisms are blatantly utilized. As the disease progresses, achievement of personal ambitions and social achievements become less important, the patient becomes increasingly self-absorbed, anxiety increases, and the recognition of personal failure may lead to depression. At this stage there may be pronounced mood swings and poor judgment, followed by diminished drive and feelings. Hallucinations and delusions may occur at any stage, and often sleep-wake cycles are altered. Extreme restlessness and wandering at night are not uncommon. As the mental deterioration progresses, anxiety and depression disappear and are replaced by complete flatness of mood. Personal cleanliness deteriorates and patients will do little, if anything, spontaneously. They may have to be led to the bathroom, dressed, and fed. It is at this stage that other neurologic dysfunctions, such as hemiparesis and seizures, may develop. Lower-level cerebral functions usually remain quite intact until very late. Once the patient has reached the point of complete flatness of mood, inability to communicate, and total dependence on others, even treatable dementias are usually irreversible.

EVALUATION AND DIAGNOSIS

The initial evaluation of a patient suspected of having dementia includes a detailed history and general medical examination, with emphasis on detecting treatable causes. The latter may range from chronic infection to liver or kidney disease to iatrogenic drug intoxication and depression. The patient may ultimately require treatment of multiple medical conditions by a multitude of physicians. Very often, relatives or close associates are unreliable observers, because deterioration of higher cortical functions frequently develops insidiously over months to years, and those close to the patient are prone to excuse even striking changes in behavior and performance as simply the result of old age. Memory deficits, which can sometimes be historically pinpointed many years before the patient sees a physician, are often totally overlooked and/or ignored. Very often, it is at the point when a major defect in memory, judgment, or behavior occurs that relatives, friends, or close associates urge the patient to seek the help of a physician.

In addition to a detailed general examination and a careful neurologic examination, the key in the evaluation of a patient with possible dementia is the mental status examination. If a patient cannot appropriately give the time of day, the day of the week, the current month, and the current year, is unable to count backwards from 20 to 1, is unable to recite the months of the year backwards, and cannot remember a name and address for 5 to 10 minutes, the likelihood of a dementing illness is high. A more detailed mental examination, as outlined in Chapter 2, should then be conducted. Such examination should also be conducted if the short mental status examination is normal but the presence of dementia is still suspected. If the detailed mental status examination is inconclusive, formal neuropsychologic evaluation should be requested. Depression is common in the elderly and may be difficult to recognize. Therefore, psychiatric consultation should be obtained freely.

Although there is a multitude of diseases that may cause dementia (Table 6–1) and the clinical examination alone may not reveal the underlying cause, certain clinical clues are helpful. For example, the patient with Alzheimer's disease (AD) will have early and profound impairment of recent memory, whereas other mental faculties may still be relatively preserved or, at least, less severely affected. At the same time, the patient with AD will retain the social graces for a long time, whereas the patient with Pick's disease in addition to dementia may lose social graces fairly early in the disease process. Accompanying choreiform movements will point to Huntington's chorea, and myoclonic jerks to Jakob-Creutzfeld disease. Patients with rigidity, instability of station and gait, and 4–5 cps flexion-extension tremors probably have Parkinson's disease. Patients with Wilson's disease will have tremor and Kayser-Fleischer rings. In patients with multi-infarct dementia, the history may suggest stepwise progression, and on examination subtle or overt neurologic abnormalities beyond impairment of cortical functions may be apparent early in the course of the illness. Early instability of gait and urinary incontinence should raise the question of normal pressure hydrocephalus. Regardless of the initial clinical impression, a complete work-up as outlined in Table 6–2 should be done to detect treatable causes of dementia. This step is important, because once patients have been labeled as demented, they will more likely than not be disposed of in nursing homes, never to be looked at again. A minimal work-up consists of an EEG, an ECG, a CT scan or MRI scan, routine hematological and serological tests, a chest x-ray, and a urinalysis. This limited work-up will provide sufficient clues in practically all situations in which a treatable dementia is encountered. Although the proper work-up of a demented patient presents no special problems, additional help from medical specialists—including neurologists, psychiatrists, and psychologists—should be readily sought. Once the correct diagnosis has been established, the course of action is usually self-evident. Patients should be reexamined after 6 months to establish the rate of progression. Close collaboration with relatives, other caregivers, and social workers and adaptability to the patient's changing requirements are important. Prompt recognition and treatment of intercurrent illnesses and other chronic debilitating medical conditions are essential. Since many elderly patients are treated by a multitude of physicians for a multitude of problems with a multitude of drugs, it is not only advisable but manda-

TABLE 6–1. Some Disorders That May Cause Dementia

1. DIFFUSE PARENCHYMATOUS DISEASE OF THE CNS

Alzheimer's disease
Pick's disease
Diffuse Lewy body disease
Huntington's chorea
Parkinson's disease
Progressive supranuclear palsy
Parkinsonian-dementia complex of Guam
Multiple system atrophy
Hallervorden-Spatz disease
Spinocerebellar degenerations
Progressive myoclonus epilepsy
Shy-Drager syndrome
Progressive subcortical gliosis
Amyotrophic lateral sclerosis with dementia
Olivopontocerebellar atrophy
Familial dementia with spastic paraparesis

2. METABOLIC DISORDERS

Hypo- and hyperthyroidism
Hypo- and hypercalcemia
Hepatic failure
Wilson's disease
Non-Wilsonian hepatolenticular degeneration
Renal failure
Dialysis encephalopathy
Hypo- and hyperglycemia
Cushing's syndrome
Hypopituitarism
Electrolyte and acid-base disturbances

3. VASCULAR DISORDERS

Multi-infarct dementia
Lacunar state
Binswanger's disease
Cortical microinfarction
Aortic arch syndrome
Vasculitis
Arteriovenous malformation

4. ANEMIA

5. HYPOXIA AND ANOXIA

6. BRAIN TUMOR

Primary intracranial
Metastatic
Menigeal carcinomatosis

7. TRAUMA

Open and closed head injuries with cerebral contusion
Subdural hematoma
Punch-drunk syndrome

8. INFECTIONS

Fungal meningitis
HIV infection
Encephalitis

Table continued on following page

TABLE 6-1. Some Disorders That May Cause Dementia *(Continued)*

Jakob-Creutzfeld disease
Progressive multifocal leukoencephalopathy
Gerstmann-Sträussler-Scheinker disease
Neurosyphilis
Behçet's syndrome
Kuru
Whipple's disease
Subacute sclerosing panencephalitis
Borreliosis (Lyme disease)

9. DEFICIENCY DISEASES

Wernicke-Korsakoff syndrome
Pellagra
B^{12} deficiency
Marchiafava-Bignami disease
Folate deficiency

10. TOXINS AND DRUGS

Alcohol
Drugs (atropine and related compounds, barbiturates, bromides, clonidine, disulfiram, fluphenazine, haloperidol, lithium carbonate, mephenytoin, methyldopa, phenothiazines, phenytoin, propranolol)
Heavy metals (arsenic, lead, mercury, thallium)
Organic compounds
Carbon monoxide

11. OTHER

Depression
Delayed effects of radiation
Multiple sclerosis
Epilepsy
Muscular dystrophy
Remote effect of carcinoma
Hydrocephalus

tory for the primary physician to know exactly what each of these colleagues is doing. All too often, patients become demented or are made worse when many different physicians, without knowledge of one another's actions, prescribe drugs that, taken together, have profound effects on patients' higher cortical functions. It is impossible to deal with the entire spectrum of diseases producing dementia. However, a few selected dementing illnesses will be discussed here, some because of their sheer numbers, some because of widespread interest in them, and some because they are treatable.

ALZHEIMER'S DISEASE

AD contributes the largest number of patients with insidiously progressing dementia. It is much more prevalent than Pick's disease. The

TABLE 6–2. Laboratory Tests in the Evaluation of Dementia

Test	Rationale
Blood tests	
Blood count	Anemia, infection
Electrolytes	Pulmonary, renal, endocrine dysfunctions
BUN, creatinine	Renal dysfunction
Liver function tests	Hepatic dysfunction
T4	Thyroid dysfunction
Serological tests for syphilis	Syphilis
Toxicology screen	Drug intoxication
B^{12}, folate levels	B^{12}, folate deficiency
Collagen-vascular disease tests	Arteritis
Sedimentation rate	Temporal arteritis
Urine examination	
Urinalysis	Renal and hepatic disease
Heavy metal screen	Heavy metal intoxication
Porphobilinogen, delta amino-levulinic acid	Porphyria
Chest x-ray	Chronic obstructive lung disease, chronic infectious diseases, primary or metastatic malignancies
ECG	Arrhythmias, recent or remote myocardial infarction
EEG	Tumor, cerebrovascular disease, epilepsy, toxic metabolic disturbances
CT scan	Focal or diffuse cerebral atrophy, infarction, tumor
MRI scan	Focal or diffuse cerebral atrophy, infarction, tumor
CSF examination	Chronic and acute infections, multiple sclerosis, meningeal carcinomatosis, subarachnoid hemorrhage
Angiography	Tumor, aneurysm, arteriovenous malformation, arteritis

clinical distinction between the two is difficult in most situations, even though pathologically they are distinctly different. One exception is that patients with Pick's disease are more likely to lose their social graces early, whereas this manifestation occurs late in patients with AD. Furthermore, the onset of Pick's disease is often earlier than that of AD. A distinction used to be made between presenile and senile dementia. Since the pathological process, the clinical manifestations, and the natural history are identical whether the onset is before age 60 or after, such distinction no longer serves a useful purpose. As indicated earlier, the incidence of AD increases significantly with advancing age, but senescence does not equal AD. Clinical and pathological observations have recently shown that AD has variable clinical and pathological expressions. In some patients, in addition to the classical pathological changes of AD, Lewy bodies are seen throughout the cerebral cortex. Clinically these patients, besides their dementia, usually have prominent rigidity and akinesia. In diffuse Lewy body disease, prominent rigidity and akinesia are present early, with dementia starting later.

The etiology of AD is unknown. Age is certainly the most important risk factor for AD. First-degree relatives of patients with AD have an increased risk of developing AD, but the extent of the estimated risk varies from 5% to 100%. The familial occurrence of AD is well established, and in different families abnormalities on chromosomes 14, 19, and 21 have been identified. In almost all of these families, the onset of AD is at a younger age than in sporadic cases. The ε4 allele of apolipoprotein E has been shown to be associated with late onset sporadic AD. In identical and fraternal twins, concordance is similar (40%–42%). The risk of AD is slightly higher in women. Many, but not all, studies have reported head trauma as a risk factor. Whether or not aluminum or other metals are risk factors is still not clear. Coronary artery disease may be a risk factor.

The pathology of AD is characterized by a shrunken brain, Alzheimer's neurofibrillary tangles (which, on electron microscopy, consist of double helical twisted tubules), senile plaques (which consist of a degenerated amyloid center and surrounding neurofibrillary tangles), and, in some patients, amyloid depositions in intracranial blood vessels. Similar but less abundant senile plaques and neurofibrillary tangles may be seen in normal, aged individuals and in some other disease entities. The abundance of these pathological changes and their widespread distribution are the hallmarks of AD. In addition, there is reduction of choline acetyltransferase in the brains of patients with AD. Somatostatin may also be decreased, frequently by as much as 50%. Recent studies have shown that one of the earliest abnormalities is selective decrease in synapses.

Early in AD, CT and MRI scans are of little help, because the degree of brain atrophy and ventricular enlargement does not correlate well with cerebral function. As a matter of fact, sometimes striking atrophy is found in individuals who have maintained a very high level of cortical functions. Similarly, nonspecific white matter changes on CT or MRI scan do not correlate with AD. Early in the course of the illness, the EEG remains normal or shows minor, nonspecific abnormalities. The spinal fluid is normal. There is no specific treatment at this time for AD or Pick's disease; care, consequently, is supportive and should take into account the patient's changing level of performance. Early supportive psychotherapy or psychotropic drugs for anxiety and/or depression may be extremely helpful. Ultimately, many patients will require institutionalization because of their total dependence on others for even the most primitive functions. Life expectancy is reduced by about 5 to 10 years after establishment of the diagnosis. Recently tacrine hydrochloride, a centrally active, noncompetitive reversible cholinesterase inhibitor, has become available for treatment of AD. Patients with mild to moderate impairment treated with tacrine had a smaller decline in activities of daily living and cognitive functions. In many patients the drug has to be withdrawn because of liver transaminase elevation and gastrointestinal complaints.

VASCULAR DEMENTIAS

Patients with vascular dementia very often will have historical evidence or findings on neurologic examination and on CT or MRI scan that will allow establishment of the appropriate diagnosis. The clinical diagnosis is usually based on the presence of dementia; evidence of two or more ischemic strokes by history, neurologic signs, and/or imaging studies; occurrence of a single stroke with documented temporal relationship to the onset of dementia; and evidence of at least one infarct on CT or T1-weighted MRI scans. Slowly progressive symptoms, psychosis, hallucinations, delusions, and seizures are not strong evidence for vascular dementia. No specific therapy is presently available except prevention of further strokes with aspirin or ticlopidine. The best prevention is long-term control of hypertension.

SUBDURAL HEMATOMA

Unilateral and, particularly, bilateral subdural hematomas may produce a dementia with only subtle or no other neurologic abnormalities. This entity should be considered very seriously in all patients subject to head trauma and in those who are on chronic anticoagulants. Although bilateral subdural hematomas are uncommon in the average adult patient, except following serious and obvious head trauma, the incidence of bilateral subdural hematomas increases with advancing age, and frequently no distinct episode of head trauma may be recalled. Elderly subjects are more likely to fall, and such an episode is only too readily ignored or forgotten. Treatment usually consists of evacuation of the clot.

INFECTION

Some of the more commonly encountered infectious processes are syphilis, fungal infection, and slow virus infection. The patient with tertiary lues of the brain rarely presents with grandiose-expansive manifestations. Most often the patient will be quiet, withdrawn, and on mental status examination will show impairment in all areas tested. Early and vigorous treatment with penicillin may halt further progression or, at times, produce dramatic improvement with return to normal. Chronic fungal infections, such as cryptococcosis, histoplasmosis, and coccidiomycosis of the CNS are not common. Nevertheless, because they are treatable entities, they should be diligently sought, even though they may require lifelong therapy. Besides the encephalopathy associated with the AIDS virus, many patients with AIDS will develop coccidiomycosis of the CNS. Representative examples of slow virus infections are Jakob-Creutzfeld disease and multifocal leucoencephalopathy, the latter usually seen in the context of an underlying malignancy. These conditions presently are not treatable but may be amenable to antiviral therapy in the future.

TRAUMA

Progressive deterioration of mental function has been known for a long time to occur in professional fighters. This possibility should always be considered in patients who have had multiple head trauma or who have engaged in activities frequently associated with such trauma. Although no specific treatment is available, further head trauma should be studiously avoided, and if posttraumatic epilepsy is present, this should be treated appropriately.

ALCOHOLISM

The recognized classical dementia of alcoholism is the Wernicke-Korsakoff syndrome. In the acute phase, this condition is characterized by moderate to severe impairment of higher cortical functions, obtundation or coma, and a variety of abnormalities of eye movements. It is also frequently accompanied by a polyneuropathy. Vigorous early treatment with thiamine may strikingly alter the course of the illness favorably in most patients. Those patients in whom treatment comes too late will exhibit profound disturbance of recent memory, evidence of variable degrees of impairment of other cortical functions, and confabulation. With time, some of these patients may improve somewhat, but many will not change. A similar clinical picture may be seen in some patients following head trauma. In addition to the Wernicke-Korsakoff syndrome, patients who chronically use alcohol may develop an insidiously progressing dementia that affects all aspects of higher cortical functions equally. This dementia is probably secondary to direct toxic effects of alcohol on cerebral neurons. Abstinence from alcohol is often followed by some improvement of cortical functions, but such improvement often falls short of the patient's former normal level of performance. Thiamine should be used in these insidiously progressing dementia patients to cover the possibility of coexisting Wernicke-Korsakoff syndrome, but not because thiamine has a direct effect on this type of dementia.

INTOXICATION

Exogenous intoxications by heavy metals such as arsenic, mercury, and lead are rare, and in most instances they are readily diagnosed by the presence of other distinct features of these intoxications. The most common form of intoxication leading to dementia, particularly in the elderly, is secondary to abuse of psychoactive drugs including barbiturates. Meticulous inquiry into a patient's pattern of drug intake, sometimes requiring information from other treating physicians and from local drugstores, may reveal that patients are ingesting an inordinate amount of different drugs, rendering them in some cases totally nonfunctional. The rather standard response by patients and relatives that they take only what their physicians prescribe is meaningless and in fact should precipitate a detailed inquiry into the patient's medications. Withdrawal from all psychoactive medications and supervision of future drug intake will restore such patients to their normal level of mental function. Accompanying ataxia and disturbance of wake-sleep cycles will also disappear. Because of inactivity, boredom, and/or physical disabilities, many elderly persons expect to sleep 12 hours or more every night and to take a few naps during the day. This expectation frequently leads to chronic abuse of sedatives, which become less effective with time, requiring even larger amounts. Most elderly subjects require no more than 6 to 7 hours of sleep per 24-hour period. Withdrawal from all sedatives, establishment of realistic sleep periods, and increase of activities during the day will very often restore such patients to a healthy pattern of living. Unfortunately, this is easier said than done because of firmly held misconceptions and convenience. Persistent efforts by the physician are essential to change such abnormal and unhealthy living patterns.

OBSTRUCTIVE HYDROCEPHALUS

Hydrocephalus means enlargement of one or several cerebral ventricles. Obstructive hydrocephalus denotes obstruction at any point from the lateral to the fourth ventricle. Obstruction at one foramen of Monroe causes lateral ventricle enlargement, aqueductal obstruction enlarges both lateral ventricles, and obstruction at the outlet of the fourth ventricle causes enlargement of all the ventricles. Evaluation of hydrocephalus is best done with the CT or MRI scan. These scans may show one of the above described patterns, as well as its cause (e.g., a mass lesion). Causes of obstructive hydrocephalus include primary and metastatic tumors; aqueductal stenosis; cerebral abscesses; hemorrhages; cysts; congenital abnormalities of the posterior fossa and ventricular system; and occasionally brain edema, which obstructs the aqueduct or fourth ventricle from strokes, trauma, meningitis, and numerous other causes. Treatment of obstructive hydrocephalus is dependent on the cause. Treatment may be aimed at removing the obstruction, such as a mass. Alternatively, a shunt may be placed in the dilated ventricles to carry the CSF to the peritoneal cavity or heart.

COMMUNICATING HYDROCEPHALUS

Communicating hydrocephalus denotes enlargement of all the ventricles and free communication from lateral ventricles to the fourth ventricle and subarachnoid space. Obstruction of the subarachnoid space either in the basilar meninges or at the superior sagittal sinus can produce communicating hydrocephalus. The CSF pressure may be markedly elevated, mildly elevated, or even normal, depending upon the relative degree of block and the acuteness of the process.

Normal pressure hydrocephalus is a form of communicating hydrocephalus in which interference with the normal flow of CSF and its absorption takes place in the subarachnoid space. The condition may be due to a previous subarachnoid hemorrhage or a meningeal infection, but very often no apparent cause is found. The patient with this condition typically presents with failing higher cortical functions, ataxia, and urinary incontinence. CT scan reveals striking enlargement of all cerebral ventricles, with or without accompanying cerebral atrophy. The EEG is usually normal or shows mild, generalized, nonspecific changes. Injection of a radiolabeled substance in the lumbar subarachnoid space will show that the radioactive material will accumulate for a prolonged period of time in the cerebral ventricles. Unfortunately, the diagnosis of this condition is difficult; none of the previously mentioned symptoms, signs, and tests is absolutely diagnostic. The patient who presents early with all of the above symptoms and signs and who has an abnormal cisternogram is the one who is most likely to respond favorably to a shunting procedure. At the time of shunting, a small cortical biopsy should be taken, which may establish that the patient has AD or some other process accounting for the dementia.

REFERENCES

Freeman FR: Evaluation of patients with progressive intellectual deterioration. Arch Neurol 1976; 33:658–659.

Wells CE (ed): Dementia, 2nd ed. Philadelphia, FA Davis, 1977.

Cummings J, Benson F, La Verme S: Reversible dementia: illustrative cases, definition, and review. JAMA 1980; 243:2434–2439.

Katzman R, Terry R, Bick K (eds): Alzheimer's Disease: Senile Dementia and Related Disorders. New York, Raven Press, 1983.

McKhann G, Drachman D, Folstein M, Katzman R, Price D, Stadlan EM: Clinical diagnosis of Alzheimer's disease: Report of the NINCDS-ADRDA work group under the auspices of Department of Health and Human Services Task Force on Alzheimer's Disease. Neurology 1984; 34:939–944.

AMA: Dementia—council on scientific affairs. JAMA 1986; 256:2234–2238.

Katzman R: Alzheimer's disease. N Engl J Med 1986; 314:964–973.

Foley J, Chairman: NIH consensus development conference statement, vol 6, no. 11. Differential diagnosis of dementing diseases. US Government Printing Office, Washington, DC, 1987, pp 1–9.

Chui HC, Victoroff JI, Margolin D, Jagust W, Shankle R, Katzman R: Criteria for the diagnosis of ischemic vascular dementia proposed by the state of California Alzheimer's disease diagnostic and treatment centers. Neurology 1992; 42:473–480.

Tacrine for Alzheimer's disease: Med Lett Drugs Ther 1993; 35:87–88.

Friedland RP: Alzheimer's disease: Clinical features and differential diagnosis. Neurology 1993; 43(Supp 4):S45–S51.

Saunders AM, Strittmatter WJ, Schmechel D, St. George-Hyslop PH, Pericak-Vance MA, Joo SH, Rosi BL, Gusella JF, Crapper-MacLachian DR, Alberts MJ, Hulette C, Crain B, Goldgaber D, Roses AD: Association of apolipoprotein E allele ε4 with late-onset familial and sporadic Alzheimer's disease. Neurology 1993; 43:1467–1472.

Winker MA: Tacrine for Alzheimer's disease. Which patient, what dose? JAMA 1994; 271:1023–1024.

7
Demyelinating Diseases

The demyelinating disorders are a broad category of diseases of the CNS in which there is destruction of normally formed myelin sheaths with relative preservation of neuronal axons. The distribution of lesions is often perivenous. The primary demyelinating diseases include multiple sclerosis (MS) and its uncommon variants: Devic's neuromyelitis optica, Schilder's encephalitis periaxialis diffusa, and Balo's concentric sclerosis. Other demyelinating diseases (see Table 7–1) include a variety of etiologically specific and nonspecific causes of demyelination such as viral infections, vaccines, and certain genetic disorders.

MULTIPLE SCLEROSIS

MS, which is the only demyelinating disorder that is frequently encountered, is a chronic neurologic disease that typically begins in early adulthood and progresses to significant disability in the majority of cases. An unpredictable course and wide variety of symptoms and signs are remarkable features of the disease. The disease is the most common progressive and disabling neurologic condition affecting young adults. There are approximately 123,000 known MS patients in the United States. Because the onset of the illness usually occurs in early adulthood, family life and job productivity are often seriously disrupted. Current theories favor an immunologic pathogenesis of MS due to a fundamental defect in the host, with or without the presence of a triggering viral agent. No virus has been isolated. The pathology consists of discrete demyelinated plaques that range in size from a few millimeters to several centimeters. They are often perivenous and in the brain cluster around the lateral ventricles. In fresh plaques an abundance of macrophages and perivenous cuffs of lymphocytes and mononuclear cells are present. Neurons and most axis cylinders are spared.

TABLE 7-1. Demyelinating Diseases

Multiple sclerosis	Relapsing and chronic progressive forms
	Acute multiple sclerosis
	Neuromyelitis optica (Devic's disease)
Diffuse cerebral sclerosis	Schilder's encephalitis periaxialis diffusa
	Balo's concentric sclerosis
Acute disseminated encephalomyelitis	After measles, chickenpox, rubella, influenza, mumps
	After rabies or smallpox vaccination
Necrotizing hemorrhagic encephalitis	Hemorrhagic leukoencephalitis
Leukodystrophies	Krabbe's globoid leukodystrophy
	Metachromatic leukodystrophy
	Adrenoleukodystrophy
	Adrenomyeloneuropathy
	Pelizaeus-Merzbacher leukodystrophy
	Canavan's disease
	Alexander's disease

Epidemiology

The mean age of onset of MS is 33 years and the mean age of diagnosis is 37 years. The condition rarely appears before the age of 10, and only in about 10% of cases does it begin after the age of 50. MS occurs most frequently in white women, having a female to male ratio of 1.7 to 1 and a white to nonwhite ratio of about 2 to 1. It is more common in the cold and temperate climates of the higher latitudes in both hemispheres. Studies of the prevalence of MS in immigrant populations indicate that a person's chance of developing the disease is correlated with having lived in these higher latitudes in the first 15 years of life. There is some evidence that genetic factors are involved. MS occurs in 1%–2% of first-degree relatives of MS patients, and MS predominantly affects individuals of northern European ancestry. Furthermore, studies of the distribution of histocompatability antigen genetic marker in MS patients have shown an overrepresentation of A3, B7, DR2, and DR3 types. The relation of these factors to the pathogenesis of the disease is unknown.

Symptoms and Signs

No two patients with MS are exactly alike, and the clinical manifestations in a particular individual are related to the distribution of lesions within the nervous system. Lesions may be found virtually anywhere within the white matter of the central neuraxis, including the white matter of the cerebral hemispheres, optic nerves, brainstem, cerebellum, and spinal cord. Although some patients have evidence of widespread lesions from the outset, others may present with isolated focal involvement of any of these structures. Symptoms and signs may disappear or may fluctuate in character and intensity. The sometimes bizarre and transient nature of the symptoms may be mistaken for a psychiatric condition.

Muscular weakness and spasticity due to corticospinal tract lesions are among the most frequent symptoms of MS. Spasticity of the lower extremities may be accompanied by painful flexor spasms. Impaired dexterity, slowness of rapid alternating movements, hyperreflexia, extensor plantar responses, and absence of abdominal reflexes may also be noted, along with hemiparesis, paraparesis, quadriparesis, or monoparesis.

Complaints of severe fatigue are common, and disabling exhaustion may be brought on by an ordinary day's activities. This symptom is remarkable, because in some patients it occurs in the presence of normal strength and without any symptoms generally associated with depression.

Visual disturbances include impaired visual acuity, impaired color vision, central scotoma, diplopia, and uncommonly such visual field defects as homonymous hemianopsia. Symptoms may be unilateral or bilateral. Optic neuritis and retrobulbar neuritis are common in MS. Visual loss progresses over days and may be mild to severe. Pain in or behind the eye, which sometimes is caused or worsened by movement of the eye, is a common complaint. Examination during the episode will show loss of visual acuity, loss of color vision, a central scotoma, and preserved peripheral vision. Examination of the fundus will show a swollen disc if the lesion is close to the optic nerve head (papillitis). During the acute phase the disc looks normal (retrobulbar neuritis) in most cases. Neurologic examination following the episode often will show residual deficits of visual acuity and color vision, together with optic atrophy manifested as a pale optic disc, particularly its temporal portion. Not all patients with optic neuritis have or will develop MS. In previously healthy patients with a first attack of optic neuritis, 40%–70% will subsequently develop symptoms and signs of MS.

Another common visual manifestation of MS is diplopia caused by an internuclear ophthalmoplegia. This is a disorder of conjugate lateral gaze, which may be unilateral or bilateral, characterized by nystagmus of the abducting eye and weakness of nasal movement of the adducting eye with preservation of convergence. Its presence in a young adult is almost pathognomonic for MS with the demyelinating lesion in the medial longitudinal fasciculus on the same side as the eye in which nasal movement is impaired.

Disturbance of sphincter control is noted in at least two thirds of patients sometime during the course of the disease. Urinary dysfunction may be due to a "failure to store" (also called hypertonic or spastic bladder), "failure to empty" (also called atonic or flaccid bladder), or a mixture of the two. Symptoms include frequency, urgency, incontinence, incomplete emptying, and urinary retention. The major bowel complaint is constipation, although fecal incontinence occurs occasionally.

Complaints of sexual dysfunction are frequent and include erectile and ejaculatory problems in men and loss of orgasmic ability in women. These problems may be compounded by depression or by urinary and fecal incontinence that may occur during intercourse.

Lesions in the cerebellar white matter or cerebellar pathways may produce nystagmus, prominent gait and extremity ataxia, and a halting or scanning quality of speech. Severe intention tremor of the upper extremities may make the simplest self-care tasks impossible, and severe ataxia of gait may prevent effective ambulation even when muscular strength is adequate.

Sensory symptoms are diverse and include numbness, tingling, impairment of temperature sensation, and abnormal sense of limb position. Vague sensory complaints in unusual distributions may mysteriously come and go and cause confusion about the diagnosis. Examination may not reveal any objective sensory deficit even in the presence of symptoms. Impairment of vibratory perception may be found without any abnormality of other sensory functions. Lhermitte's phenomenon, which is provoked by flexion of the neck, is usually described as an electric shock sensation that radiates down the spine or into the extremities. This unusual symptom is often due to MS but may also occur with other disorders affecting the posterior columns of the cervical spinal cord. Approximately 5%–10% of MS patients experience either typical trigeminal neuralgia or a pseudoradicular pain of the extremities or trunk.

Some form of mental disturbance eventually occurs in half of MS patients. Depression is common. An inappropriate euphoria is seen on occasion. Mild dementia and organic psychosis due to cerebral involvement occur frequently. These disorders may be severe in patients with advanced disease.

Precipitating and Exacerbating Factors

Although the cause of MS is unknown, certain factors sometimes precipitate attacks in known MS patients. Trauma, infection, and surgery have all been associated with worsening of MS. There may be a slight increase in risk of exacerbation during and in the 6 months following pregnancy. There is no evidence that immunization is a precipitating factor. Elevation of body temperature has a different effect. Fever, heavy physical exertion, hot weather, a hot shower or bath, and exposure to sunlight may all cause a transient and reversible worsening of existing symptoms. For example, weakness may become worse to the point where a normally ambulatory patient is unable to get out of the bathtub after a hot bath. Neurologic function will then return to baseline within minutes to several hours of when the patient is helped out of the bath. Similarly, a person who can usually transfer independently may require assistance in this activity during very hot weather. Occasionally a symptom such as visual difficulty in one eye may be present only during exposure to heat. Interestingly, lowering of body temperature by swimming in a cold pool or taking a cold shower may result in a temporary improvement of function.

Course of MS

The natural progression of MS is unpredictable. In approximately 40% of MS patients, the disease is initially exacerbating-remitting, with or without complete recovery between episodes. After several years, there is then a transition to a slow and relentless chronic progression. In another 20%–30% of patients, the disease maintains an exacerbating-remitting course. In 10%–20% of patients, the course from the outset is chronically progressive, a pattern that is seen most often in patients who are older at the time of onset of the illness. Finally, in about 20% of MS patients, the course is benign, with the patient suffering only one or two mild exacerbations and no permanent functional disability. The rate of progression of MS is variable, ranging from the occasional malignant course with death within weeks or months after onset to lifelong benign disease with minimal symptoms and disability. In general, those who have either chronic progression or frequent severe relapses from the outset of the illness have a less favorable long-term prognosis. Patients who have been in the chronic progressive stage of the illness for a number of years may experience decline in the rate of deterioration. In general patients with a primary progressive course experience the most severe course. In the intermittent type a relatively favorable prognosis is associated with few exacerbations, a low number of affected neurologic systems, high degree of remissions, and mild neurologic impairment.

Over the last half century, advances in antibiotic therapy and in the management of complications have resulted in an increase in the life span of MS patients. In 1936, only 8% of patients were reported to survive beyond 20 years after the onset of illness. By 1961, survival had increased tenfold, with over 80% of patients surviving for 20 years after onset of illness. Of those patients surviving for 20 years or more, approximately 30% remained gainfully employed. These statistics indicate that the long-term prognosis in MS is more favorable now than in the past.

Clinical Diagnosis

The diagnosis of MS remains a clinical one; there is no specific laboratory test for the disease. The clinician generally makes the diagnosis of MS when there is evidence of multiple lesions in time and space. The diagnosis of clinically definite MS requires two attacks and clinical findings compatible with two separate lesions; or two attacks, clinical evidence of one lesion, and evidence of another lesion on CT, MRI, or evoked potentials. The diagnosis of definite MS is supported by the presence of oligoclonal bands in the CSF or increased synthesis of IgG. If the age of onset is between 10 and 50 years, the patient has lived in the higher latitudes during part of the first 15 years of life, and the symptoms worsen transiently with exposure to heat, the diagnosis is more likely. There must be no better neurologic explanation for the patient's symptoms and signs. Often the diagnosis cannot be made at the time of presentation. In the young person with a single attack consisting of a single lesion in space, laboratory tests may fail to show evidence of other subclinical lesions. MS can then only be suspected. Similarly, in the older patient with a gradually progressive deficit that can be explained by one lesion at a specific location, MS is a diagnosis of exclusion.

Laboratory Examinations

There is no specific laboratory test for MS. Such tests are, however, important for ruling out other nervous system diseases that may mimic MS. They are also invaluable for demonstrating evidence of a second lesion that is subclinical and therefore not detectable by history or neurologic examination. The demonstration of the second lesion is generally the key to making the diagnosis of MS in the patient with early disease. Laboratory tests are also important in the patient who has symptoms suggestive of MS but lacks objective physical signs of nervous system disease. One or more definite lesions of the nervous system may be shown to be present.

The hot bath test may be done in the clinic or on the hospital ward. The patient is immersed in a bathtub of hot water and then examined neurologically for the transient appearance of additional deficits. A patient with subclinical optic neuritis may develop an abnormality of visual acuity or color vision. In other patients, an internuclear ophthalmoplegia, nystagmus, or ataxia may become apparent. Weakness, hyperreflexia, and Babinski signs may also develop. Visual, auditory, and somatosensory evoked responses are sensitive electrophysiologic procedures that can identify clinically silent lesions. If all three tests are performed, approximately 80%–85% of patients with a clinically definite diagnosis will have an abnormality on at least one of the tests. The visual and auditory evoked response tests are especially useful in identifying a second subclinical lesion in patients who have clinical evidence of only a single spinal cord lesion. In this instance, the demonstration of a second lesion remote from the spinal cord may help establish the diagnosis of MS.

MRI of the brain and spinal cord has become the most important tool in the diagnosis and follow-up of patients with MS. CT of the brain is of limited usefulness, because only 20% of patients with clinically definite MS will have radiographic abnormalities. MRI is useful in excluding other CNS diseases that may mimic MS. In patients with only one known lesion, the MRI may demonstrate a second lesion, thereby making MS the likely clinical diagnosis. MS lesions appear as areas of increased signal on spin-echo images and of decreased signal on inversion-recovery images. Unfortunately, MRI abnormalities do not correlate too well with clinical symptomatology and findings. Patients who appear clinically stable may develop new lesions on MRI. Some patients with only one clinical exacerbation during a 12-month period may develop 5 or more new lesions on MRI. In patients with an acute clinically isolated syndrome suggestive of MS, the presence of 4 or more lesions on MRI is associated with a high rate of progression to MS.

Nonspecific abnormalities present in the CSF are frequently useful in supporting the diagnosis of MS by suggesting the presence of an inflammatory CNS lesion. The CSF cell count commonly shows a modest increase in mononuclear cells. The total CSF protein is mildly or moderately elevated in less than half of MS patients. In approximately 60%–75% of patients, there is an abnormal elevation of the CSF IgG. Furthermore, 85% of patients with clinically definite MS have abnormal oligoclonal bands in the IgG zone on CSF electrophoresis. If IgG and oligoclonal bands are both measured, 90% of such MS patients will have abnormalities. One limitation of these tests is that they are less frequently abnormal in early or very mild cases of MS. Additionally, abnormalities of the more sensitive tests may also be produced by other CNS inflammatory processes and by chronic CNS infections.

In summary, the patient with reliable historical or clinical evidence of two separate CNS lesions should have a CSF examination to rule out infection. In addition, an MRI scan of the brain and, in some cases, of the spinal cord should be obtained to rule out other pathological processes that may mimic MS. Patients suspected of having MS who have only one established lesion or no definite CNS lesions should undergo these tests together with the hot bath test and evoked responses. In these patients, the laboratory tests are done in an attempt to rule out other CNS pathology and to demonstrate the presence of at least two separate CNS lesions required to make the clinical diagnosis of MS.

Differential Diagnosis

The differential diagnosis (see Table 7–2) of MS depends on the syndrome of CNS dysfunction present at the time of diagnosis. When an isolated optic neuritis is secondary to local orbital or sinus infection, the causative process can generally be demonstrated with CT or MRI. Similarly, serology and spinal fluid exam will show whether the optic nerve lesion is due to a meningeal process such as neurosyphilis or carcinomatous meningitis. A presentation that can be entirely explained by a single posterior fossa lesion could be produced by a benign or malignant tumor, basilar impression of the skull, developmental diseases such as Arnold-Chiari malformation, or occasionally by cerebrovascular disease. MRI scan will generally rule out these conditions. The uncommon chronic meningeal process that began in the posterior fossa would be ruled out by an examination of the spinal fluid for infection or tumor. If an isolated spinal cord lesion is caused by spondylosis, tumor, or syrinx, it will be seen with MRI or CT myelography. When no cause is found for an isolated spinal cord lesion, and both the history and spinal fluid are suggestive of a mild acute or subacute inflammatory process, an idiopathic transverse myelitis is the probable diagnosis. Only a few percent of these patients will go on to develop MS.

On the rare occasions when MS presents clinically as a subacute or chronic intracerebral mass lesion, low-grade glioma will generally be suspected. MRI scan or, if necessary, brain biopsy will reveal the true cause of the lesion. In any patient with remitting-relapsing neurologic illness, collagen vascular disease, sarcoidosis, and Behçet's syndrome must be considered. All three commonly have associated involvement of other organ systems. MS in contrast, is a strictly neurologic disease.

TABLE 7–2. Differential Diagnosis of Multiple Sclerosis

Transverse myelitis secondary to viral or bacterial infections
Acute disseminated encephalomyelitis
Leber's optic atrophy
Spinocerebellar degeneration
Hereditary ataxias
Tropical spastic paraparesis
HIV paraparesis
Compressive myelopathies
Brainstem and cerebellar tumors
Collagen vascular disease, including arteritides
Neurosyphilis
Lyme disease
Progressive multifocal leukoencephalopathy

In the patient with collagen vascular disease, there may also be abnormal rheumatologic blood tests. Many patients with sarcoidosis will have an abnormal angiotensin converting enzyme.

Neuroimaging tests will rule out mass lesions, particularly tumor or spondylosis, in the patient with a gradually progressing illness. Neurodegenerative diseases may also present in this fashion and may sometimes be demonstrated by family history or actual examination of family members. Patients with established MS are not exempt from developing other neurologic diseases, including cervical spondylosis with cord compression, and it is far better to obtain too many additional tests than to assume that everything is related to MS.

The diagnosis of possible or probable MS is made after ruling out the appropriate conditions in the differential diagnosis. Except for the rare cases in which the diagnosis is proved pathologically, the diagnosis is—and remains—presumptive. For this reason, future changes in neurologic status will generally warrant reconsideration of the differential diagnosis at a number of times during the course of the disease.

Therapeutics

The management of MS can be divided into four categories: (1) treatment aimed at modification of the disease course, including treatment of the acute exacerbation and treatment directed at long-term suppression of the disease; (2) treatment of the symptoms of MS; (3) prevention and treatment of medical complications; and (4) management of secondary personal and social problems. The short-term use of either adrenocorticotropic hormone (ACTH) or oral corticosteroids is the only specific therapeutic measure available for the treatment of the patient with an acute exacerbation of MS. Controlled studies of such therapy have shown that patients treated with ACTH (80 units in 500 ml dextrose and water given intravenously daily for 3 days) have a faster recovery, although there is no difference in the final amount of recovery. This treatment is followed by intramuscular injections of ACTH gel (40 units twice daily for 7 days). The dose is then decreased by 10 units every 3 days. If symptoms recur, some neurologists advocate using ACTH gel (40 units every other day) for several weeks or even months. In most cases this parenteral therapy has to be administered in the hospital. Pretreatment evaluation should include a search for tuberculosis, uremia, high blood pressure, diabetes, electrolyte disturbance, and peptic ulcer, which are relative contraindications to the use of ACTH. Because ACTH produces a variable amount of salt and water retention, weight and blood pressure should be checked regularly during treatment, and a low sodium diet with oral potassium supplementation should be prescribed. The occurrence of complications necessitating early discontinuation of therapy are infrequent, although intensification of preexistent depression or euphoria, emotional lability, insomnia, and frank psychosis are among the most common troublesome side effects. Intravenous methylprednisolone (500–1000 mg daily for 3 to 5 days) may be as effective as ACTH. Some prefer to prescribe oral prednisone. The total daily dose is determined by weight: 50 mg twice daily for weight greater than 180 pounds, 40 mg for patients weighing 110 to 180 pounds, and 30 mg for patients weighing less than 110 pounds. This weight-adjusted dose is given for 7 consecutive days. On the eighth day the total daily amount is given as a single morning dose, and the dosage is thereafter gradually tapered to 0 mg at the rate of 10 mg per day. Lower doses of prednisone are probably ineffective.

There is no established treatment that will suppress MS on a long-term basis. Chronic ACTH or prednisone therapies have not proved beneficial in either reducing the number of exacerbations or in slowing gradually progressive disability. High-dose cyclophosphamide (80–100 mg/kg intravenously for 10 to 14 days) or azathioprine (1–2.5 mg/kg/per day), often in conjunction with prednisone, has been shown to have some favorable effect on the course of patients with progressive and intermittent-progressive disease. However, these therapies are potentially quite toxic, and retreatment is necessary because the majority of patients regress. The role of plasmapheresis is unclear. Recently, interferon beta-1b has been shown to reduce the exacerbation rates, severity of exacerbations, and accumulation of MRI abnormalities in patients with the relapsing-remitting form of MS. In preliminary trials cladribine (2-chlorodeoxyadenosine; 2-CdA) had promising results in patients with progressive MS.

Effective symptom management and assistance in coping with the problems of everyday living can improve the quality of life for the MS patient. For example, spasticity may be alleviated by drug therapy. Baclofen (40–80 mg/per day in divided doses) is usually of value in reducing severe spasticity and involuntary flexor spasms. Mild spasticity generally should not be treated, but most patients with moderate to severe spasticity warrant a trial of therapy. Increased weakness and deterioration in gait are, unfortunately, a limiting side effect of baclofen in some ambulatory patients. Such weakness clears up within 24 to 48 hours after reduction in dose or discontinuation of therapy. This side effect is especially prominent in patients who are relying on their spasticity as a support during standing or walking. Dantrolene sodium is an alternative antispasticity drug that offers no major advantage over baclofen and has the disadvantage of potential hepatotoxicity. Diazepam is also effective in reducing spasticity, but the dosage required for relief of spasticity often produces an unacceptable degree of sedation. In some patients, a bedtime dose of 10 mg of diazepam may quiet nighttime flexor spasms and allow for uninterrupted sleep.

Gait difficulties in MS are often due to combinations of weakness, spasticity, and incoordination. Evaluation by a physical therapist with instruction in the use of walking aids and, in some instances, customized braces may be beneficial for ambulatory patients. Bladder dysfunction in MS is common. Referral to a urologist for urodynamic studies and measurement of post void residual urine are often required to define the type of bladder dysfunction and to determine the proper therapy. The failure to store urine may produce simple urinary urgency and occasional accidental incontinence. These symptoms can be effectively managed by intermittent restriction of fluid intake and/or small intermittent doses of oxybutynin chloride. When there is severe urgency and frequent incontinence, the failure to store urine may be converted to a failure to empty the bladder by the regular administration of oxybutynin chloride (5 mg, 2 to 3 times a day). Treatment then proceeds as described below. The failure to empty the bladder produces frequent overflow incontinence, recurrent infection, or symptoms of urinary retention. The use of chronic indwelling catheters for treatment should be avoided where possible because complicating infection will invariably develop. Intermittent self-catheterization is a far safer and surprisingly well-tolerated therapy. It is, however, possible only in patients who have reasonably well-preserved dexterity in the hands. Constipation is frequent in patients with spinal cord involvement and should be treated by conventional methods.

Pain, as a direct result of MS lesions within the CNS, may occur as a typical trigeminal neuralgia or as pseudoradicular pain—usually in one leg, sometimes in an arm or part of the trunk. The trigeminal neuralgia may be treated with carbamazepine, although such treatment can be associated with undesirable transient weakness similar to that occasionally encountered with baclofen. Surgical procedures such as percutaneous rhizotomy have been employed in refractory cases of trigeminal neuralgia, although the long-term effectiveness of such procedures in MS patients is not well established. When pseudoradicular pain is chronic, it is usually refractory to treatment. Low back pain related to weak trunk muscles and poor posture is common in wheelchair patients or in those who have gait disturbance. Conventional therapeutic measures for low back strain are usually effective. For example, patients with spastic, tight hamstring muscles may need physical therapy to stretch these muscles and thus relieve tension on the lumbosacral spine. A firm bed, proper wheelchair posture, and regular swimming, along with physical therapy, are also usually beneficial for low back pain.

Intention tremor due to cerebellar dysfunction unfortunately responds very little to drug therapy. Surgical cryothalamotomy is reserved for treatment of severe incapacitating intention tremor; useful function in one extremity can sometimes be restored in patients who are otherwise totally helpless. Diplopia is often temporary and can be managed simply by the use of an eye patch. Impaired visual acuity, deafness, and vertigo are often temporary, which is fortunate, since there is no effective treatment for these symptoms. When fatigue and lassitude are severe and disabling, a trial with antidepressant drugs such as imipramine or amitriptyline is worthwhile and may be surprisingly beneficial in some patients. Placement of a penile prosthetic device should be considered in carefully selected patients who are impotent. Penile prostheses should not be implanted in men with a significant degree of sensory impairment of the penis or perineum because the penis may be painlessly traumatized during intercourse.

All of the major medical complications of MS are either preventable or treatable. These include contractures of limbs, pressure sores, and pulmonary and urinary tract infections. Every wheelchair and bedridden patient should be involved in a regular program to prevent contractures and pressure sores. Wheelchair patients with good arm function should be taught how to press down on the arms of the chair at frequent intervals in order to relieve pressure on the sacrum and buttocks. Bedridden patients require special air or water flotation mattresses and should be carefully positioned and turned every 2 to 3 hours. Pressure points must be examined frequently, and nursing care efforts must be intensified at the earliest sign of a developing sore. The smallest ulceration should be considered as a potentially life-threatening complication and treated vigorously. Patients with progressing pressure sores may require surgical treatment for debridement or skin grafting.

The secondary complications of MS cover a broad spectrum of personal and social difficulties that include marital, occupational, psychosexual, recreational, legal, and financial problems. Most physicians are not traditionally prepared to deal in depth with many of these problems, but it is often in this area that most can be done to help some patients. In order to deal effectively with these problems, the physician must become familiar with resources in the community and enlist the help of psychologists, social workers, marriage counselors, vocational rehabilitation counselors, and lawyers. The local chapter of the National Multiple Sclerosis Society may be able to help directly or recommend referral to people who are qualified and experienced in working with MS patients. The patient can also be encouraged to participate in support groups, which are often sponsored and organized by the local Multiple Sclerosis Society.

The physician's attitude may have a powerful psychological impact on the MS patient. Sometimes both physicians and patients have a tendency to view the disease as incurable and untreatable. Such a view is excessively negative and unwarranted. A positive but realistic approach by a knowledgeable and sympathetic physician can greatly improve the patient's sense of well-being and perhaps even have a beneficial effect on the course of the disease. Hope is a powerful elixir that should be encouraged. Helplessness should be discouraged. Many patients gravitate toward unproven popular therapies, such as special diets. If the putative therapy is both low risk and affordable, then the physician can be most helpful by taking a tolerant position. An additional benefit of this approach is that the patient thereby learns that the physician is open-minded and eager to support the patient's search for legitimate therapy. At a later date the patient will be more likely to follow the physician's advice against some other therapy that might be unreasonably expensive or potentially harmful.

DIFFUSE CEREBRAL SCLEROSIS

Schilder's disease is representative of this group and shares many features with MS. It is more likely to occur in childhood and adolescence, but onset may occur at any age. The disease often progresses very rapidly to severe disability in weeks or months. Large, sharply defined demyelinating foci, often involving an entire lobe or even hemisphere, are characteristic in this disease. Progressive multifocal leucoencephalopathy should be considered in the differential diagnosis; but the presence of a known lymphoma, lymphatic leukemia, other malignancies, or AIDS, will clarify the diagnosis.

ACUTE DISSEMINATED ENCEPHALOMYELITIS

This disorder develops over a period of hours to days in the context of viral exanthematous diseases, after rabies or smallpox vaccination, and following other rare viral infections. While some patients die acutely, most survive, and some make an excellent clinical recovery. The initial symptoms often consist of fever, headache, confusion, and seizures. When cord involvement is present, there is flaccid weakness of legs, upgoing toes, and urinary retention. The CSF may show pleocytosis with a normal protein content. Even though corticosteroids are used, there is little evidence that they alter the course of this disease.

NECROTIZING HEMORRHAGIC ENCEPHALITIS

This disease may occur in an acute fulminating fashion or may progress over 1 to 2 weeks. It affects mainly adults who have recently had a respiratory infection. Acutely, there are often seizures, severe hemiplegia, and a CSF pleocytosis with up to 3000 cells and an increased protein but normal sugar. No virus has ever been isolated from CSF or brain tissue. The pathological picture consists of perivascular inflammation, demyelination, many small hemorrhages, and inflammation of the meninges. Steroids have been reported to be beneficial.

LEUKODYSTROPHIES

These disorders occur sporadically and in families. Because they are characterized by defective myelination, they are not strictly demyelinative. The cause of most is unknown. Onset is usually in childhood but may occur later in life. The course is variable, but all cases progress, and most end fatally.

REFERENCES

Poser CM (ed): The Diagnosis of Multiple Sclerosis. New York, Thieme-Stratton, 1984.

Sibley WA: Management of the patient with multiple sclerosis. Seminars in Neurology 1985; 5:134–145.

Smith CR, Scheinberg LC: Clinical features of multiple sclerosis. Seminars in Neurology 1985; 5:85–93.

Ebers GC: Optic neuritis and multiple sclerosis. Arch Neurol 1985; 42:702–704.

Kurtzke JF: Optic neuritis or multiple sclerosis. Arch Neurol 1985; 42:704–710.

Paty DW, Asbury AK, Herndon RM, McFarland HF, McDonald WI, McIlroy WJ, Prineas JW, Scheinberg LC, Wolinsky JS: Use of magnetic resonance imaging in the diagnosis of multiple sclerosis: Policy statement. Neurology 1986; 36:1575.

Gonzalez-Scarano F, Frossman RI, Galetta S, Atlas SW, Silberberg DH: Multiple sclerosis disease activity correlates with gadolinium-enhanced magnetic resonance imaging. Ann Neurol 1987; 21:300–306.

Weiner HL, Hafler DA: Immunotherapy of multiple sclerosis. Ann Neurol 1988; 23:211–222.

Matthews WB, Acheson ED, Batchelor JR, Weller RO (eds): McAlpine's Multiple Sclerosis, 2nd ed. New York, Churchill Livingstone, 1991.

Smith ME, Stone LA, Albert PS, Frank JA, Martin R, Armstrong M, Maloni H, McFarlin DE, McFarland HF: Clinical worsening in multiple sclerosis is associated with increased frequency and area of gadopentetate dimeglumineenhancing magnetic resonance imaging lesions. Ann Neurol 1993; 33:480–489.

Arnason BGW: Interferon beta in multiple sclerosis. Neurology 1993; 43:641–643.

The IFNB multiple sclerosis study group: Interferon beta-1b is effective in relapsing-remitting multiple sclerosis. I. Clinical results of a multicenter, randomized, double-blind, placebo-controlled trial. Neurology 1993; 43:655–661.

The IFNB multiple sclerosis study group: Interferon beta-1b is effective in relapsing-remitting multiple sclerosis. II. MRI analysis results of a multicenter, randomized, double-blind, placebo-controlled trial. Neurology 1993; 43:662–667.

Runmaker B, Andersen O: Prognostic factors in a multiple sclerosis incident cohort with twenty-five years of follow-up. Brain 1993; 116:117–134.

Morrissey SP, Miller DH, Kendall BE, Kingsley DPE, Kelly MA, Francis DA, MacManus DG, McDonald WI: The significance of brain magnetic abnormalities at presentation with clinically isolated syndromes suggestive of multiple sclerosis. Brain 1993; 116:135–146.

8

Amyotrophic Lateral Sclerosis and Other Motor System Diseases

The motor system diseases are characterized by progressive, selective degeneration of motor neurons in the spinal cord, brainstem, and brain. The clinical picture reflects which part of the motor system is affected. Involvement of spinal cord anterior horn cells (lower motor neuron) is accompanied by asymmetrical weakness, muscle atrophy, fasciculations, hypo- or areflexia, and — early in the course of the disease — muscle cramps. In the brainstem (bulb), nuclei that innervate extra-ocular muscles (cranial nerve nuclei III, IV, and VI) are practically never diseased. Involvement of the other motor neurons of the brainstem produces weakness, atrophy, and fasciculations in facial, tongue, palatal, masticatory, laryngeal, and neck muscles. When the cells of origin of the corticospinal tract (upper motor neuron) are involved, the clinical presentation often is that of impaired fine, coordinated movements; weakness is usually less severe than in lower motor neuron disease; and often a characteristic pattern of weakness can be discerned (see Table 8–1). In addition, hyperreflexia, spasticity, loss of abdominal reflexes, and the Babinski sign are often present. Predominant involvement of corticobulbar neurons will produce spastic dysarthria, poor volitional face, tongue, and palatal movements with an increased gag reflex. This is referred to as pseudobulbar palsy because it is not the brainstem nuclei themselves that are involved but the cortical cells of origin of axons projecting to them. Usually a motor system disease starts in one system, but as the disease progresses, varying combinations of lower motor neuron (spinal cord and brainstem) and upper motor neuron symptoms and signs occur.

TABLE 8–1. Lower Motor Neuron Versus Upper Motor Neuron Muscle Weakness

Lower motor neuron	Upper motor neuron
Weakness, usually severe	Weakness, usually less severe
Marked muscle atrophy	Minimal disuse muscle atrophy
Fasciculations	No fasciculations
Decreased muscle stretch reflexes	Increased muscle stretch reflexes
Clonus not present	Clonus may be present
Flaccidity	Spasticity
No Babinski sign	Babinski sign
Asymmetric and may involve one limb only in the beginning to become generalized as the disease progresses.	Often initial impairment of only skilled movements. In the limbs the following muscles may be the only ones weak or weaker than the others: triceps; wrist and finger extensors; interossei; iliopsoas; hamstrings; and foot dorsiflexors, inverters and extroverters.

The temporal course of motor system diseases ranges from subacute and fatal to chronic and disabling. Since the etiology in most cases is unknown, the diseases are usually classified by age of onset, whether or not the disease is sporadic or inherited, and the pattern of neurologic involvement. The value of classification is that it permits the outline of a prognosis. There is, however, considerable variability in the course of these diseases.

POLIOMYELITIS

Poliomyelitis vaccines have practically eliminated the disease. Paralytic poliomyelitis can be prevented by immunization with an oral vaccine administered to infants in 2 doses 8 weeks apart. Boosters are given at 1 and 4 years of age. The disease follows vaccination in 0.02 to 0.04 cases per 1 million doses.

Occasional cases still occur in unvaccinated children and adults exposed to a recently vaccinated child. The latter happens because the commonly used vaccine employs a live, attenuated virus that may be transmitted to other individuals. Other enteroviruses (Coxsackie A and B) and echoviruses may produce a similar but usually milder disease. Poliomyelitis is an acute infectious disease caused by one of three types of polioviruses that have a predilection for the anterior horn cells of the spinal cord and motor nuclei of the brainstem, sparing the extra-ocular muscle nuclei. The disease is highly contagious and in the initial phase cannot be distinguished from other viral infections. Paralytic cases occur in less that 10% of infected individuals. Clinically, fever, nausea and vomiting, and aching of muscles is followed in 3 to 4 days by pain in the neck and back with stiffness of the neck and weakness of muscles supplied by cranial nerves and spinal segments. Paralysis usually reaches its maximum severity within 48 hours. The pattern of weakness is highly variable. Common presentations are weakness in one or both legs and an arm and both legs. Purely bulbar forms with respiratory paralysis occur. Tendon reflexes in paralyzed limbs are lost. Even though paresthesias and pain are frequent complaints, sensory abnormalities cannot be demonstrated. Bladder and bowel are usually spared. CSF examination demonstrates an increased pressure; 50–250 white cells per cc; predominantly polymorphonuclear cells initially; and subsequently lymphocytes, elevated protein, normal glucose, and negative bacterial cultures. The differential diagnosis of acute polio includes acute bacterial and tuberculous meningitides. In these cases, weakness is rarely a prominent feature, and spinal fluid examination shows low glucose with positive stain and culture for the responsible organism. Treatment of acute paralytic poliomyelitis is purely symptomatic and supportive. Many patients recover, and almost all at least improve. The residuals are atrophic and weak muscles. Weakness may improve for up to two years because of sprouting of undamaged axons, which innervate denervated muscle fibers.

Twenty to 30 years after an episode of paralytic poliomyelitis, about 10%–20% of patients develop a syndrome of excessive fatigue and progressive weakness of previously paralyzed muscles. Progression is very slow and may stop. This post-polio syndrome is not related to amyotrophic lateral sclerosis (ALS), upper motor neuron symptoms and signs do not occur, and no active virus or virus particles have ever been identified. The etiology of this syndrome is unknown, but age and fatigue appear to be factors in its development.

AMYOTROPHIC LATERAL SCLEROSIS

ALS is a progressive disease of both upper and lower motor neurons with adult onset anywhere from 20 to 90 years. The median age of onset is 65 years. The etiology is unknown, but in about 5% of cases the disease is inherited as an autosomal dominant trait. The familial type does not differ from the sporadic type. The incidence is 1.0 to 1.76 cases per year per 100,000 people worldwide. On the island of Guam, on the Kii peninsula (Japan), and in Irian Jaya (West New Guinea) the prevalence of ALS has been reported as 50 to 100 times that of the incidence seen in the United States. The clinical picture in these areas is indistinguishable from elsewhere, except that the median age of onset is two decades earlier. In the last 40 years the incidence of ALS in these geographic isolates has drastically decreased, and the age of onset has increased considerably. In Guam ALS can also occur as part of a syndrome of ALS, Parkinson's disease, and dementia.

Pathologically, ALS is characterized by atrophy and loss of cells in the anterior horns of the spinal cord, motor nuclei of the lower brainstem, and Betz cells in the motor cortex, with secondary degeneration of corticospinal tracts.

In the classic form of ALS, symptoms and signs begin asymmetrically with weakness and wasting of hand muscles, followed by cramping and fasciculations in arm and then shoulder girdle muscles. Less often the earliest manifestations are in one leg. When upper and lower motor neurons are affected simultaneously, muscle stretch reflexes may be quite brisk in atrophic and weak muscles. Progression is relentless; before long weakness, atrophy, fasciculations, and hyperreflexia can be detected in arms and legs. Bulbar or pseudobulbar symptoms and signs, or both, may develop concurrently or after progression of limb weakness is well established. Mentation remains intact, bladder and bowel control are normal, and there are no abnormalities of volitional eye movements or of the sensory system.

ALS often presents with one of four characteristic forms, which are determined by where in the motor system the degeneration of motor neurons begins. Patients will sometimes continue to manifest one of these forms of ALS for months or years before more widespread involvement of the motor system occurs. In predominantly lower motor neuron involvement in the spinal cord, extremity weakness—with loss of muscle tone, atrophy, fasciculations, and hyporeflexia—is present. This presentation is labeled spinal muscular atrophy. Progressive bulbar palsy is the form in which predominantly lower brainstem nuclei are involved. The clinical picture is that of flaccid dysarthria, dysphagia, and sometimes facial weakness, with depressed jaw jerk and gag reflexes. The label primary lateral sclerosis is applied when there is predominant involvement of the upper motor neurons in the motor cortex, which innervate spinal cord anterior horn cells. The patient will show initially mild to moderate extremity weakness with spasticity, hyperreflexia, and Babinski signs. Finally, pseudobulbar palsy is present when upper motor neurons in the motor cortex, which innervate lower brainstem motor nuclei, are predominantly involved. The clinical expression includes spastic dysarthria, dysphagia, sometimes facial weakness, and hyperactive jaw and gag reflexes.

The clinical course of ALS is almost always one of relentless worsening. In most patients, upper and lower motor neurons in the spinal cord, brainstem, and cortex are eventually involved. The patient becomes severely disabled and dies of respiratory failure or an infection. Although the median survival from time of onset is 22 months, it varies greatly and depends on the predominant location of neuropathological involvement. Patients with bulbar palsy have the worst prognosis, while some patients with primary lateral sclerosis may survive for over 20 years. Patients with the other two forms of the disease have intermediate life expectancies. However, a patient with one form of the disease who develops bulbar palsy then has the poor median survival for that group.

Rare patients have been described with fairly widespread, but more often focal, amyotrophy in the distribution of several cervical or lumbosacral spinal cord segments, which may progress for 2 to 3 years and then arrest or even improve. It appears to be most common in young adults. Whether or not this amyotrophy represents a benign form of ALS or an entirely different disease is unknown.

EMG is the one laboratory test of value in the diagnosis of ALS. The diagnosis is reasonably certain if there is evidence of acute and chronic denervation in several muscles innervated by several nerves and roots in at least three extremities, or in two extremities and brainstem-innervated muscles. Except for low-amplitude motor responses, mild slowing of motor nerve conduction velocities in association with very low-amplitude responses, and an occasional decrementing response to repetitive stimulation, the sensory and motor conduction studies are normal. All other laboratory tests, including CSF examination, are normal. Rarely, serum creatine kinase is slightly elevated.

The differential diagnosis depends on the stage of the disease and on the pattern of neurologic involvement. If the patient has difficulty primarily with swallowing, polymyositis and myasthenia gravis, as well as neoplastic and vascular diseases affecting the brainstem, should be considered. If the patient presents with findings in muscles innervated by the cervical segments, with or without associated upper motor neuron dysfunction in the legs, then focal lesions of the cervical cord—such as tumor, syringomyelia or cervical spondylosis—should be considered. An MRI study of the neck is the most cost-effective way to rule out such other diseases. If the symptoms begin with predominantly lower motor neuron findings in one extremity, then lesions of peripheral nerves, plexi, and spinal nerve roots—including painless disc protrusions—should be considered. EMG is valuable in this setting because it may detect evidence of subclinical involvement of muscles in other extremities. If the patient presents with prominent fasciculations, this may be a sign of metabolic disorder such as hyperthyroidism. Fasciculations also occur in normal individuals. They are commonly seen in athletes. In contrast to the fasciculations seen in ALS (which are rarely felt), healthy individuals feel them. In normal individuals these fasciculations most commonly occur in the orbicularis oculi, deltoid, and quadriceps muscles. Minimal contraction of normal muscles may produce fasciculations. Therefore, fasciculations should be looked for with the muscle examined completely relaxed.

Since there is no treatment for ALS, only supportive measures can be used. As weakness progresses, orthotic aids to counter wrist and foot drop may restore usefulness of grip and the ability to walk. Crutches, cane, and eventually wheelchair may be required for ambulation later in the disease. In a patient with neck muscle weakness, a neck brace will keep the head from falling forward while the patient is sitting. A few patients with electromyographic evidence of a defect of neuromuscular transmission may have some increase in strength when they take anticholinesterase medication. Amitriptyline (75 mg at bedtime), a few drops of tincture of belladonna under the tongue as needed, or the use of a bedside suction device may eliminate drooling and reduce the risk of aspiration. For patients with severe dysarthria, electronic speech devices, writing boards, and word boards may enhance the ability to communicate. Mild dysphagia may be treated with a blended diet. Severe dysphagia and frequent aspirations in a patient with an otherwise slowly progressive disorder may be alleviated by use of a nasogastric tube, gastrostomy, or cervical esophagostomy. Whether the patient with failing strength of respiratory muscles should have mechanical ventilatory assistance is a decision that must be made by patient, family, and physician. The depression that occurs in the setting of an incurable disease must be recognized and appropriately treated. Psychological support for patient and family is imperative throughout the course of the disease. Several experimental drug therapies are being tested, but none has so far shown conclusive evidence of being effective in arresting or slowing the disease process.

INFANTILE MUSCULAR ATROPHY (WERDNIG-HOFFMANN DISEASE)

There are two forms of this syndrome; both have an incidence of about 5 cases per 100,000 births and shown an autosomal recessive form of inheritance. In the first form, the onset of symptoms is during the first 3 months of life. Such children are never able to sit, stand, or walk and rarely survive more than 2 or 3 years because of dysphagia and respiratory insufficiency. In the second form, onset is after age 3 months but before age 15 months, and the course is marked by survival into adulthood. The illness may present in the last months of pregnancy when the mother notes that the normal kicking movements weaken or disappear entirely. At birth, the baby may be limp, have a weak cry and respiratory distress, and display generalized weakness of arms and legs. In other cases, the infant is normal for the first few weeks, and then generalized weakness of the skeletal musculature follows. The weakness of the hip adductors and flexors is manifested by a spreading of the legs at the hip, similar to the position of a frog's legs. Weakness of the abdominal and thoracic musculature is manifest during inspiration, with inward movement of the thoracic wall and protuberance of the abdomen. Fasciculations of the tongue may be seen in about 50% of patients.

Diagnosis can generally be made on the basis of the combination of clinical and electromyographic examination, both of which show findings similar to those described for ALS. The serum creatine kinase (CK) may be slightly elevated, probably due to widespread muscle fiber degeneration. A muscle biopsy demonstrates group hypertrophy and group atrophy, which are characteristic of neuropathic disease. Death usually ensues following development of pneumonia. It is important to confirm the diagnosis with appropriate studies in order to be able to prognosticate the course of the disease and to assist in genetic counseling. The differential diagnosis includes other forms of hypotonia, including cerebral palsy, myotonic dystrophy, benign congenital hypotonia, and congenital myopathies.

JUVENILE MOTOR NEURON DISEASE (KUGELBERG-WELANDER)

This is a form of spinal muscle atrophy that begins between the ages of 5 and 15 years and generally is inherited in an autosomal recessive manner. Because proximal muscles are involved early in this disease, it is easily mistaken for a primary muscle disease. The muscles first involved are frequently about the hips, so that the child shows a waddling gait and difficulty climbing stairs. Subsequently there is difficulty rising from a chair and from the recumbent position. Calf muscles may appear hypertrophied compared to the atrophic thigh muscles. Shoulder and arm muscle weakness occurs later, and ultimately all the muscles of the body are involved. Occasionally, bulbar musculature weakness develops, particularly in the facial muscles. Progression is usually slow and may be stepwise. In the case of adult onset spinal muscular atrophies, life expectancy is not appreciably reduced. Modes of inheritance of these syndromes include autosomal dominant, autosomal recessive, and sex-linked traits.

EMG shows changes of diffuse motor neuron disease and is the most helpful test in distinguishing this juvenile motor neuron disease from the muscular dystrophies and myopathies that it may clinically resemble. Muscle biopsy will confirm the presence of a lower motor neuron lesion and demonstrate the absence of primary muscle pathology. In addition, serum CK is only mildly elevated, in contrast with the high elevations commonly seen in Duchenne's dystrophy. Because of the difference in prognosis between this spinal muscular atrophy and Duchenne's dystrophy, EMG, muscle biopsy and serum CK determinations are all recommended to confirm the diagnosis.

OTHER MOTOR SYSTEM DISEASES

Rarely, a progressive bulbar muscle atrophy may begin in a child or young adult and lead to a syndrome known as Fazio-Londe disease. Facial and extra-ocular muscles may be involved. EMG can generally distinguish this condition from myotonic dystrophy and facioscapulohumeral dystrophy.

The syndrome of familial spastic paraplegia usually has its onset in the fourth or fifth decade of life, progresses very slowly, and does not shorten life expectancy. In the most common form, only cortical motor neurons degenerate. In other types the spastic paraplegia may be associated with optic atrophy, pigmentary retinal degeneration, polyneuropathy, extrapyramidal manifestations, cerebellar abnormalities, or dementia.

Vasculitis and organophosphate poisoning each occasionally cause a motor neuron disease. Additionally, there are some reports of motor neuron disease being produced as a remote effect of cancer and as a postinfectious condition.

REFERENCES

Juergens SM, Kurland LT, Okazaki PHH, and Mulder DW: ALS in Rochester, Minnesota, 1925–1977. Neurology 1980; 30:463–470.

Janiszewski DW, Caroscio JT, Wisham LH: Amyotrophic lateral sclerosis: A comprehensive rehabilitation approach. Arch Phys Med Rehab 1983; 64:304–307.

Rowland LP (ed): Advances in neurology, vol 36: Human Motor Neuron Diseases. New York, Raven Press, 1982.

Mitsumoto H, Hanson MR, Chad DA: Amyotrophic lateral sclerosis: Recent advances in pathogenesis and therapeutic trials. Arch Neurol 1988; 45:189–202.

Pestronk A, Chaudhry V, Feldman EL, Griffin JW, Cornblath DR, Denys EH, Glasberg M, Kuncl RW, Olney RK, Yee WC: Lower motor neuron syndromes defined by patterns of weakness, nerve conduction abnormalities, and high titers of antiglycolipid antibodies. Ann Neurol 1990; 27:316–326.

Armon C, Kurland LT, Daube JR, O'Brien PC: Epidemiologic correlates of sporadic amyotrophic lateral sclerosis. Neurology 1991; 41:1077–1084.

9

Toxic-Metabolic Encephalopathies and Coma

DEFINITION

Encephalopathy refers to any dysfunction of the CNS due to generalized failure of neuronal or glial metabolism. The cause may be intrinsic, as in degenerative CNS disorders, or extrinsic, secondary to systemic diseases or toxins. Brain metabolism is almost entirely dependent on oxygen and glucose, with high metabolic demands for both. Brain damage occurs if either is lacking. When cerebral venous pCO2 decreases below 25 mm Hg, the brain shifts to anaerobic metabolism, which is less efficient than oxidative metabolism. If cerebral oxygen consumption is reduced by more than 30%, neurologic impairment occurs. In general, gray matter has a higher metabolic rate than white matter and cortex a higher rate than brainstem. When cerebral blood flow is reduced, ischemic damage to the brain can occur. Cerebral perfusion pressure (CPP) is defined as the mean arterial pressure minus the intracranial pressure. The CPP should be greater than 50 mm Hg to maintain adequate blood flow to brain tissue. If it falls below that, brain metabolism is compromised. If CPP is reduced to 30 mm Hg or less, neuronal death occurs. Ischemia is caused by any process that decreases cardiac output. Ischemia will also occur if intracranial pressure is greatly increased (e.g., because of cerebral edema secondary to Reye's syndrome, hepatic encephalopathy, or lead poisoning). Thus, anything that impairs cerebral blood flow or otherwise depletes glucose and oxygen can alter cerebral function and produce an encephalopathy. Depletion of an essential cofactor (e.g., thiamine or pyridoxine) will also interfere with cerebral metabolism.

SYMPTOMS AND SIGNS

Development of metabolic encephalopathy is often insidious. An encephalopathy may be acute or chronic. Early symptoms may be subtle and include slowed mentation, indifference, confusion, depression, and disorientation. As the encephalopathy progresses, symptoms become more severe and include agitation, hallucinations, seizures, stupor, and coma. Chronic forms of encephalopathy resemble other forms of organic brain syndromes and are characterized by poor memory, confusion, indifference, and other impairment of cognitive functions.

The neurologic examination in patients with metabolic encephalopathy typically has no focal features, but mental status changes are prominent. Cranial nerves are unaffected unless the patient is in deep coma. Muscle stretch reflexes may be hyperactive, and the patient may have Babinski signs. Periodic loss of muscle tone (asterixis) in the outstretched hands and/or arms may be present. Coordination may be affected early. Seizures are a frequent problem. They may be generalized, tonic-clonic, or—less commonly—focal. Myoclonus, either focal or generalized, is particularly common with certain types of metabolic encephalopathy.

Abnormal respiratory patterns are common in metabolic encephalopathy and are of two types. Nonspecific abnormalities are the result of the level of coma, e.g., periodic, Cheyne-Stokes respirations in light coma, central neurogenic hyperventilation in deeper coma, and irregular gasping respirations with severe brainstem dysfunction. Patients with metabolic coma exhibit respiratory patterns that reflect the body's attempt to correct the metabolic derangement (Table 9–1).

TABLE 9–1. Respiratory Abnormalities in Metabolic Encephalopathies

Hyperventilation
  Compensation for metabolic acidosis
    Uremia   Lactic acidosis
    Diabetes mellitus   Toxin ingestion (salicylates)
  Primary stimulation of respiratory center (respiratory alkalosis)
    Salicylism   Sepsis
    Hepatic coma   Reye's syndrome
    Pulmonary disease   Psychogenic hyperventilation
Hypoventilation
  Respiratory compensation for metabolic alkalosis
    Excessive ingestion of alkali
    Excessive loss of acid
  Respiratory depression
    Severe pulmonary or neuromuscular disease
    Depression of respiratory centers

ELECTROENCEPHALOGRAPHIC ABNORMALITIES

The EEG often shows generalized, nonspecific abnormalities. In light stages of coma generalized theta activity is predominant, while in deeper coma diffuse delta waves prevail. Triphasic waves are common in moderately severe hepatic encephalopathy but may be seen in other metabolic encephalopathies. Occasionally, superimposed epileptiform activity is present. Focal EEG abnormalities always suggest coexisting structural lesions.

SPECIFIC CAUSES

Anoxic Encephalopathy

Total lack of oxygenation of the brain is caused by failure of the heart, circulation, or lungs and respiration. Cerebral neurons cannot store oxygen and will die when their oxygen supply is cut off for longer than 5 minutes. When oxygenation is reduced but not abolished (hypoxia) patients may just be confused, inattentive, lack judgment and have motor incoordination. If consciousness is preserved, patients usually recover without sequelae. The period and degree of oxygen deprivation is usually difficult to measure. Resuscitation should therefore be instituted promptly, because even in the absence of pulse, blood pressure, and respiration, there may still be some blood flow to the brain; and complete recovery may occur after apparent anoxia of longer than 5 minutes.

In the most severe anoxia the patient rapidly lapses into coma and may reach a state of brain death within a short period of time. With progressive anoxia, the course of the encephalopathy is rostral to caudal. Impaired judgment is an early symptom, followed by perceptual and visual difficulties. The disorder then progresses to unconsciousness, decorticate posturing, and then decerebrate posturing, with progressive paralysis of cranial nerves. Finally, respiratory failure occurs as medullary function is depressed. Recovery from anoxic encephalopathy follows the opposite path. Complicating the course of anoxic encephalopathy is the development of cerebral edema, usually about 48 hours after the anoxic episode. In such cases the patient may appear to be improving but then deteriorates, with seizures and deepening coma supervening. The clinical course is variable after anoxic brain damage. Some patients have a course of progressive deterioration and death. Others appear to be recovering well but then, several days to weeks after the anoxic episode, suffer neurologic deterioration and may die or be left with permanent brain damage. Still other patients show a course of gradual improvement. Generalized seizures may occur in the first few days after the anoxic insult. Patients who recover with only brainstem structures functioning may live for years in a vegetative state. Prognosis of anoxic encephalopathy is quite variable, but in general, the younger the patient, the better the prognosis. It is very difficult to determine prognosis immediately after an anoxic event. A few patients may remain comatose for many days but eventually recover with little or no sequelae. If brainstem function is intact soon after the anoxic episode, the prognosis is somewhat more favorable. If pupils are fixed and dilated and there is no evidence of brainstem function, cerebral death has most likely occurred. An EEG showing electrocerebral silence will corroborate the clinical suspicion. In general, the longer the duration of coma, the worse the prognosis.

The treatment for anoxic encephalopathy is adequate oxygenation, good fluid and electrolyte balance, dexamethasone and mannitol for cerebral edema, and controlled hyperventilation if necessary to reduce intracranial pressure. Some patients who at least partially recover from anoxic encephalopathy develop a syndrome of postanoxic myoclonus, a movement disorder that is worsened by intentional movements. These patients have multifocal myoclonus with voluntary movements, which can be quite debilitating. It does respond in some cases to treatment with clonazepam.

Hypertensive Encephalopathy

Patients with chronic hypertension who have a rapid rise in blood pressure are most at risk for development of hypertensive encephalopathy. Typical symptoms include headache, focal or generalized seizures, and obtundation. Neurologic examination may show focal abnormalities, changes in mental status, diffuse hyperreflexia, and Babinski signs. Ophthalmoscopic examination shows papilledema, retinal arterial spasms, and exudates. Intracranial pressure is elevated acutely, and CSF protein may be elevated. Treatment consists of rapidly reducing systemic arterial blood pressure. When blood pressure is controlled symptoms usually abate within a few days, and the majority of patients have no neurologic sequelae.

DISORDERS OF GLUCOSE HOMEOSTASIS

Hypoglycemia

Acute, severe hypoglycemia produces direct effects on the cerebral cortex. The brain has a limited glucose reserve of about 1 to 2 g per 100 g of tissue and cannot tolerate hypoglycemia for longer than 90 minutes.

Onset of symptoms occurs 30 to 40 minutes after a drop in blood glucose concentration. By then the brain has depleted its glucose reserve. Several different manifestations of acute hypoglycemia are found. When blood glucose levels have fallen to about 30 mg/dl, symptoms include sweating, pallor, confusion, syncope, tachycardia, tremors, and anxiety. Focal or generalized seizures may be the initial or only symptom of hypoglycemia. Such seizures are difficult to control with anticonvulsants alone and require intravenous glucose infusions to abate. At blood glucose levels of 10 mg/dl or less, rapid onset of coma is accompanied by shallow respiration, bradycardia, dilated pupils, and generalized hypotonia. Focal abnormalities such as hemiparesis and aphasia may be part of the neurologic picture of hypoglycemia, particularly in elderly patients. Chronic low-grade hypoglycemia may produce insidious symptoms such as subtle changes in mental status. Causes of hypoglycemia are listed in Table 9–2.

Treatment consists of correcting the glucose deficiency as quickly as possible with intravenous glucose infusion (50% dextrose in water, 50 ml administered over 5–10 minutes). Since the symptoms of hypoglycemic encephalopathy are not specific, it is important to draw blood for glucose determination prior to giving glucose. If treated promptly, encephalopathic symptoms are totally reversible. Persistent neurologic deficits, including seizures and dementia, may occur with prolonged or recurrent hypoglycemic attacks.

Hyperglycemia

A significant increase in serum glucose concentrations, as is seen in diabetes mellitus, produces extracellular hyperosmolality with resultant cellular dehydration. Significant dehydration of brain cells will result in hallucinations, coarse flapping tremors, coma, and focal or generalized seizures. In nonketotic hyperglycemia, blood glucose levels may be greater than 1000 mg/dl. Treatment consists of decreasing glucose con-

TABLE 9–2. Causes of Hypoglycemia

Adult-onset
   Prediabetic state
   Insulin overdose
Neonatal and Juvenile Onset
   Hereditary fructose intolerance
   Leucine sensitivity
   Insulinoma
   Infant of diabetic mother
Postmaturity
   Glucose-6-phosphatase deficiency

Beta-cell adenoma
Chronic liver disease

Galactosemia
Panhypopituitarism
Ketotic hypoglycemia
Beckwith syndrome

centrations to normal levels with insulin, followed by cautious rehydration. Rapid rehydration produces excessive fluid shifts into cells and may cause cerebral edema with added neurologic deficits.

Diabetic Ketoacidosis

Diabetics have excessive breakdown of adipose tissue due to low levels of circulating insulin, resulting in an increase of serum-free fatty acids and keto acids. These patients are also hyperglycemic. The hyperglycemia produces an osmotic diuresis, with dehydration and electrolyte imbalance. Usually blood glucose is greater than 400 mg/dl, pH less than 7.2, and pCO2 10 meq/L or less. Coma may be the result of the acidosis, cellular dehydration, electrolyte disturbance, or a combination of all three. Hyperventilation is common in diabetic ketoacidosis and reflects the body's attempt to compensate for the metabolic acidosis. Neurologic examination is nonfocal, and brainstem function is usually intact. Cerebral edema may complicate the course of diabetic coma and produce central herniation and death. Treatment consists of administration of insulin (both intravenous and subcutaneous) to reduce serum glucose levels to normal, as well as rehydration and restoration or maintenance of electrolyte balance.

DISORDERS OF FLUID AND ELECTROLYTE BALANCE

Hyponatremia

Decreased serum concentrations of sodium result from excessive intake or abnormal retention of hypotonic fluids (i.e., water intoxication). Causes of water intoxication include the syndrome of inappropriate antidiuretic hormone secretion (which can be idiopathic or a complication of meningitis), pituitary tumors, and head trauma. Water intoxication is also caused by excessive ingestion of water, as seen in infants given diluted formula. Patients with water intoxication have an increase in extracellular and intracellular water levels, and this results in cerebral edema. Serum osmolality is low. Symptoms include confusion, lethargy, anorexia, headache, nausea, and vomiting. Coma and seizures may develop. Treatment consists of fluid restriction and cautious hypertonic saline administration in severe cases.

Central Pontine Myelinolysis

This syndrome occurs most commonly in alcoholics but is also seen in association with severe, extensive burns, following liver and kidney transplantation, and in a variety of other systemic illnesses. Pathologically it is characterized by symmetric demyelination of the center of the basis pontis and, occasionally, other parts of the brain. MR scanning allows visualization of the lesion in many patients, but it may not show until several days or weeks after the onset of symptoms. When the lesion is extensive, the patient is quadriplegic and has only vertical eye movements, but remains fully conscious (locked-in syndrome). Common to most cases is severe hyponatremia, less than 120 meq/L. Hyponatremia in itself does not cause central pontine myelinolysis, but rapid correction of it probably is responsible for the development of the syndrome in many patients. The optimal method to correct severe hyponatremia is to increase serum sodium by 12 meq or less in the first 24 hours and by 20 meq or less during the first 48 hours. Central pontine myelinolysis used to be a postmortem diagnosis, but with aggressive, supportive therapy patients survive and occasionally recover without residual neurologic deficits.

Hypernatremia

Increases in serum sodium concentrations occur (1) secondary to excess water loss (dehydration) from vomiting, diarrhea, and fever or (2) as a result of ingesting hypertonic solutions. (They are seen particularly in infants given concentrated formula and home remedies for diarrhea.) In either case, a hyperosmolar state exists and water is pulled out of cells, resulting in cell shrinkage. With severe dehydration, brain shrinkage occurs. Occasionally this produces tearing of cortical veins with resulting subarachnoid and cerebral hemorrhages. Venous sinus thromboses and cerebral infarctions may also complicate the clinical picture. Symptoms of hypernatremia include somnolence, muscular rigidity, opisthotonus, and decerebrate rigidity. There is a high mortality rate (approximately 30%), and of the survivors, 50% have permanent neurologic sequelae, including hemiparesis, mental retardation, and seizure disorders. Treatment consists of slow rehydration over 48 to 72 hours. Rapid hydration results in sudden shifts of fluid into cells and can cause severe cerebral edema and death. Seizures may occur during rapid rehydration.

Hypomagnesemia

The causes of hypomagnesemia are listed in Table 9–3. Symptoms occur when serum magnesium drops below 1.5 meq/dl. Neurologic abnormalities consist of mental confusion, irritability, agitation, hallucinations, and coma. Motor abnormalities include muscle twitching, myoclonic jerks, tremors, and choreoathetosis. Muscle stretch reflexes are nomas. Excess vitamin ingestion should be discontinued. For severe hypercalcemia, a chelating agent such as ethylene diamine tetraacetic acid (EDTA) can be used parenterally or orally. Mild hypercalcemia may respond to a low-calcium diet.

COFACTOR DEFICIENCIES

Thiamine

Thiamine (vitamin B^1) is a necessary cofactor in carbohydrate metabolism. Deficiency of this vitamin creates a block in normal cerebral metabolic pathways and produces metabolic encephalopathy. Causes of thiamine deficiency are listed in Table 9–6. The Wernicke-Korsakoff syndrome is associated with acute thiamine deficiency and is usually, but not exclusively, found in alcoholics. Acutely, the classical clinical triad is ophthalmoplegia, ataxia, and dementia. Ataxia and ocular abnormalities usually precede the mental changes. The ataxia is primarily truncal, with wide-based gait and truncal instability. Ocular findings include bilateral lateral rectus palsies and horizontal and vertical nystagmus. Pupillar light reaction is normal and ptosis is usually absent. The remainder of the cranial nerve examination is normal. Mental status changes are characterized by disorientation, somnolence, poor concentration, and impairment of recent memory. Diagnosis is based on a history of alcoholism or malnutrition, plus evidence of the clinical triad on neurologic examination. Once the diagnosis is made or suspected, treatment should be given promptly to prevent death or permanent neurologic impairment. Treatment consists of initial administration of 100 mg thiamine hydrochloride intravenously, followed by 100 mg thiamine hydrochloride twice a day intravenously or intramuscularly, until the patient can consume a full regular diet. Oral multivitamins, particularly of the B complex, should be given as well. Early treatment may reverse the symptoms totally. However, when the encephalopathy is prolonged, the ataxia and ophthalmoplegia may still respond to ther-

TABLE 9–6. Causes of Thiamine Deficiency

Alcoholism
Starvation
Malnutrition
Hyperemesis gravidarum
Carcinoma of the stomach
Gastrointestinal and liver disease

apy, but the dementia, with severe impairment in recent memory and confabulation (Korsakoff syndrome), may be permanent. It is an excellent policy to give thiamine to any patient who may have even a remote chance of being an alcoholic, regardless of symptomatology.

Pyridoxine

For all practical purposes, pyridoxine (vitamin B^6) deficiency is found only in infants fed inadequate diets. This situation may occur, for example, if parenteral vitamin supplements are not given to premature infants who are not able to maintain adequate oral intake. Adults on chronic isoniazid or hydralazine therapy can develop B^6 deficiency if not given supplemental pyridoxine. Vitamin B^6 deficiency causes generalized and myoclonic seizures that are, at times, refractory to anticonvulsant therapy. The EEG eventually develops a hypsarrhythmic pattern. Untreated chronic deficiency can lead to mental retardation. Diagnosis depends on awareness that pyridoxine deficiency is a cause of neonatal and infantile seizures and abolition of electrical seizure activity with pyridoxine (50–100 mg intravenously) during recording of the EEG. Excess doses of pyridoxine may lead to a sensory polyneuropathy.

Pyridoxine dependency is a state in which the infant's requirements for this vitamin are significantly greater than normal. It is related to an inherited deficiency of glutamic acid decarboxylase. On a regular diet, the infant develops myoclonic seizures (infantile spasms) at 3 to 4 months of age, with a severely abnormal (hypsarrhythmic) pattern on EEG. Persistence of this problem leads to mental retardation. Seizures are refractory to anticonvulsants. Diagnosis is dependent on recognition of the fact that pyridoxine dependency is one cause of infantile spasms. A therapeutic trial should be performed by administering intravenous pyridoxine while the EEG is being recorded. The doses should be at least 100 mg, but some infants require much higher doses (200–500 mg) before seizures stop and EEG abnormalities reverse. Once the diagnosis of pyridoxine dependency is made, long-term therapy with high doses of pyridoxine (10–15 mg/kg/per day) should be initiated.

Vitamin B^{12}

Vitamin B^{12} deficiency almost always occurs as a result of malabsorption of the vitamin due to absence of intrinsic factor in the gastric mucosa. Neurologic symptoms of B^{12} deficiency are of two types. In one, mental changes are prominent and include irritability and forgetfulness, which may progress to frank dementia. The other type is subacute combined degeneration of the spinal cord. The clinical findings are decreased or absent position and vibratory senses in the legs, ataxia of gait, limb weakness, hyperreflexia, and Babinski signs. A macrocytic normochromic anemia occurs only in the most severely B^{12}-depleted patients, and neurologic abnormalities may occur before serum B^{12} levels are low. It has recently been suggested that the cutoff for diagnosing B^{12} deficiency should be raised from 148 pmol/L to 258 pmol/L. The most sensitive method of detecting B^{12} deficiency is determination of serum metylmalonic acid and homocysteine levels. Diagnosis consists of documenting low serum B^{12} levels. An oral Schilling test to measure urinary excretion of labeled B^{12} will usually show abnormally low values. Treatment consists of intramuscular administration of B^{12} (100 mcg/per day) initially. Neurologic symptoms, including dementia, may revert rapidly, especially in the early stages. Daily treatment should be continued until the anemia disappears. The patient should then be placed on a maintenance dose (100 mcg of B^{12} per month) given intramuscularly.

ORGAN FAILURE

Hepatic Encephalopathy

Both acute and chronic forms of hepatic encephalopathy occur. In acute cases, the patient may show indifference, somnolence, and paucity of speech. Asterixis may be the only finding on neurologic examination. More severe cases progress to coma, with hyperventilation and nonfocal neurologic examination. Asterixis disappears as coma deepens. Decerebrate rigidity and respiratory arrest may follow. Chronic hepatic encephalopathy may develop on the background of repeated episodes of acute hepatic encephalopathy or independently and can manifest itself in two ways. The first is as a neuropsychiatric disorder, with intermittent confusion and depression alternating with euphoria. The second is as a syndrome known as acquired (non-Wilsonian) hepatolenticular degeneration, with dementia, rigidity, and a coarse proximal (wing-beating) tremor. The latter syndrome is usually irreversible. Patients with chronic hepatic encephalopathy may have periods of exacerbation with coma. This is often a terminal event.

Liver disease results in a variety of metabolic disturbances, including hyperammonemia, hyperaminoacidemia, short-chain fatty acidemia, abnormalities of carbohydrate metabolism, and imbalance of neurotransmitters. The diagnosis of hepatic encephalopathy rests on finding evidence of abnormal liver functions, including increased serum bilirubin and serum transaminases. Blood ammonia may be elevated and hypoglycemia is occasionally found. The EEG shows progressive generalized slowing of background rhythms. Often bilaterally synchronous triphasic delta waves are present. LP produces normal findings, although the CSF may be yellow in color due to bilirubin and CSF pressure may be increased.

Treatment of acute hepatic encephalopathy is difficult because of the multiple metabolic abnormalities. With mild encephalopathy (precoma) careful attention should be paid to correcting electrolyte imbalance and hypoglycemia. A low-protein diet should be provided to prevent worsening of hyperammonemia; and fluid and electrolyte balance should be maintained. In addition, the following therapeutic approaches should be considered. High concentrations of glucose (15–20% solutions intravenously) will provide calories, prevent hypoglycemia, and help to combat accumulation of short-chain fatty acids. Neomycin (1–2 gm every 6 hours by nasogastric tube or enema) will help to decrease serum ammonia concentrations. Lactulose (60–160 gm per day by nasogastric tube) may also help to reduce ammonia accumulation. Administration of levodopa (l-dopa) (500–1000 mg every 6 hours by nasogastric tube) is recommended. Some patients respond quite dramatically to this therapy with improved levels of consciousness. Exchange blood transfusions, plasmapheresis, or hemodialysis can be used to correct multiple metabolic abnormalities and improve abnormal clotting. Anticerebral edema agents should be employed to lower increased intracranial pressure. Mannitol (1–2 gm/kg intravenously over 5 to 10 minutes) is effective in reducing intracranial pressure. Glycerol is less effective with this type of cerebral edema. The value of dexamethasone in treating cerebral edema in hepatic coma is unclear. Use of an intracranial pressure monitoring device is extremely helpful in controlling increased intracranial pressure. However, insertion of such a monitor (either epidural, subdural, or intraventricular) carries potential risks in patients with abnormal blood-clotting studies. If an intracranial pressure monitor is used, clotting studies should first be corrected by exchange transfusion or plasmapheresis. Thereafter, repeated exchanges may be necessary to maintain satisfactory clotting indices. There is a high mortality rate in acute hepatic encephalopathy. Many patients who die have massive cerebral edema on postmortem examination, and this may be the immediate cause of death. Some patients who survive the acute episode return to normal neurologic function; others develop chronic hepatic encephalopathy with dementia and movement disorders.

Renal Failure

UREMIC ENCEPHALOPATHY. Renal failure causes a multitude of metabolic abnormalities—including uremia, hyperkalemia, hypocalcemia, hyperphosphatemia, and acidosis. Each of these is capable of producing changes in the CNS, but retention of urea is primarily responsible for the encephalopathy associated with renal failure. The probability of incurring uremic encephalopathy is related to the length of time renal failure is present and to the degree of uremia. Focal abnormalities are not uncommon with uremic encephalopathy. Early symptoms include lethargy, restlessness, and agitation. There may be diffuse muscle weakness and fasciculations. Dysarthria and dysphagia are often initial complaints. Asterixis is frequently seen in patients in the early stages. Symptoms progress to delirium, stupor, and coma. Seizures are common and may be focal or generalized. Extrapyramidal abnormalities, including rigidity and tremor, may also be present. Uremic encephalopathy is usually a feature of acute, severe renal failure. Chronic uremia may not produce CNS alterations, unless an acute exacerbation of the uremia occurs. Patients with chronic renal failure often have peripheral nervous system involvement, with mixed sensorimotor neuropathies. The blood urea nitrogen (BUN) is elevated, as is serum creatinine. Serum concentrations of potassium and phosphate are also increased, and calcium may be decreased. The EEG shows diffuse high-amplitude slowing; at times triphasic waves are seen.

Treatment consists of reducing urea levels by peritoneal or hemodialysis and correcting concomitant metabolic abnormalities. Uremic encephalopathy is reversible if treated early. Clinical improvement may lag behind correction of measurable metabolic and electrolyte abnormalities by days.

DIALYSIS ENCEPHALOPATHY. A peculiar syndrome has been recognized in patients on chronic hemodialysis. Dialysis encephalopathy is characterized by aphasia, dysarthria, speech apraxia, dementia, behavioral disturbances, and myoclonic and generalized seizures. Initially there is often a stuttering course, with waxing and waning of symptoms over a course of hours to days. Elevated aluminum concentrations in serum and body tissues have been documented, and these may represent a possible etiology. The EEG is profoundly abnormal, with generalized slowing in the theta and delta range, as well as multifocal spike discharges. Dialysis encephalopathy is frequently fatal. This encephalopathy has been practically eliminated by the use of purified dialysis water.

DISEQUILIBRIUM SYNDROME. This syndrome develops in uremic patients during the third and fourth hours of dialysis or sometimes after completion of dialysis. These patients have headaches, agitation, muscle cramps, convulsions, and drowsiness. The cause is probably brain edema secondary to water intoxication and inappropriate antidiuretic hormone secretion.

PULMONARY ENCEPHALOPATHY. Severe parenchymal lung disease, severe weakness of respiratory muscles, and failure of respiratory centers may all lead to hypoxemia and hypercapnia. The neurologic manifestations are primarily the result of hypercapnia and intracellular acidosis. Onset may be insidious, with headache, slowed mentation, and confusion. These symptoms progress to stupor and coma. Asterixis and multifocal myoclonus are common. Muscle stretch reflexes tend to be depressed, and plantar responses are extensor. Papilledema and increased intracranial pressure are frequent findings. Seizures and focal neurologic abnormalities are rare. A patient with chronic pulmonary disease with marginal compensation may have sudden onset of encephalopathy during or after infection or administration of sedative drugs that cause rapid decompensation. Diagnosis is made by arterial blood gas determination with a pCO2 > 50 mm Hg and respiratory acidosis. Treatment with mechanical ventilation produces rapid improvement in the encephalopathy. Administration of oxygen without mechanical ventilation may be harmful, because low arterial oxygen may be the only stimulus to the respiratory centers, no longer sensitive to CO^2.

Thyroid Dysfunction

CONGENITAL HYPOTHRYOIDISM. Severe thyroid insufficiency in utero produces the clinical picture of cretinism. Signs of cretinism in the infant include large head size, coarse dry skin, hoarse cry, large protruding tongue, persistent patent posterior fontanel, large abdomen, and an umbilical hernia. Severe mental retardation results if untreated. Diagnosis is made on the basis of clinical observations and low values on thyroid function tests. Early treatment with oral thyroid supplements will prevent mental retardation. However, once mental deficiency is apparent, it is unlikely to revert to normal even with treatment.

JUVENILE HYPOTHYROIDISM. Onset of thyroid deficiency in childhood is usually the result of Hashimoto's thyroiditis. Children with hypothyroidism are sluggish and apathetic; mental retardation is not a feature of juvenile hypothyroidism. At times muscle weakness is the only symptom of thyroid deficiency.

ADULT-ONSET HYPOTHYROIDISM. Thyroid function can be impaired by chronic thyroiditis, surgical removal, effects of drugs (para-aminosalicylic acid, iodides, thiocyanates), and pituitary dysfunction, with deficient thyroid stimulating hormone production. Patients with severe thyroid deficiency typically have marked psychomotor retardation, hoarse voice, cold intolerance, dry skin, brittle hair, frontal baldness, and muscular weakness. Physical examination shows bradycardia, subnormal temperature, and slow relaxation phase on eliciting muscle stretch reflexes ("hung" reflexes). Encephalopathic manifestations of hypothyroidism include dementia, personality changes with psychotic behavior, and severe psychomotor retardation. Coma may develop with severe myxedema. Other neurologic complications of hypothyroidism include myopathy, peripheral neuropathy, truncal ataxia, and carpal tunnel syndrome. Diagnosis is based on finding decreased serum levels of thyroid hormones and an increase in serum cholesterol. LP provides normal results, although CSF protein may be elevated. The EEG shows generalized slowing. EMG may demonstrate myopathic changes, and nerve conduction velocities may be slowed.

Treatment consists of thyroid replacement. This should be instituted cautiously and should be preceded by giving adrenal corticosteroids. All of the neurologic complications of hypothyroidism respond to replacement therapy, and they may revert completely by 6 to 8 weeks following institution of treatment.

HYPERTHYROIDISM. The general features of hyperthyroidism include hyperactivity, restlessness, insomnia, increased sweating, heat intolerance, warm and moist skin, sinus tachycardia, weight loss, and diarrhea. Exophthalmos and lid lag are usually found on examination. Neurologic manifestations consist of personality changes, irritability, and psychosis. Muscle stretch reflexes are hyperactive, and a fine, rapid tremor of the hands is common. Thyroid crisis may be accompanied by psychosis, seizures, and hyperpyrexia. Diagnosis is based on elevated serum thyroid hormone levels, in association with the clinical picture. The EEG is nonspecific and may show diffuse slowing.

Treatment of thyroid crisis is a medical emergency. The patient may require sedation with barbiturates. A cooling blanket will reduce excessive body temperature. Careful fluid and electrolyte balance should be maintained. Intravenous hydrocortisone should be administered until the patient is stable. Treatment with a thyroid blocking agent such as propylthiouracil (PTU) should be initiated early, since it takes several days before any effect is seen in decreasing thyroid function. Milder cases of hyperthyroidism can be treated with thyroid blocking agents and sedation as needed.

ACQUIRED METABOLIC AND TOXIC ENCEPHALOPATHIES

Reye's Syndrome

Reye's syndrome is a disease confined primarily to children, although cases have been reported in young adults. The clinical picture is that of a biphasic illness. The initial phase is an antecedent viral illness, usually an upper respiratory infection or gastroenteritis, from which the patient is recovering. However, persistent vomiting develops and progresses to irritability, confusion, and coma, with decorticate and then decerebrate posturing. Death may occur rapidly (within 24 to 48 hours) in some cases. Mortality may be as high as 60%. Generalized seizures occur at any time during the course of the encephalopathy. Liver function tests are abnormal, and blood ammonia concentrations are increased. Massive increases in intracranial pressure are common. Pathological changes consist of extensive small droplet fatty accumulation in liver, kidney, and heart. Diagnosis rests on the clinical history of a biphasic illness with protracted vomiting. Toxic ingestions (e.g., salicylates) must be ruled out. Serum transaminase, prothrombin time, creatine phosphokinase (CPK), and ammonia concentrations are elevated, whereas bilirubin is normal. Hypoglycemia occurs in 40% of patients, and more often in children under 2 years of age. Reye's syndrome is related to aspirin ingestion. Numerous viruses have been associated with the antecedent illness. The most common are influenza A and B and varicella. However, no virus has been cultured from brain tissue, and the disease is not due to active viral infection. Treatment is directed toward providing intensive supportive care, correcting metabolic abnormalities, and reducing intracranial pressure. Children who are awake or lethargic should be given intravenous fluids with hypertonic glucose and watched carefully. Patients who are unresponsive to verbal stimuli and who exhibit decorticate or decerebrate posturing require aggressive treatment in a pediatric intensive care unit with physicians knowledgeable in the treatment of Reye's syndrome.

Lead Poisoning

Both acute and chronic forms of lead poisoning produce encephalopathy. Lead intoxication is most frequent in children. Sources of ingested lead include old house paint, improperly glazed pottery, leaded jewelry, inhalation of fumes from burned storage batteries, lead contamination in the water supply near industrial plants, industrial crayons and old paints, lead toy soldiers, and inhalation of leaded gasoline. There is no "normal" lead concentration in blood, but poisoning is thought to occur with blood lead levels greater than 40 mg/dl. Acute lead encephalopathy begins with vomiting, abdominal pain, paresthesias, and generalized weakness. These symptoms progress to lethargy, coma, and seizures, without focal abnormalities. Cerebral edema with massive increases in intracranial pressure is present. Chronic lead poisoning can result in hyperactive behavior, mental retardation, epilepsy, and neuropathy. Laboratory abnormalities include a microcytic, hypochromic anemia with basophilic stippling of red blood cells, metaphyseal densities in long bones on x-ray, and presence of coproporphyrins in urine. Blood lead levels are elevated. CSF pressure is elevated, and CSF protein may be increased. Treatment of acute encephalopathy is based on reducing intracranial pressure and controlling seizures. Fluid restriction should be instituted at two-thirds maintenance. Continuous intracranial pressure monitoring is important. Mannitol and controlled hyperventilation can be used to decrease intracranial pressure. Methods to increase urinary excretion of lead should be instituted early. British anti-Lewisite (BAL) (2,3-dimercaptopropanol) 4 mg/kg is given intramuscularly every 4 hours for 5 to 7 days. Calcium EDTA (50 mg/kg per day as an intramuscular injection) can be used simultaneously for 5 days. Parenteral EDTA administration is used to treat chronic encephalopathy as well. Anticonvulsant medications may also be needed to control seizures. Acute and chronic forms of lead encephalopathy have a mortality rate of 25%. Of the survivors, most have permanent brain damage, including mental retardation, behavior abnormalities, and seizure disorders.

Salicylism

Salicylate poisoning occurs from either prolonged excessive ingestion or accidental or intentional ingestion of a single toxic dose. Initial symptoms are vomiting, sweating, paresthesias, and confusion. Respiratory abnormalities are present early, with hyperventilation causing a respiratory alkalosis. Coma and dehydration ensue. Either hypo- or hyperglycemia may be found. A metabolic acidosis is superimposed on the respiratory alkalosis. A salicylate level of 35 μg/dl or greater confirms the diagnosis of salicylism. Treatment consists of adequate intravenous fluid replacement with twice the normal maintenance amount. Correction of the acidosis with bicarbonate may be indicated. Acetazolamide (5 mg/kg every 8 to 12 hours) increases excretion of salicylates. In severe cases, exchange transfusion, peritoneal dialysis, or hemodialysis is necessary to clear salicylates more rapidly. Vitamin K (5 mg intramuscularly) should be administered initially to correct clotting abnormalities. Severe salicylate poisoning can be fatal. In cases in which therapy can be instituted early, the symptoms are potentially reversible.

Bromism

Bromide intoxication is quite rare, since bromide-based medications are seldom used. However, some nonprescription sedative preparations (e.g., Nervine, Miles Laboratories) still contain bromides. Symptoms of bromide intoxication are hallucinations, delusions, confusion, irritability, and impaired thought processes. Dysarthria and cerebellar signs may also be present, with tremors and incoordination. A maculopapular skin rash may appear in a generalized fashion. Diagnosis is made by a serum bromide level of 18 meq/L or greater. Treatment consists of vigorous hydration with normal saline. Thiazide diuretics will increase the excretion of bromide. Symptoms usually reverse when the bromide level falls below the toxic range.

Barbiturate Poisoning

Both deliberate and accidental overdoses of barbiturates are common and should be considered in the differential diagnosis of anyone in coma. Mild symptoms of intoxication include lethargy, ataxia, slurred speech, and nystagmus. Severe intoxication results in coma, depressed muscle stretch reflexes, cardiorespiratory depression, and shock. Barbiturate overdose may produce electrocerebral silence (flat EEG), which is reversible. For this reason the presence of barbiturates in the blood precludes the ability to diagnose brain death. The diagnosis of barbiturate intoxication is based on finding elevated barbiturate levels in blood. The quantity of drug needed to produce encephalopathy is quite variable. For example, in the management of patients with seizures, the therapeutic phenobarbital level is 1–2 mg%. With acute ingestion, intoxication may occur with a serum phenobarbital level of only 3–4 mg%, whereas patients with chronic ingestion may show no signs of intoxication at that level. The immediate goal of treatment is to maintain adequate blood pressure and respiration. Patients may need mechanical ventilation. Gastric lavage should be performed to remove any undigested drug. If patients are in deep coma with life-threatening complications, peritoneal dialysis or hemodialysis can be used to clear barbiturates rapidly. Milder cases can be treated with intensive supportive care alone.

Methyl Alcohol

Ingestion of methyl alcohol (rubbing alcohol) results in blurred vision, restlessness, delirium, coma, and metabolic acidosis within 8 to 36 hours. Papilledema and increased intracranial pressure may develop. Laboratory tests show evidence of a metabolic acidosis with low serum pH and bicarbonate. Methanol and formic acid can be detected in blood and urine. Treatment is aimed primarily at correcting the metabolic acidosis through administration of bicarbonate, as well as careful fluid and electrolyte balance. Encephalopathic symptoms are usually reversible, but permanent visual impairment with optic atrophy may occur.

Neuroleptic Malignant Syndrome

The neuroleptic malignant syndrome occurs infrequently in patients who receive any of the D2 dopamine-receptor antagonist neuroleptics, most commonly haloperidol or thiothixene, or who are withdrawn from dopaminergic indirect agonistic drugs. Mortality ranges from 10% to 35%. The syndrome may develop early or several weeks after treatment with a neuroleptic was started or a dopaminergic drug withdrawn. Once symptoms have begun, though, the course is quite rapid. The cardinal manifestations are high fever, stupor or coma, rigidity, autonomic instability with unstable blood pressure, cardiac arrhythmias, and diaphoresis, and high serum CK levels. Treatment has to be initiated promptly with bromocriptine (5 mg 3 times a day by mouth or by nasogastric tube). Dosage of bromocriptine may have to be increased to as much as 20 mg 4 times a day. If the patient responds to this treatment, bromocriptine is continued for 10 days and then gradually withdrawn. Dantrolene (0.25 mg/kg of body weight intravenously 4 times a day) has also been used effectively, but it will not control the CNS symptoms. Controversy exists in the literature as to the optimal treatment methods. Patients who have suffered from neuroleptic malignant syndrome have a high probability of suffering subsequent episodes on rechallenge with neuroleptics. In rare patients taking a combination of monoamine oxidase (MAO) inhibitors and tricyclics, delirium, hyperpyrexia, convulsions, coma, and death have been reported.

COMA

The comatose patient is unarousable, has lost awareness, and is unable to respond to internal or external stimuli. If coma persists, the outcome is often fatal or the patient may recover with a neurologic deficit. Different degrees of coma can be recognized that allow the clinician to assess a patient's course. In deep coma the patient does not respond to even the most painful stimuli. In semicoma the patient may respond to pinching by groaning, restlessness, increased respirations, or momentary eye opening. In stupor the patient will respond to manipulation or loud voice by opening of the eyes or some simple response but will not speak. An obtunded patient may respond intermittently to simple commands, open the eyes, and utter a few simple words. The confused patient may appear drowsy, and it will be apparent that orientation and the ability to have a meaningful discussion are impaired. When the patient is unable to respond but is alert, this condition is referred to as "locked-in," a syndrome seen with lesions in the basis pontis. In this state descending motor pathways are impaired, but ascending sensory tracts and structures responsible for wakefulness and arousal are functioning. In akinetic mutism, often seen with bilateral medial orbitofrontal lesions, the patient is not paralyzed but lacks the impulse to move, is unaware of the surroundings, needs to be fed, and is incontinent. Some patients survive an episode of coma only to progress to a persistent vegetative state. In this condition the patient is awake but has no awareness, does not respond except with blinking to threat, has primitive reflex and postural movements, and retains all autonomic functions.

Arousal and consciousness are dependent on an intact and functioning reticular formation, and its connections, in the thalamus and midbrain. Bilateral, widespread structural cortical lesions will render a patient comatose, but unilateral hemispheric lesions do not produce coma, unless there is herniation with compression of the upper brainstem. Destructive lesions in the midbrain tegmental reticular formation are invariably associated with coma. Drugs and metabolic disturbances lead to coma by suppressing reticular and/or cortical functions.

Causes of Coma

The cause and mechanism (see Table 9–7) of coma is usually obvious in patients with head trauma, except that elderly patients and small children may have bilateral traumatic subdural hematomas without obvious evidence of trauma. Nontraumatic coma is caused by drug intoxication in about one third of patients, metabolic derangements in one third, and cerebrovascular disease in another third of patients in coma. These proportions will vary depending on the medical setting. Meningitis, brain abscess, and encephalitis are rare causes of coma.

Examination and Management

Maintaining vital functions takes precedence, and neurologic (see Chapter 2) and general examinations are performed only after ade-

TABLE 9–7. Mechanisms of Coma

Generalized seizure
Head trauma
Toxic-metabolic disturbance
Destructive lesion with extensive involvement of both hemispheres
Destructive lesion involving hypothalamus or upper brainstem and thalamic reticular formation
Hypotension, systolic blood pressure below 70 mm Hg in normotensive individuals
Psychogenic unresponsiveness

quate respiration and cardiac functions are assured. The primary concern in the evaluation of a comatose patient is to determine if a structural lesion is the cause. The history will often provide information about the etiology of the coma. If no history can be obtained, the head, ear canals, nasal passages, and pharynx should be carefully examined for evidence of bleeding from head trauma. The head and neck in patients suspected of trauma should not be manipulated but stabilized until there is evidence that there is no cervical spine fracture or displacement of cervical vertebrae. Fever alone or fever and a stiff neck suggest the possibility of intracranial infection, and after a CT scan of the head, an LP should be performed as soon as possible. If the neurologic examination of the comatose patient does not show focal or unilateral signs, the patient most likely suffers from toxic-metabolic coma. Besides depth of coma, the Glasgow coma scale (Table 9–8) may serve as a tool in assessing progression of coma and in predicting outcome. Patients in psychogenic coma usually appear healthy; they have normal respirations, blood pressure, and pulse; they have no abnormalities on neurologic examination; all laboratory tests are normal; and an EEG shows normal electrical activity of the brain.

Management of comatose patients (Table 9–9) is difficult and is best provided by a team of experienced physicians and nurses. Ideally, PaO_2 should be greater than 100 mm Hg and $PaCO_2$ between 30 to 35 mm Hg. Mean arterial pressure should be maintained at approximately 100 mm Hg, and dopamine is preferred over levophed because it causes less

TABLE 9–8. Glasgow Coma Scale

Eyes open	
Spontaneous	4
To verbal command	3
To pain	2
No response	1
Best verbal response	
Oriented and converses	5
Disoriented and converses	4
Inappropriate words	3
Incomprehensible sounds	2
No response	1
Best motor response	
Obeys verbal commands	6
Localizes pain	5
Flexion withdrawal	4
Flexion abnormal	3
Extension	2
No response	1
Total	3–15

TABLE 9-9. Management of the Comatose Patient

Assure oxygenation.
Maintain circulation.
Restore electrolyte and acid-base balance.
Administer thiamine and glucose.
Stop seizures.
Treat infection.
Control body temperature.
Use specific antidotes.
Perform gastric lavage.
Lower increased intracranial pressure.
Control agitation.

damage to kidneys. Fifty ml of a 50% solution of glucose is given with 100 mg thiamine. Seizures can be controlled acutely with diazepam (2.5 to 10 mg intravenously) followed by phenytoin (500 to 1000 mg, infusion rate less than 50 mg per minute). In patients with sedative overdosage, Naloxone (0.4 mg every 5 minutes) should be given. This may produce acute withdrawal symptoms and signs, because its effects last 2 to 3 hours, which is shorter than that of many sedatives. Physostigmine (1 mg intravenously) counteracts the effects of tricyclics with anticholinergic properties. Gastric lavage is useful in removing remaining unabsorbed intoxicants. Patients with increased intracranial pressure can initially be hyperventilated to reduce $PaCO_2$ by about 20 to 25 mm Hg, which leads to vasoconstriction. Its effect is rapid but transient. Mannitol as a bolus (1.5 to 2.0 gm/kg of body weight) rapidly reduces pressure and its effects last 4 to 6 hours, at which time another dose may be given. Dexamethasone (16 mg initially and 4 mg at 6-hour intervals) is often effective in reducing intracranial pressure in patients with mass lesions and cerebral edema. Bacterial infections of the CNS should be promptly treated: the earlier treatment is initiated, the better the prognosis. A cooling blanket may be required to control hyperthermia.

Prognosis

The prognosis of coma depends on the underlying etiology, the age of the patient, the presence of certain neurologic abnormalities, and the duration of the coma. In severe head trauma 55% of those less than 20 years of age make a moderate to good recovery, while only 5% of those over age 60 do. Coma that lasts longer than 6 hours carries a poor prognosis, with a 95% mortality rate for patients who are still in coma after 6 hours and have nonreacting pupils or absent oculocephalic reflexes.

Decorticate and decerebrate posturing and flaccidity carry a poor prognosis. The mortality of patients in deep coma from depressant drug poisoning is 5%. In hepatic coma the prognosis is worse in patients with acute fulminating hepatic failure, in the elderly, and in those with severe liver damage. In subarachnoid hemorrhage the initial mortality is 15% to 40%. Any degree of altered consciousness reduces the probability of a good outcome in patients with acute stroke, particularly in those suffering from intracerebral hemorrhages. After cardiac arrest one rarely knows the exact duration of cerebral hypoxic ischemia. Some patients reawaken quickly and make a satisfactory recovery. Others suffer brain injury and will be in coma for variable periods of time. At 6 hours after cardiac arrest, persistent coma and absence of pupillary light reflexes, corneal reflexes, and oculovestibular reflexes correlate with a high probability of an outcome of death or severe neurologic disability, including the vegetative state.

Brain Death

In comatose patients surviving for longer than 12 hours the question of brain death invariably arises. Considerations in the diagnosis of brain death are absence of cerebral functions; absence of brainstem functions, including respiration, irreversibility, and absence of CNS depressants, hypothermia (temperature less than 32.2 degrees centigrade), high cervical cord injury, and pharmacological neuromuscular blockade. Absence of cerebral functions is present when the patient is unreceptive and unresponsive (coma). Spinal reflexes may be present. Absence of brainstem functions is evidenced by midposition of the eyes; absence of spontaneous or induced eye movements (oculocephalic and oculovestibular reflexes); dilated or midposition fixed pupils; absence of facial movements and of gag, cough, corneal, and sucking reflexes; and absence of spontaneous respiratory movements. In patients with adequate cardiac and pulmonary function, apnea is established when no spontaneous respirations occur after ventilating the patient with oxygen concentrations of 100% at normocapnia for 10 minutes, then disconnecting the respirator and administering oxygen at 8 to 12 L/M via tracheal cannula for 10 minutes. At this time arterial blood should be drawn, and $PaCO_2$ should be greater than 60 mm Hg. The respirator is reconnected at the end of the 10-minute period. If hypotension and/or arrhythmia develops, the respirator is immediately reconnected. Electrocerebral silence on EEG is a useful confirmatory test. Except in cases of acute, traumatic massive brain injury, the cessation of all brain function must be established by two examinations at least 6 hours apart. Independent confirmation of the diagnosis of brain death by another physician is mandatory.

REFERENCES

Farmer TW: Neurologic complications of vitamin and mineral disorders. *In* Baker AB, Baker LH: Handbook of Clinical Neurology, vol 3, chapter 42. Hagerstown, MD, Harper. 1979.

O'Doherty DS, Canary JF: Neurologic aspects of endocrine disturbances. *In* Baker AB, Baker LH: Handbook of Clinical Neurology, vol 3, chapter 43. Hagerstown, MD, Harper, 1979.

Plum F, Posner JB. Diagnosis of Stupor and Coma, 3rd ed. Philadelphia, FA Davis, 1980.

Laureno R. Central pontine myelinolysis following rapid correction of hyponatremia. Ann Neurol 1983;13:232–242.

Chugani HT, Menkes JH. Neurologic manifestations of systemic disease. *In* Menkes JH, (ed): Textbook of Child Neurology, 3rd ed. Philadelphia, Lea and Febiger, 1985, pp 720–763.

Levy DE, Caronna JJ, Singer BH, et al: Predicting outcome from hypoxic-ischemic coma. JAMA 1985;253:1420–1426.

Victor M: Neurologic disorders due to alcoholism and malnutrition. *In* Baker AB, Joynt RJ, (eds): Clinical Neurology, chapter 61. Philadelphia, JB Lippincott, 1986.

Caronna JJ: Neurological syndromes following cardiac arrest and cardiac bypass surgery. *In* Barnet HJM et al (eds): Stroke. New York, Churchill Livingstone, 1986, pp 707–719.

Fraser CL, Arieff AI: Nervous system complications of uremia. Ann Int Med 1988;109:143–153.

McKee AC, Winkelman MD, Banker BQ: Central pontine myelinolysis in severely burned patients: Relationship to serum hyperosmolality. Neurology 1988; 38:1211–1217.

Victor M, Adams RD, Collins GH: The Wernicke-Korsakoff Syndrome and Other Disorders Due to Alcoholism and Malnutrition. Philadelphia, FA Davis, 1989.

Massey EW: Neurological manifestations of hematological disease. Neurol Clin 1989;7:549–561.

Kaminski J, Ruff RL: Neurological complications of endocrine disease. Neurol Clin 1989;7:489–508.

Rothstein JD, Herlong HF: Neurological manifestations of hepatic disease. Neurol Clin 1989;7:563–578.

Drugs for psychiatric disorders: Med Lett Drugs Ther 1989;31:13–20.

Victor M, Rothstein J: Neurologic complications of hepatic and gastrointestinal disease. *In* Asbury AK, McKhann G, McDonald WI (eds): Diseases of the Nervous System, 2nd ed. Philadelphia, WB Saunders, 1992, pp 1442–1445.

Caroff SN, Mann SC: Neuroleptic malignant syndrome. Med Clin North Am, Contemp Clin Neurol 1993;77:185–202.

Allen LH, Casterline J: Vitamin B^{12} deficiency in elderly individuals: Diagnosis and requirements. Am J Clin Nutr 1994;60:12–14.

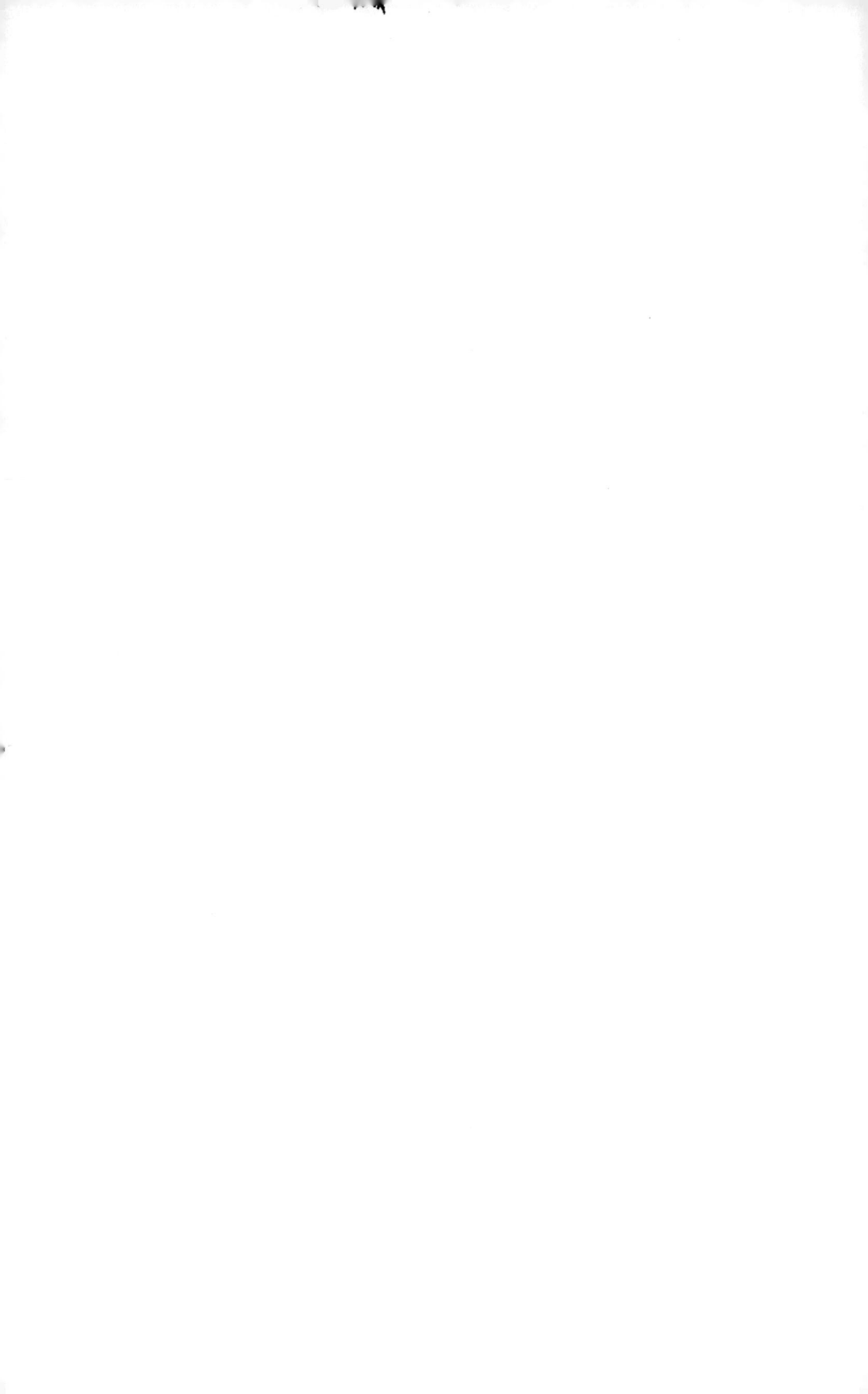

10
Muscle Diseases and Disorders of Neuromuscular Transmission

MUSCLE DISEASES

The muscle diseases, or myopathies, are a diverse group of degenerative, inflammatory, toxic, metabolic, and endocrine disorders of striated muscle. Proximal muscles are usually more severely affected than distal muscles; therefore, patients generally complain of difficulty with activities that require use of the shoulder and pelvic muscles, such as lifting an object from a shelf, carrying a heavy object, rising from a chair or from the floor, and climbing or descending stairs. Complaints of diplopia, ptosis, dysarthria, and dysphagia are less common but may be present in some patients. Pain is a rare complaint in primary muscle disease but occurs in dermatomyositis, and shoulder pain may be an early complaint of patients with some forms of proximal muscular dystrophy. In the latter condition the pain is due to excessive stress on ligamentous structures at the shoulder due to weakness of muscles that normally keep the arm attached to the chest. Many patients complain of weakness when they really mean fatigue, and many nonmuscular diseases produce muscle weakness. Therefore, detailed muscle strength testing is needed. Neurologic examination shows greater proximal than distal muscle weakness in most primary muscle disorders, sensory examination is normal, and muscle stretch reflexes are reduced in proportion to loss of muscle function. Muscle atrophy is present in proportion to muscle tissue destruction. In some disorders the lost muscle tissue is replaced by fat, and the involved muscle may look hypertrophied (pseudohypertrophy).

The clinical pattern of neurologic involvement at presentation, together with the time course, presence or absence of family history, and presence or absence of associated abnormalities of other organ systems, will generally permit classification of a muscle disease into a broad category and will sometimes permit identification of the exact pathologic process responsible. Thus, familial myopathies that are slowly and relentlessly progressive are generally classified as muscular dystrophies. Familial or sporadic muscle disorders that present at an early age with hypotonia and delay of motor milestones (but are not associated with significant progression over time) are usually classified as congenital myopathies. Subacute, occasionally painful, proximal muscle weakness in an adult without family history is the typical picture of the inflammatory myopathies. Finally, the toxic, metabolic, and endocrine myopathies generally present as acute, subacute, or insidiously progressive proximal weakness.

The serum CK and aldolase levels are frequently elevated in patients with myopathy, particularly in those with rapid progression or significant destruction of muscle fibers. Thus, these muscle enzymes are likely to be elevated in the muscular dystrophies, inflammatory myopathies, and acute toxic myopathies.

Electromyographic studies often show characteristic "myopathic" abnormalities, thereby confirming primary muscle pathology. The additional presence of acute "denervation" or fibrillation and positive wave activity indicates that the muscle disease is inflammatory or associated with significant muscle fiber necrosis. Unfortunately, the EMG examination is frequently normal in patients with congenital myopathies, as well as in those with subacute or chronic, toxic, or endocrine myopathies.

Needle or open muscle biopsy will almost always confirm the presence of primary muscle pathology and may indicate the specific myopathy. The muscle biopsied should be one that is weak but not severely involved, so as to maximize the likelihood of making the diagnosis and minimize the risk of finding only loss of muscle fibers with replacement by connective tissue. The differential diagnosis of myopathy depends on the clinical presentation. The patient with proximal weakness usually has a myopathy but may have a predominantly proximal motor neuron disease, multiple mononeuropathy, or polyneuropathy. Guillain-Barré syndrome in particular may present as progressive proximal rather than distal weakness. The patient with prominent dysphagia may have a pharyngeal muscular dystrophy but may also have myasthenia gravis or a structural brainstem lesion.

Table 10–1 lists the muscle diseases that are included in the categories of muscular dystrophies; congenital myopathies; inflammatory myopathies; and toxic, metabolic, and endocrine myopathies. The eval-

TABLE 10–1. Muscle Diseases

Muscular dystrophies
  Duchenne
  Becker
  Emery-Dreifuss
  Myotonic
  Facioscapulohumeral
  Scapuloperoneal
  Limb-girdle
  Ocular
  Oculocraniosomatic
  Distal
Congenital myopathies
  Central core
  Nemaline
  Mitochondrial
  Other
Inflammatory myopathies
  Polymyositis
  Dermatomyositis
  Inclusion body myositis
  Sarcoid myopathy
  Lupus
  Polyarteritis nodosa
  Rheumatoid arthritis
  Mixed connective tissue disease
  Scleroderma
  Sjoegren's syndrome
  Paraneoplastic syndrome
Infectious myopathies
  Toxoplasmosis
  Trichinosis
  Cysticercosis
  Viral myositis
  HIV
Toxic, metabolic, and endocrine myopathies
  Alcohol
  Emetine
  Chloroquine
  Vincristine
  McArdle disease (muscle phosphorlyase deficiency)
  Mitochondrial encephalomyopathy
  Several glycogen and lipid storage diseases
  Periodic paralyses
  Paroxysmal myoglobinuria
  Corticosteroid excess or deficiency
  Thyroid hormone excess or deficiency
  Acromegaly
Other
  Fibromyalgia

uation of the patient with suspected myopathy or with myopathy of unknown etiology is detailed in Table 10–2.

Muscular Dystrophies

Muscular dystrophies are progressive hereditary myopathies marked by progressive weakness and atrophy of the affected muscles. They are classified in terms of the pattern of selective muscle involvement, the type of inheritance, the age of onset, and the mode of progression.

MYOTONIC DYSTROPHY. This disorder is the most common of the muscular dystrophies, and it is also one of the few with prominent involvement of distal extremity muscles. It is inherited in an autosomal dominant fashion, but the degree of penetrance is variable, and some patients reach old age with minimal symptoms. Progression is usually slow. The defective gene segregates as a single locus on chromosome 19. The DNA fragment increases in size in successive generations and is paralleled clinically by earlier occurrence and increasing severity. The disease can be recognized prenatally. The characteristic clinical picture includes a thin, narrow face; droopy eyelids; and weakness of face, neck, hand, and other extremity muscles. Also generally present is myotonia, which is demonstrated by difficulty of grip relaxation and by persistent contraction of thenar or tongue muscles following percussion. The EMG is diagnostic with myopathic changes and typical myotonic discharges. Because myotonic dystrophy is a systemic disor-

---

TABLE 10–2. Laboratory Tests in the Evaluation of Muscle Diseases

Tests to confirm muscle disease; may also identify specific diseases
   DNA testing
   Blood CK, aldolase
   EMG
   Muscle biopsy
Tests to identify specific muscle disease
   Blood potassium, free T4, cortisol
   Blood alcohol level, red-cell MCV, liver function tests
   Angiotensin converting enzyme (ACE)
Tests for evidence of cardiac or smooth muscle involvement
   ECG
   Holter monitor
   Cardiac echo
   Chest x-ray
   Barium swallow
Tests to rule out diseases that mimic muscle disease
   Nerve conduction studies
   Repetitive nerve stimulation studies

MUSCLE DISEASES

der, numerous other clinical features may be present. These include mild mental retardation, frontal baldness, cataracts, gonadal atrophy, diabetes, and conduction abnormalities on the ECG, which may be associated with symptomatic cardiac arrhythmias. Although the dystrophy cannot be treated, quinine, (300 mg, 2 or 3 times a day) or diphenylhydantoin (300 mg a day) often reduces the symptoms of myotonia. Periodic ECG and Holter monitor examinations are recommended to detect the development of treatable cardiac conduction abnormalities.

A very rare but potentially lethal form of the disease may be present at birth. It is almost always inherited from the mother. Sucking and swallowing are impaired and bronchial aspiration and pneumonia are common. Myotonia usually does not develop until later in childhood. Surviving infants often have mental retardation and arthrogryposis.

Congenital myotonia is distinctly different from myotonic dystrophy. Patients do not develop muscle weakness but have tonic spasms that develop after forceful muscle contractions. In some patients enormous muscle hypertrophy occurs due to work hypertrophy.

DUCHENNE DYSTROPHY. This disorder is a severe sex-linked recessive form of muscular dystrophy passed to boys from their unaffected mothers. Up to one third of the cases are felt to represent new mutations. Incidence ranges from 13 to 33 per 100,000 per year. The abnormal gene is located at Xp21 on the short arm of the X chromosome. The gene product, dystrophin, is absent in Duchenne dystrophy. Diminished amounts or truncated forms of dystrophin result either in a less severe form of muscular dystrophy or in a variety of different phenotypes. The child has normal or slightly delayed early motor developmental milestones but by 4 to 5 years of age develops signs of proximal muscle weakness such as waddling, hyperlordotic gait, and difficulties when rising from the floor. Pseudohypertrophy of calf muscles is frequently present. Ambulation is usually lost early in the second decade of life, and the patient dies 5 to 10 years after becoming wheelchair-bound. Complications include kyphoscoliosis and cardiomyopathy. About one third of boys with Duchenne dystrophy are mildly mentally retarded. The serum CK is usually strikingly elevated, and the EMG exam and muscle biopsy confirm the diagnosis.

There is no specific treatment for this or any of the other muscular dystrophies. Prednisone has been shown to improve strength. The addition of azathioprine does not have a beneficial effect, and the effect of prednisone is probably not due to immunosuppression. Specific gene therapy is in the experimental stages. A number of orthopedic surgical maneuvers — including tendon release operations at the hip, knee, and ankle — are often valuable in preserving ambulation for a number of years. In addition, leg splints may be used. The female carrier can often be identified by slight enlargement of calf muscles, mild muscle weakness, elevation of serum CK, minimal abnormalities on EMG examination, and mild pathologic features on muscle biopsy. Serum CK is elevated in carriers during their first decade of life and may be slightly elevated after this. Genetic counseling of young women who have been identified as carriers is recommended. Amniocentesis and therapeutic abortion of male fetuses is presently the only means of preventing the occurrence of this devastating neurologic illness.

BECKER DYSTROPHY. This disorder is also passed to boys from their unaffected mothers. The patient's presentation is that of proximal weakness late in the first decade, with loss of ambulation at about 10 years and survival into the fourth or fifth decade. Mental and cardiac abnormalities are rarely observed. The serum CK is elevated, but usually not as much as in Duchenne dystrophy. The incidence of this disorder is about one-tenth that of Duchenne dystrophy. Dystrophin is present but is structurally abnormal.

EMERY-DREIFUSS DYSTROPHY. This is another sex-linked dystrophy with a generally benign course. A severe cardiomyopathy is commonly seen in these patients. Sudden death is a frequent occurrence. Variants of the disease exist, as do phenotypically similar but genetically different dystrophies.

FACIOSCAPULOHUMERAL AND SCAPULOPERONEAL MUSCULAR DYSTROPHIES. Most cases of facioscapulohumeral (FSH) dystrophy are inherited in an autosomal dominant fashion. The onset of weakness in the face and shoulders usually occurs in the second decade. The weakness may be asymmetrical. Proximal leg muscles are involved later and usually to a lesser degree. The rate of progression is variable but usually slow, and there may be periods of apparent arrest. The disease is compatible with survival to old age. In more severe cases, truncal musculature and the muscles of the anterior compartment of the leg are affected as well. The serum CK is usually elevated, and the EMG and muscle biopsy show changes common to the dystrophies. Scapuloperoneal dystrophy, which presents with shoulder girdle and lower leg weakness, is a variant of FSH.

LIMB GIRDLE DYSTROPHIES. This is a heterogeneous group of familial myopathies with various patterns of inheritance, ages of presentation, and rates of progression. The clinical picture is generally one of gradually progressive shoulder and pelvic girdle weakness. CK is often elevated. Most cases show EMG and muscle biopsy changes typical for the dystrophies.

OCULAR, OCULOPHARYNGEAL, AND OCULOCRANIOSOMATIC DYSTROPHIES. The ocular dystrophies are relatively uncommon disorders affecting the extra-ocular muscles. If the pharyngeal musculature is also affected, the disorder is termed oculopharyngeal dystrophy. If there is additional involvement of the girdle muscles, the dystrophy is called oculocraniosomatic. The combination of short stature, ophthalmoplegia, retinitis pigmentosa, heart block, and elevated CSF protein—called the Kearns-Sayre syndrome—is a widespread mitochondrial disorder.

DISTAL MUSCULAR DYSTROPHY. This uncommon disorder is inherited in an autosomal dominant fashion and has its onset in the fifth or sixth decade of life. Since it is manifested by weakness and atrophy of distal muscles of the arms and legs, it can be mistaken for a predominantly motor polyneuropathy. EMG and muscle biopsy show features typical for muscular dystrophy.

Congenital Myopathies

Congenital myopathies are inherited disorders that are generally characterized by onset during infancy with little or no subsequent progression, but adult-onset cases have been reported. An affected infant is often hypotonic. Motor milestones such as the ages at which the infant sits and walks are typically delayed. Throughout childhood, physical abilities remain somewhat behind those of other children of the same age. Nevertheless, the child continues to develop motor skills and never loses a skill once it is developed. The adult with a congenital myopathy generally exhibits mild impairment of motor abilities, though this may not be recognized as a neurologic impairment. Because of this, an infant suspected of having a congenital myopathy may be found to have a parent who was a late walker and who has always had below-average physical abilities. Clinical and laboratory evaluations of infant and parent may then demonstrate that both have the same congenital myopathy.

Because the serum CK and EMG are often normal, the diagnosis is made by muscle biopsy. The most common forms of congenital myopathy are central core disease and nemaline myopathy, but there are many other types that are defined by characteristic patterns of abnormality seen on muscle biopsy. Cerebral palsy, congenital and acquired neuropathies, and disorders of neuromuscular transmission may present a similar picture of infantile weakness and hypotonia. There is no specific treatment for these myopathies, although physical therapy is sometimes helpful. Parents should expect affected children to have delayed motor milestones and reduced motor skills. The degree of disability present in the child and in affected relatives should determine expectations for the ultimate adult level of physical ability.

Inflammatory Myopathies

The inflammatory myopathies are characterized by subacute or acute proximal weakness, with evidence of muscle inflammation on biopsy.

POLYMYOSITIS AND DERMATOMYOSITIS. Both polymyositis and dermatomyositis are marked by a subacute onset and progression of proximal muscle weakness, which may include dysphagia and, occasionally, respiratory insufficiency. Less commonly, the onset is acute or insidious. These diseases affect individuals of all ages and both genders, but middle-aged and elderly individuals are somewhat overrepresented. The weakness may be focal, although it is most commonly diffuse and asymmetrical, or diffuse and relatively symmetrical. Distal muscles may be affected. Muscle pain and tenderness are generally absent, except in the cases with acute onset. Dermatomyositis is diagnosed when this pattern of weakness is associated with a skin rash, which may take several forms and may appear before, after, or at the same time as the weakness. There may be a blotchy flush over the cheekbones that blanches on pressure, the eyelids may be discolored and assume a purple color, or an erythematous rash may appear on the chest or neck, as well as over the knuckles and interphalangeal joints. At times the myocardium is affected.

Most patients with polymyositis and dermatomyositis have an elevation of serum CK and/or aldolase. The erythrocyte sedimentation rate is only occasionally abnormal, and in these cases the degree of elevation does not correspond to the severity of the disease. EMG is abnormal in 90% of patients. It generally shows nonspecific myopathic changes and often shows acute "denervation" activity. This pattern of abnormality on EMG, together with the clinical picture described here, is highly suggestive of the diagnoses of polymyositis or dermatomyositis. The muscle biopsy confirms the presence of a myopathy in about 90% of patients and demonstrates the inflammatory character in 75%.

The treatment of polymyositis and dermatomyositis is prednisone (1–2 mg/kg of body weight daily for at least 1–2 months). If the patient is significantly improved and serum CK has decreased, the dose is gently tapered at approximately 5 or 10 mg every other week until the minimum effective dose is found. At a dose of 20 mg per day, 40 mg may be given on alternate days. The lowest possible dose should be continued for 6 to 12 months. If a relapse occurs, the dose is increased again. Potassium supplements are given with prednisone. In cases where steroids cannot be used or are not tolerated, (and in steroid-resistant cases), azathioprine (up to 150–300 mg per day) or methotrexate (25–30 mg intravenously each week) are of value. The advantage of combining other drugs with prednisone is that lower steroid doses can then be used. The therapeutic value of cyclosporine, intravenous immunoglobulin, and plasmapheresis are being investigated. Prognosis for survival is usually good, except in those with malignant tumors. Some patients may need continual therapy.

There are a number of variants of these two inflammatory myopathies. Childhood dermatomyositis presents like the adult form but may be clinically more benign. About 20% of cases of polymyositis and dermatomyositis are found in association with another collagen vascular disease such as systemic lupus erythematosus, progressive systemic sclerosis, mixed connective tissue disease, or rheumatoid arthritis. In these cases, the patient independently meets diagnostic criteria for both conditions, and both disorders must be treated. Polymyositis and dermatomyositis are associated with carcinoma in about 10% of cases, with the incidence rising to 20% in patients over the age of 50. In women carcinoma of the breast and ovary are most frequently seen, while carcinoma of the lung and gastrointestinal tract are most frequently present in men. For this reason, any adult with one of these inflammatory muscle diseases should have a careful physical examination for possible occult malignancy, stool exam for occult blood, chest x-ray, urine exam for occult blood, blood count, and liver function tests. Further tests to search for underlying malignancy should be done if indicated by history or by abnormalities found on any of these screening tests.

Inclusion body myositis is a special type of inflammatory myositis. The diagnosis can be made only by muscle biopsy. The disorder is more frequent in men and affects distal muscles more severely than proximal ones. Dysphagia is rarely present, CK is only slightly elevated, and the disease does not respond to corticosteroid therapy.

SARCOID MYOPATHY. Sarcoidosis may involve muscle and cause proximal muscle weakness. It is estimated that approximately 50% of patients with generalized sarcoidosis have abnormal muscle biopsies, but far fewer of these patients have symptomatic muscle weakness. The serum CK and EMG may be abnormal, but definitive diagnosis depends on muscle biopsy evidence of characteristic noncaseating granulomas. If the patient is weak, it is reasonable to give steroid treatment similar to that for polymyositis and dermatomyositis.

Infectious Myopathies

Trichinosis is the best known of the parasitic infections of the muscle. The patient generally presents with malaise, fever, and myalgia along with periorbital edema, skin rash, and muscle weakness. In addition to elevation of the serum CK, there may be eosinophilia related to the allergic nature of the infection. If the patient is in pain or quite weak, therapy with prednisone (60 mg per day) is recommended, along with thiabendazole, (50 mg/kg of body weight per day for about 2 weeks). Cysticercosis and other parasites may also affect muscle, resulting in localized muscle masses with evidence of calcification on soft tissue x-rays. Definitive diagnosis is made by biopsy.

Viral myositis presents as a syndrome of myalgias and fever with rapid onset and resolution, usually over 2 to 3 weeks, often with elevation of the serum CK. It has been related to a variety of viral muscle infections. Therapy is limited to supportive measures, including analgesics for pain.

Toxic, Metabolic, and Endocrine Myopathies

This heterogeneous group of muscle diseases is listed in Table 10–1. The most common members of this group are discussed below.

TOXIC MYOPATHIES. In contrast to peripheral nerves, muscle is remarkably resistant to damage by toxins. The major exceptions are the acute and chronic myopathies produced by alcohol abuse, such as acute alcoholic myopathy, in which the patient generally complains of painful progressive weakness. Clinical examination shows proximal muscle weakness, CK is elevated, and EMG exam shows myopathic motor units and signs of acute "denervation." Rest and abstinence from alcohol are generally associated with improvement of the weakness. Chronic alcoholic myopathy presents as painless, gradually progressive proximal weakness in patients with prolonged alcohol abuse. Dysphagia may also be found in these patients. Examination shows proximal weakness, CK may be mildly elevated, and EMG is often normal. The treatment is supportive measures combined with the patient's cessation of alcohol consumption.

Emetine abuse, particularly in the patient with anorexia nervosa, may also produce a progressive proximal weakness. Supportive therapy and discontinuation of this medicine generally result in considerable improvement.

The eosinophilia-myalgia syndrome (EMS) was first reported in 1989 and is felt to be secondary to ingestion of l-tryptophan. The clinical presentation is similar to the toxic oil syndrome, which appeared in Spain in 1981 and was attributed to the ingestion of adulterated rapeseed oil. EMS is also similar in clinical presentation to eosinophilic fasciitis. Patients present with arthralgias, myalgias, and scledermalike skin changes. Neuropathies are not uncommon. Muscle biopsy may show perivascular inflammatory cells.

METABOLIC MYOPATHIES. A number of rare, autosomal recessive metabolic disorders that present as adult-onset myopathies can be diagnosed only by muscle biopsy with special histochemical stains. Acid maltase deficiency, a glycogen storage disease, may present as a gradually progressive proximal weakness, which may also involve the diaphragm. Myophosphorylase deficiency (McArdle disease) and phosphofructokinase deficiency are glycogen storage diseases that may present as fatigue, together with attacks of muscle pain, cramps, and occasionally myoglobinuria—particularly with exercise. Eventually, patients with these disorders may develop permanent proximal weakness. Carnitine and carnitine palmityltransferase deficiencies are lipid storage disorders that present as progressive proximal weakness.

The periodic paralyses may also be thought of as metabolic myopathies. Clinically, this group of disorders is characterized by episodes of weakness that usually begin in the legs and ascend over a period of hours to the muscles of the trunk and upper extremities. The eyes and diaphragm are spared. Serum potassium levels taken during the episode of paralysis may be normal, elevated, or reduced—leading to the diagnoses of normokalemic, hyperkalemic, or hypokalemic periodic paralysis. In addition, disorders may be classified as primary (hereditary) or secondary (due to endogenous or exogenous toxins). For example, hyperkalemic periodic paralysis may occur secondary to hyperthyroidism and respond to treatment with propranolol. Hypokalemic periodic paralysis may be caused by abuse of diuretics or excessive ingestion of licorice, which contains a potent mineralocorticoid. Unlike the primary periodic paralyses, the secondary forms of periodic paralysis are usually marked by abnormal potassium levels between the episodes of paralysis. The most common of the primary periodic paralyses is hypokalemic periodic paralysis. In this form, the paralysis usually occurs following heavy physical exercise or after a heavy carbohydrate meal. During the attack the serum potassium level may fall as low as 1.8 meq per liter but without increased secretion in the urine. Potassium enters muscle fibers, which on biopsy show marked vacuolation with an increased water content. During the paralysis virtually no muscle action potentials are present. The attack can be terminated by 10 g of KCL. In primary hyperkalemic paralysis the attacks are usually brief, lasting a half hour to an hour. They occur when the serum potassium level rises above 6 to 6.5 meq/l. Two grams of oral KCL will provoke an attack. Regardless of the change in serum potassium level during the attack, the primary forms of periodic paralysis are all generally responsive to acetazolamide (250 mg, 2 to 3 times per day). In addition, the patient should avoid excessive ingestion of carbohydrates and excessive exercise when fatigued.

ENDOCRINE MYOPATHIES. A number of endocrine disorders may cause myopathy. An elevated corticosteroid level produced by Cushing's syndrome or by steroid therapy is a common cause of gradually progressive, painless proximal muscle weakness. In these cases, the CK is generally normal and the EMG is also normal or shows only mild, nonspecific myopathic changes. A similar syndrome may be seen with steroid deficiency, thyroid hormone excess or deficiency, and acromegaly. In all cases, improvement of the weakness with normalization of endocrine status is the best evidence that the weakness was due to the hormone excess or deficiency.

Fibromyalgia Syndrome

Some physicians do not believe that fibromyalgia is a discrete condition, but rheumatologists report that it is one of the most common disorders seen in primary care practices. Prevalence figures range from 3 to 6 million in the United States. The condition is most common in women between the ages of 20 and 50. The etiology is unknown. Criteria for the diagnosis of fibromyalgia include chronic, generalized aches, pain, or stiffness involving three or more anatomic sites and present for 3 or more months; absence of other conditions that can account for the symptoms; and pain at a minimum of 11 of 18 tender point sites on digital palpation (occiput, lower cervical, trapezius, supraspinatus, second rib, lateral epicondyle, gluteal, greater trochanter, knee). Patients also often complain of waking without feeling rested, frequent awakenings during the night, chronic fatigue, morning stiffness and aching, frequent episodes of abdominal pain, subjective swelling of hands and feet, numbness in hands and feet, and anxiety and depression. Fibromyalgia may occur in association with osteoarthritis, rheumatoid arthritis, and hypothyroidism. Except for tender points the examination is normal. Laboratory tests are needed only to rule out other conditions. EMG examination is normal. Fibromyalgia is a chronic condition, and most patients continue to be symptomatic for many years, if not decades. Reassurance appears to be the most important therapeutic modality. Physical therapy has its champions, but in most patients it provides little, if any, relief in the long run. Anti-inflammatory agents are of benefit in an occasional patient. Amitriptyline (10–25 mg at night) helps to control pain in some patients and in many cases promotes sleep. Most patients use their favorite analgesic to remain reasonably functional.

Chronic fatigue syndrome, which has never been shown to be a discrete condition, has, if it should exist, nothing to do with muscles. The best one can say about this nonexistent syndrome is that it satisfies the need of some patients and physicians to attach a label to one of many forms of human suffering for which no ready explanation exists.

DISORDERS OF NEUROMUSCULAR TRANSMISSION

Disorders of the neuromuscular junction may affect the presynaptic nerve terminal or the postsynaptic muscle end-plate. In either case, neuromuscular transmission occasionally fails to generate an end-plate potential sufficient to produce a muscle action potential and subsequent muscle contraction. The patient affected by these disorders generally has weakness that is worsened with exercise and improved by rest. The more common conditions that affect neuromuscular transmission are listed in Table 10–3.

Myasthenia Gravis

Myasthenia gravis (MG) is an autoimmune disorder that is caused by antibodies to the acetylcholine receptor of skeletal muscle. In the United States it has an incidence of 1 per 20,000. Familial cases are uncommon. The disease is most prevalent in the third decade of life for women and in the fifth and sixth decades for men. On muscle biopsy of affected muscles the postsynaptic folds are markedly decreased but presynaptic structures are normal. The number of postsynaptic acetylcholine receptors is decreased, and immune complexes (IgG and complement components) are deposited. The primary manifestation of MG is weakness—particularly of ocular, bulbar, pharyngeal, respiratory and proximal extremity muscles. This weakness is often conspicuously worse following exercise and may improve following rest. Thus, ptosis may worsen noticeably after 1 to 3 minutes of sustained upgaze or may transiently improve following 1 to several minutes of resting the eyelids with the eyes closed. Similarly, the strength of abduction at the shoul-

---

TABLE 10–3. Disorders of Neuromuscular Transmission

Myasthenia gravis
Myasthenic (Eaton-Lambert) syndrome
Congenital myasthenia
Botulism
Arthropod envenomation (tick, scorpion, black widow spider)
Snake envenomation (cobra, mamba, viper, sea snake, South American rattlesnake)
Induced by aminoglycoside antibiotics
Induced by anesthetic agents
Induced by organophosphate insecticides
Associated with polymyositis
Associated with amyotrophic lateral sclerosis

ders may significantly decrease following a period of holding the arms outstretched. There are no sensory findings.

The onset of MG may be gradual or surprisingly sudden. The initial symptom may be ptosis or diplopia (50%), dysarthria or dysphagia (30%), or limb weakness (20%). In 20% of cases, termed "ocular" MG, weakness begins in and remains confined to ocular muscles. In the remainder of cases, there is initially or eventually some weakness of muscles other than ocular, and the disease is called "generalized" MG. A clinical classification of the disease, introduced by Osserman in 1958, is widely used and shown in Table 10–4. Symptoms may be intermittent initially, and the clinical course is generally marked by remissions and exacerbations. About one third of the patients, particularly those who have ocular MG, improve spontaneously and have long-standing remissions. On the other hand, those with generalized MG may develop potentially fatal respiratory failure.

The diagnosis of MG can sometimes be made on clinical grounds alone. In most cases, however, the edrophonium (Tensilon) test, electrophysiologic examination, and measurement of acetylcholine receptor antibodies will be required to confirm the diagnosis. The edrophonium test is positive if an improvement of muscle weakness or fatigability occurs following the injection of this cholinesterase inhibitor. The ability to perform a particular task (such as rising from a squatting position or swallowing), the duration of sustained arm abduction, the length of time a patient can look up before developing ptosis, or the quantification of the maximum inspiratory or expiratory force may be followed by improvement with edrophonium. The test is performed in the following manner. Two solutions are used: a placebo (1 ml saline) and edrophonium (10 mg in 1 ml), both prepared and labeled by a third party (double-blind test). If 0.3 ml of the first solution injected rapidly intravenously produces no change within 2 minutes, then 0.5 ml is injected. After 2 minutes, the second solution is tried in the same fashion. To avoid side effects, the test with each solution is

---

TABLE 10–4. Classification of Clinical Types of Myasthenia Gravis

I. Ocular myasthenia
II. A. Mild generalized with slow progression; no crisis; drug responsive
   B. Moderate generalized; severe bulbar and some skeletal involvement; no crisis; drug response less satisfactory
III. Fulminant; rapid progression to severe weakness with respiratory crises; poor drug response; high incidence of thymoma and high mortality
IV. Late-onset severe; same degree of weakness as under III; progression over 1 to 2 years from I to II.

stopped if improvement is seen after the initial injection. After writing down the examiner's impression, the third party is asked to break the code. If no improvement is seen with either solution, or if a better effect is seen with the placebo, the test is negative. An initial injection of the full 1 ml (10 mg) of edrophonium should be avoided, since it can cause significant gastrointestinal distress, even in the myasthenic. The dose should be scaled down appropriately when the test is used in children.

Repetitive stimulation studies may document a defect of neuromuscular transmission in patients with myasthenia gravis. A decremental response will be found in up to 90% of cases if proximal as well as distal muscles are tested, if the patient takes no anticholinesterase medication for 12 to 24 hours before the test, and if the muscle to be tested is warmed prior to the test. Some patients who do not show a decremental response with repetitive stimulation studies may show, with single fiber recording, increased variability in the firing rate of individual muscle fibers.

Serum antibodies to acetylcholine receptors can be obtained through commercial laboratories. If antibody is demonstrated to be present, one can be fairly certain of the diagnosis. However, 50% of patients with ocular MG and 20% of patents with generalized MG do not have detectable levels of circulating antibody. For this reason a negative antibody test does not rule out the diagnosis of MG.

When the diagnosis of MG has been made, the patient should then be evaluated for associated disorders. The MG patient should have a CT or MR scan of the chest to rule out thymoma, which occurs in 10% of MG patients. Every MG patient should also have thyroid function tests, and if there is clinical suspicion of pernicious anemia, the patient should have a Schilling test.

The differential diagnosis of MG depends on the clinical presentation. Ocular MG may be confused with brainstem neoplasm, stroke, or dysthyroid eye disease. MG affecting predominantly the bulbar muscles may be difficult to distinguish from polymyositis, ALS, or pharyngeal dystrophy. MG with prominent proximal extremity weakness must be distinguished from myopathy, myasthenic syndrome, proximal motor neuropathy, and proximal motor neuron disease. In each case, the demonstration of weakness that worsens with fatigue and improves with rest will suggest the diagnosis of MG. The positive edrophonium test, a decrementing response with repetitive stimulation of affected muscles, and presence of antibodies to the acetylcholine receptor will confirm the diagnosis.

The patient with MG should be managed according to the scheme presented in Table 10–5. If a thymoma is present, it should be removed through a median sternotomy. The transcervical approach is generally less desirable. Radiation therapy may be required in conjunction with

TABLE 10–5. Treatment of the Patient with Myasthenia Gravis

Patient with thymoma
  Thymectomy*
Patient without thymoma, generalized disease
  Thymectomy*
  Pyridostigmine or neostigmine
  Alternate-day steroids in gradually increasing doses
  Immunosuppressive therapy
  Plasmapheresis
Patient without thymoma, with ocular disease only
  Lid crutches, eye patch
  Alternate-day steroids in gradually increasing doses

* Treatment prior to surgery with pyridostigmine, steroids, or plasmapheresis is advisable, and patients may have to continue medication after surgery for variable periods of time.

surgery. The patient who has generalized MG without thymoma should also have thymectomy. Patients over the age of 50 were previously considered unsuitable candidates for thymectomy, but now patients at any age who are in reasonably good health are at least considered for this procedure. In about 30% to 40% of patients who undergo thymectomy, the disease will remit. An equal or greater percentage will have a partial remission of their symptoms. Although some patients improve significantly within a few days to a few weeks of surgery, others do not demonstrate full benefit until 1 to 2 years after the operation. Patients who have thymectomies must often be treated with the standard medical therapies described below prior to and for some time following surgery. Some patients, unfortunately, do not respond to thymectomy at all and have to be managed medically.

The mainstay of medical therapy, regardless of the presence or absence of receptor antibodies, is pyridostigmine (60–180 mg, every 3 to 4 hours), together with sustained-release pyridostigmine (180 mg at bedtime). Therapy must be adjusted for each patient, and the effective regimen varies considerably from one to another. Prednisone is begun if the patient does not respond adequately to this anticholinesterase therapy. Prednisone is started at 10 mg every other day and gradually increased to 80 to 100 mg every other day. Many patients will experience considerable relief of symptoms within a few weeks of starting this therapy. An attempt should be made to keep the prednisone at the minimum effective dose. The patient who fails corticosteroid treatment is a candidate for immunosuppressive therapy, such as azathioprine. Plasmapheresis is generally reserved for treating serious exacerbations, or for preparing patients for surgical therapy.

The MG patient who does not have a thymoma and whose disease is confined to ocular muscles generally responds well to conservative management. An eye patch will prevent double vision, and a lid crutch attached to glasses will keep the ptotic lid up so that the patient can see. If this therapy does not provide adequate symptomatic relief, the patient is then treated with steroids on alternate days in gradually increasing doses.

The syndrome of transient neonatal MG is found in 15% of infants born of mothers with MG. The disorder arises from the transplacental interaction of the mother's antibodies with the infant's acetylcholine receptors. The infant recovers spontaneously over 2 to 3 months as these antibodies are eliminated from the circulation and carries no greater risk of subsequently developing MG than the general population. The baby usually presents with hypotonia, feeding difficulty, and respiratory distress. The diagnosis of transient neonatal MG is made by the same tests employed in the diagnosis of adult MG. Treatment involves the administration of appropriate doses of an anticholinesterase drug.

The syndrome of congenital MG is probably a heterogeneous group of autosomal recessive metabolic disorders of neuromuscular transmission. Affected infants present with hypotonia and other signs of weakness. The treatment of choice is oral anticholinesterase medication, and there is no role for the other therapies employed in adult MG.

Myasthenic Syndrome

The myasthenic syndrome, or Eaton-Lambert syndrome, is a disease related to a presynaptic defect of neuromuscular transmission. It is usually found in association with oat-cell carcinoma of the lung or with another malignancy, but it sometimes occurs in otherwise normal individuals. Patients complain of limb stiffness and easy muscle fatigue, particularly during activities requiring use of shoulder and hip muscles. Both paresthesias in the feet and a dry mouth are also common. Neurologic examination demonstrates mild to moderate weakness—particularly of proximal muscles—and hypoactive muscle stretch reflexes. Occasionally, it is possible clinically to demonstrate an increase in strength of a muscle with repeated use. The diagnosis, however, may only be made with certainty by the electrophysiologic examination. Motor nerve stimulation studies demonstrate low-amplitude motor responses at rest, which, after maximum voluntary effort or a train of repetitive stimuli, are multiplied in amplitude several times over. Circulating antibodies to acetylcholine receptors are absent. Other disorders that may clinically resemble this syndrome include polymyositis, thyrotoxicosis, and limb-girdle dystrophy.

The patient with myasthenic syndrome should have a careful clinical and laboratory examination for possible occult malignancy. If this evaluation is negative, repeat tests may be needed at a future date. Oat-cell carcinoma in particular may not become otherwise symptomatic or be detectable by chest x-ray for up to two years after the onset of the myasthenic syndrome.

The management of myasthenic syndrome includes pharmacologic therapy together with treatment of any underlying malignancy. Guanidine is given orally (5–10 mg/kg per day in divided doses), and acts by facilitating release of acetylcholine from the presynaptic nerve terminal. Because of hematologic, liver, and renal toxicity, guanidine therapy must be carefully monitored.

Botulism

Botulism is caused by the exotoxin of the bacteria clostridium botulinum, which blocks the release of acetylcholine from presynaptic vesicles at the neuromuscular end-plate, at all autonomic ganglia, and at postganglionic parasympathetic nerve endings on smooth and cardiac muscle and exocrine glands. Clostridium botulinum is an anaerobic bacteria that may contaminate canned food and may also thrive in the intestine of susceptible infants. Botulism most commonly presents as a progressive descending paralysis. Paralysis of accommodation and convergence progresses over hours to external ophthalmoplegia and then to weakness of facial, bulbar, extremity, and respiratory muscles. It may be initially misdiagnosed as Guillain-Barré syndrome. Infantile botulism, in contrast to the adult form, is caused by production of the toxin within the intestine of the affected infant and evolves over several days to weeks. The clinical diagnosis of botulism is confirmed by electrophysiologic tests that demonstrate a presynaptic defect of neuromuscular transmission. Further confirmation may be obtained by means of a bioassay for the presence of toxin. Therapy is generally supportive, with particular attention to respiratory assistance. With appropriate treatment, the prognosis is generally good.

Tick Paralysis

Tick paralysis is related to a neurotoxin discharged by a feeding gravid female tick. The tick may feed unnoticed in hair-covered areas, and paralysis of limb musculature may be followed by bulbar and respiratory symptoms; weakness of extra-ocular muscles rarely occurs. Removal of the tick is usually followed by prompt reversal of symptoms. The condition may clinically resemble the Guillain-Barré syndrome. The presence of the tick, or the electrophysiologic demonstration that there is a defect in neuromuscular transmission with normal nerve conduction studies, distinguishes tick paralysis from the Guillain-Barré syndrome.

Other Disorders of Neuromuscular Transmission

The aminoglycoside antibiotics and the organophosphate insecticides may each cause a defect of neuromuscular transmission in some individuals. A clinical picture similar to MG will transiently develop. Polymyositis and motor neuron disease occasionally have some degree of associated myasthenic phenomenon. In these cases treatment with pyridostigmine may produce some improvement of myasthenic symptoms.

REFERENCES

Osserman KE: Myasthenia Gravis. New York, Grune and Stratton, 1958.

Seybold ME: Myasthenia gravis: A clinical and basic science review. JAMA 1983; 250; 2516–2521.

Mastaglia FL, Ojeda VJ: Inflammatory myopathies. Ann Neurol 1985; 17:215–227 and 317–323.

Brooke MH: A Clinician's View of Neuromuscular Diseases, 2nd ed. Baltimore, Williams and Wilkins, 1986.

Engel AG, Banker BQ (eds): Myology. New York, McGraw-Hill, 1986.

Goldenberg DL: Fibromyalgia syndrome: An emerging but controversial condition. JAMA 1987; 257:2782–2787.

Walton JN (ed): Disorders of Voluntary Muscle, 5th ed. Edinburgh, UK, Churchill Livingstone, 1988.

Thompson JM: Tension myalgia as a diagnosis at the Mayo Clinic and its relationship to fibrositis, fibromyalgia, and myofascial pain syndrome. Mayo Clin Proc 1990; 65:1237–1248.

Sagman DL, Melamed JC: L-tryptophan–induced eosinophilia-myalgia syndrome and myopathy. Neurology 1990; 40:1629–1631.

Kamb ML, Murphy JJ, Jones JL, Caston JC, Nederlof K, Horney LF, Swygert LA, Falk H, Kilbourne EM: Eosinophilia-myalgia syndrome in L-tryptophan–exposed patients. JAMA 1992; 267:77–82.

Griggs RC, Moxley RT, Mendell JR, Fenichel GM, Brooke MH, Pestronk A, Miller JP, Cwick VA, Pandya S, Robison J, King W, Signore L, Schierbecker J, Florence J, Matheson-Burden N, Wilson B. Duchenne dystrophy: Randomized, controlled trial of prednisone (18 months) and azathioprine (12 months). Neurology 1993; 43:520–527.

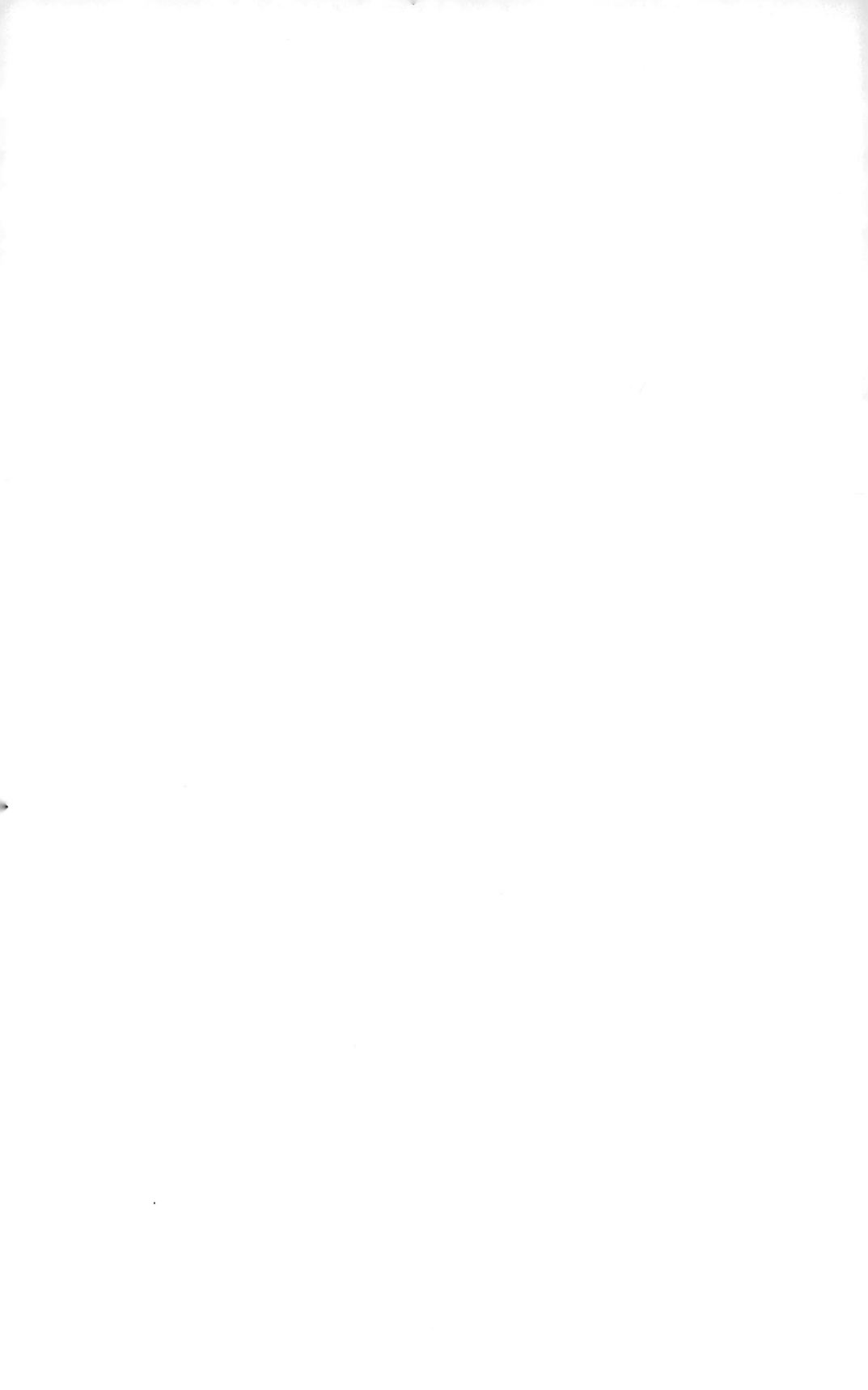

11

Diseases of Peripheral and Cranial Nerves

The peripheral nervous system includes all neural elements lying outside the pia of the spinal cord and brainstem. Cells of origin of efferent axons—somatic, visceral, and branchial—lie within the spinal cord and brainstem. Cells of origin of afferent axons, with few exceptions, lie outside the spinal cord and brainstem. Spinal and cranial nerve roots are those parts of the peripheral nervous system that lie in the subarachnoid space and are lacking epineurial membranes. Most peripheral nerves are made up of motor, sensory, and postsynaptic visceral axons. Axon diameters vary widely. The larger the diameter, the faster the transmission of electrical impulses. All nerve fibers are enclosed in epineurial and perineurial membranes. Each axon is contained within at least one layer of a process from a Schwann cell. Multiple layers wrapping around an axon are referred to as myelin sheath. Motor and discriminatory sensory axons are in general of large diameter and highly myelinated, while autonomous nervous system axons are small in diameter and poorly myelinated or unmyelinated. Disease processes can affect the function of the nerve cell body and its axon (axonal neuropathy), attack the Schwann cell or the myelin sheath directly (demyelinating neuropathy), or affect both axon and myelin sheath. The latter situation is present in vascular disease and direct trauma to peripheral nerves. The primary disease process may be in the subarachnoid space, connective tissue, or blood vessels. There are three principal pathologic processes. In Wallerian degeneration both the axon and the myelin sheath degenerate distal to the site of injury, with the proximal cell body showing chromatolysis. In axonal disease the axon degenerates, usually starting distally and in the longest nerve fibers, with myelin degeneration taking place secondarily. In segmental demyelination axons are preserved, and function is restored when remyelination occurs. In demyelinating neuropathies nerve conduction is slowed; but in primary axonal disease the amplitude of the evoked potential is reduced in proportion to the number of axons lost, while conduction velocities are normal or only minimally slowed. Diseases of the peripheral and cranial nerves may be caused by metabolic, toxic, vascular, infectious, inflammatory, immunologic, neoplastic, traumatic, hereditary, and idiopathic factors.

The presenting symptoms of a neuropathy are either weakness, sensory complaints, or a combination of both. In visceral neuropathies patients may have postural hypotension, difficulties with micturition, intermittent diarrhea, and impotence. In certain neuropathies pain is a prominent feature; some of these conditions are listed in Table 11-1. The pain is often burning but may be lancinating or aching. Prickling sensations, according to Dr. Peter Dyck, occur in only 17% of inherited neuropathies but in more than 60% of acquired neuropathies. Many patients with neuropathies involving sensory fibers will report distortion of sensation (e.g., coldness when the skin is actually warm), band-like feelings, or a sensation of water running between toes or fingers when these are quite dry. Commonly used medical terms in relation to neuropathies are paresthesia, dysesthesia, hyperpathia, allodynia, and causalgia. Paresthesia refers to an abnormal sensation, spontaneous or evoked, while dysesthesia defines a sensation that is similarly abnormal but also unpleasant. Hyperpathia refers to an increased reac-

TABLE 11-1. Painful Neuropathies

Mononeuropathies
  Compressive neuropathy (carpal tunnel, meralgia paresthetica)
  Trigeminal neuralgia
  Ischemic neuropathy
  Polyarteritis nodosa
  Diabetic mononeuropathy
  Herpes zoster
  Idiopathic and familial brachial plexopathy
Polyneuropathies
  Diabetes mellitus
  Paraneoplastic sensory neuropathy
  Nutritional neuropathy
  Multiple myeloma
  Amyloid
  Dominantly inherited sensory neuropathy
  Toxic (arsenic, thallium, metronidazole)
  AIDS-associated neuropathy
  Tangier disease
  Fairy disease

tion to a sensory stimulus, particularly in the setting of an increased sensory threshold. Allodynia is characterized by pain resulting from a normally painless sensory stimulus. Causalgia refers to sustained burning pain, allodynia, and hyperpathia after nerve injury. The pain usually spreads well beyond the cutaneous innervation of the injured nerve.

With over 100 known neuropathies, the task of arriving at a specific diagnosis is daunting. In many cases a specific diagnosis cannot be made; nevertheless, in the majority of patients the neuropathy can be appropriately characterized by using a certain framework of thinking. The important points are (1) the anatomical pattern of symptoms and signs (mononeuropathy, with abnormalities in the distribution of a single peripheral nerve; multiple mononeuropathies; or a polyneuropathy with relatively symmetrical and generally distal pattern of involvement); (2) the temporal profile (acute, subacute, chronic, or relapsing); (3) large versus small fiber involvement; (4) primary involvement of neurons and axons, Schwann cells and myelin sheath (this differentiation can often be made by nerve conduction studies), connective tissue, or blood vessels; (5) family history; (6) preceding or concurrent infections; (7) associated diseases; (8) drug use; and (9) laboratory abnormalities. The work-up of a patient with a neuropathy includes a detailed neurologic examination, EMG, and other pertinent laboratory studies to search for associated diseases. Nerve biopsy often is helpful in defining the type of neuropathy but may not provide specific etiological clues. Nerve biopsy may be diagnostic in some diseases, such as amyloidosis, sarcoidosis, hereditary neuropathies, vasculitis, neurofibromatosis, leprosy, metachromatic leukodystrophy, Krabbe's disease, vincristine neuropathy, and some toxic neuropathies.

MONONEUROPATHIES

Common Mononeuropathies of the Extremities

Lesions of an individual nerve produce symptoms and signs in the distribution of the involved nerve. Pain is a common symptom and may be confined to the sensory distribution of the nerve or may radiate for a considerable distance proximal to the level of the lesion. Palpation of the nerve may show focal tenderness at the site of abnormality. Sensory complaints (numbness and tingling) often appear before motor symptoms. Common causes of mononeuropathy are listed in Table 11–2. Ulnar and peroneal compression neuropathies can occur in neurologically normal patients on prolonged bed rest. These neuropathies are avoidable by using padding at the elbows and knees.

TABLE 11-2. Common Causes of Mononeuropathy and Multiple Mononeuropathy

Mononeuropathy
  Compression
  Trauma
  Diabetes
  Vasculitis (systemic or nonsystemic)
  Other vascular
  Postinfectious or inflammatory
  Herpes zoster or herpes simplex
  Tumor
Multiple mononeuropathy
  Multiple compressions
  Demyelinating with conduction block
  Necrotizing vasculitis
  Diabetes
  Sarcoidosis
  Postinfectious or inflammatory
  Neurofibromatosis
  Leprosy
  Wegener's granulomatosis
  Lymphomatoid granulomatosis
  Malignant infiltration

MEDIAN NEUROPATHY AT THE WRIST (CARPAL TUNNEL SYNDROME). Entrapment of the median nerve at the level of the wrist is the cause of the carpal tunnel syndrome. Pain in the hand and forearm is a frequent complaint. Along with pain, there may be symptoms of intermittent or persistent numbness and/or tingling. The sensory complaints are particularly bothersome at night and may awaken the patient from sleep. These symptoms are usually confined to the sensory distribution of the median nerve, although a more diffuse and poorly localized subjective numbness of the hand and forearm is sometimes encountered. Weakness of the hand may be noted and is often manifested by difficulty in unscrewing bottle tops, turning a key, or other maneuvers that involve opposition of the thumb. Activities involving flexion of the wrist make the symptoms worse. Sensory examination of a symptomatic hand may be normal, or there may be an objective sensory deficit in the distribution of the median nerve distal to the wrist. Motor examination may reveal atrophy of the thenar eminence and selective weakness of the abductor pollicis brevis and opponens pollicis muscles. Extreme flexion or extension of the affected hand by the examiner for a minute or two may precipitate or worsen the patient's sensory symptoms.

Congenitally small carpal tunnel, remote trauma to the wrist, rheumatoid arthritis, and extensive use of the fingers and hands may contribute to the development of a median neuropathy at the wrist. Hypothyroidism and pregnancy may be associated with bilateral symptoms. The diagnosis of median neuropathy at the wrist is usually not difficult. The differential diagnosis includes cervical plexopathy, cervical radiculopathy, and, occasionally, CNS disorders such as MS. Not infrequently, carpal tunnel syndrome is incorrectly diagnosed as a C6 radiculopathy. A C6 radiculopathy is differentiated by dermatomal sensory loss (which includes part of the dorsal surface of the hand and often extends proximal to the level of the elbow); weakness of the biceps, brachioradialis, and other C6-innervated muscles; reduction or loss of the biceps and brachioradialis reflexes; and pain with movement of the neck.

EMG and nerve conduction studies are a useful means of confirming a suspected median neuropathy at the wrist. Only a small percentage of patients with a typical clinical picture will have a completely normal electrophysiological study. EMG is also useful in distinguishing between cervical radiculopathy and median neuropathy, as well as in detecting contralateral asymptomatic median neuropathy or underlying polyneuropathy. It is important to realize that a median neuropathy at the level of the wrist is not necessarily a progressive problem, because many patients have a self-limited course. For this reason, a conservative, "wait and see" approach to management is indicated unless there is severe pain, significant neurological deficit, or EMG evidence of denervation at the initial examination. Underlying medical conditions such as hypothyroidism should be treated when present, and if occupational trauma is suspected to be a factor, the patient should be advised to avoid excessive use of the symptomatic fingers and hands as far as possible. A wrist splint for support of the wrist in a neutral position often alleviates symptoms, especially if the splint is worn at night. If significant symptoms persist or progress despite a period of conservative management and observation, surgical decompression of the carpal tunnel is a highly effective treatment.

ULNAR NEUROPATHY AT THE ELBOW. The ulnar nerve is particularly vulnerable to damage at the elbow as it passes through the ulnar groove behind the medial epicondyle and enters the cubital tunnel. Chronic compression due to positional or occupational habits is the most common cause of trouble at this site. Sensory symptoms with numbness and tingling in the distribution of the ulnar nerve are frequently the initial symptoms. Pain may be present at the level of the elbow with radiation down the medial aspect of the forearm. Weakness of the ulnar-innervated muscles may be manifested by loss of dexterity of the fingers. On examination, palpation may show thickening of the nerve within the ulnar groove and focal tenderness. The sensory deficit characteristically involves the medial aspect of the palmar and dorsal surfaces of the hand, splits the ring finger, and does not extend proximal beyond the wrist. Motor examination may show weakness and atrophy of the following muscles: abductors and adductors of the fingers (interossei), adductor pollicis, and ulnar lumbricales.

The major considerations in the differential diagnosis include lesions of the C8 nerve root or of the lower portion of the brachial plexus. In both of these conditions, the distribution of muscular weakness is more widespread and includes the median-innervated thenar musculature. Additionally, the sensory deficit usually extends proximal above the wrist along the medial surface of the forearm. EMG and nerve conduction studies are helpful in confirming the diagnosis of a suspected ulnar neuropathy and in ruling out cervical plexopathy or radiculopathy. The electrophysiological study may also demonstrate an asymptomatic contralateral ulnar neuropathy at the elbow or a predisposing polyneuropathy.

The therapeutic approach to the ulnar neuropathy at the elbow is similar to that previously outlined for median neuropathy at the wrist. A period of conservative management and observation is indicated, unless there is severe pain or a significant neurologic deficit present on the initial examination. The patient should be advised to avoid prolonged flexion or compression of the elbow. An elastic elbow pad may protect the nerve to some extent. If the symptoms and signs are progressive despite conservative management, or if there is significant neurologic deficit present at the outset, surgical decompression, sometimes with transposition of the nerve out of the ulnar groove, is the treatment of choice. However, the degree of recovery of ulnar nerve function following surgery is generally less satisfactory than with surgical decompression of the median nerve at the wrist.

RADIAL NEUROPATHY AT THE MID-HUMERUS. The radial nerve is especially vulnerable to injury as it passes along the spiral groove in the posterior aspect of the mid-humerus. Injury at this level produces a characteristic wrist drop. On examination, the most obvious clinical feature is weakness of the extensor muscles of the wrist, fingers, and thumb. The triceps muscle, which is innervated by a branch of the radial nerve proximal to the spiral groove, is normal, whereas the brachioradialis and other muscles in the forearm extensor compartment are weak. The sensory component of the radial nerve is relatively minor, and sensory symptoms and signs are restricted to the lateral aspect of the dorsal surface of the hand.

The differential diagnosis includes proximal radial nerve injury in the axilla, such as that caused by compression due to improper use of a crutch. In this case there will be weakness of the triceps in addition to weakness of the more distal radial-innervated muscles. If a radial palsy accompanies blunt trauma to the arm, the arm should be x-rayed to exclude fracture of the humerus with entrapment of the nerve. The polyneuropathy of lead poisoning may also present as a prominent wrist drop, although there will invariably be some degree of bilateral involvement. An EMG and nerve conduction studies generally confirm the diagnosis of radial mononeuropathy at the spiral groove.

Treatment of an acute compressive injury of the radial nerve is entirely conservative. Further compression of the nerve should be avoided, and the wrist and hand may be supported by a splint. The prognosis for spontaneous recovery is related to the severity of the focal injury. In the majority of instances, radial nerve function will either partially or completely recover. If there is significant denervation on the EMG, the prognosis for recovery is less favorable.

PERONEAL NEUROPATHY AT THE KNEE. The peroneal nerve is vulnerable to injury just below the knee as it passes around the lateral aspect of the head of the fibula. Leg crossing is a common postural habit that can lead to peroneal nerve damage. The nerve is also subject to traction injury caused by severe ankle sprains with sudden inversion of the ankle. Single or repeated episodes of blunt trauma and repeated tension from working in the squatting position are also causes of injury to the nerve in this location. A foot drop is the usual clinical presentation. On examination, there is weakness of the muscles that extend the ankle and toes and evert the foot. The anterior compartment muscles and extensor digitorum brevis, located dorsally and laterally on the foot, may be atrophic. Frequently, the only sensory abnormality is found in the distribution of the deep branch of the peroneal nerve, which is a small triangle on the distal dorsum of the foot and the proximal portion of the first two toes. Rarely, the sensory loss may extend to the lateral surface of the calf. Manipulation of the nerve as it passes around the head of the fibula may elicit pain or tingling.

The important differential diagnostic consideration is an L-5 radiculopathy. In this case, there will be weakness not only of the above-mentioned peroneal-innervated muscles but also of the muscles of foot inversion and thigh abduction. An EMG and nerve conduction studies generally confirm the involvement of the peroneal nerve and localize the lesion to the fibular head. The management of a foot drop due to a peroneal neuropathy is conservative. Ambulation may be improved by a foot brace, which may also prevent an accidental inversion sprain of the ankle and further nerve damage. The foot brace should be properly fitted so that the proximal portion of the brace does not compress the nerve at the level of the fibular head. The majority of patients with an acute compressive peroneal neuropathy will have significant spontaneous recovery of function. If there is significant denervation on the EMG, the prognosis for recovery is less favorable.

LATERAL FEMORAL CUTANEOUS NEUROPATHY. The lateral femoral cutaneous nerve is a pure sensory nerve, which is vulnerable to damage as it passes laterally under the inguinal ligament. The clinical syndrome produced by a neuropathy of this nerve is called meralgia paresthetica. The symptoms include burning pain, numbness, tingling, and increased sensitivity to cutaneous stimuli in the anterolateral and lateral thigh. Patients may complain bitterly about unpleasant dysesthesias that are triggered by contact of the lateral surface of the thigh with clothing. Obesity with a large abdominal fat pad, pregnancy, tight-fitting clothing, chronic low back pain with diffuse muscle spasm, and diffuse polyneuropathy predispose to this particular mononeuropathy. Examination shows normal motor and reflex function in the leg, with a sensory deficit in the distribution of the lateral femoral cutaneous nerve. Firm pressure to the nerve at the inguinal ligament just medial to the superior iliac crest may elicit local pain and/or distal tingling.

The important differential diagnostic consideration is a radiculopathy of one of the upper lumbar nerve roots. The lateral femoral cutaneous nerve lesion may be distinguished by the fact that it is confined to a discrete nonradicular sensory distribution without any motor or reflex changes. Needle EMG examination is normal.

The symptoms of meralgia paresthetica are difficult to treat, but they often subside spontaneously. If the patient is obese, weight reduction may be beneficial. Patients should be discouraged from wearing tight-fitting garments. If chronic low back pain with spasm and stiffness of the muscles of the lower spine and pelvis is present, appropriate treatment for this problem may also be helpful. Application of a topical counterstimulant such as 3% menthol cream to the dysesthetic area may provide some relief. Simple analgesics are rarely helpful. Sometimes excellent results are obtained by treatment with amitriptyline, gradually increased from 25 mg to 150 mg in the evening, together with fluphenazine (1 mg 3 times daily and as needed) for pain. Surgical decompression or resection of the nerve at the level of the inguinal ligament has been employed in refractory cases, although the efficacy of such treatment is not established.

Common Cranial Mononeuropathies

OCULOMOTOR, TROCHLEAR, AND ABDUCENS NEUROPATHIES. A lesion of cranial nerve III, IV, or VI will produce a disorder of ocular motility, causing the patient to complain of double vision. In addition, a lesion of cranial nerve III may cause ptosis and pupillary enlargement. Most cases of dysfunction of these nerves are caused by vascular lesions, trauma, or tumor. There are a variety of other identifiable causes, but about one quarter will be idiopathic. Vascular disease is a frequent cause of acquired ocular palsies. Acute dysfunction of cranial nerve III associated with pain, oculomotor paralysis, and ptosis with usually spared pupillary function is typically associated with diabetes. Diabetics may also develop an isolated neuropathy of cranial nerve IV or VI. These diabetic cranial mononeuropathies are presumably due to occlusion of vasa nervorum and generally improve or recover spontaneously. Hypertensive patients without diabetes and patients with vasculitis may develop similar ocular mononeuropathies, which are also felt to be vascular in origin. The differential diagnosis of painful acute third-nerve palsy includes an enlarging aneurysm at the junction of the internal carotid and posterior communicating arteries. In this instance the ocular motility defect is practically always accompanied by pupillary enlargement and impairment of the pupillary light reflex. Head trauma, with or without brain injury or concussion, can also produce mononeuropathies of the nerves that control eye movements. The fourth cranial nerve is especially vulnerable to the effects of trauma. Intracranial, locally invasive, or metastatic neoplasms can affect these ocular nerves. Cranial nerve VI may be affected by increased intracranial pressure due to tumor or other mass lesion. Congenital abnormalities; meningeal lesions such as meningitis, carcinomatosis, or sarcoidosis; and certain polyneuropathies are less common causes of mononeuropathy of these cranial nerves. Dysthyroid eye disease can produce dysfunction of extra-ocular muscles, but this is usually bilateral.

TRIGEMINAL NEURALGIA. The common cause of mononeuropathy of the fifth cranial nerve is trigeminal neuralgia, also known as tic douloureux. Brief, severe lancinating pains occur in the distribution of one of the branches of the trigeminal nerve. There is often an accompanying trigger zone, where pressure or another stimulus will cause an attack of neuralgia. Neurologic examination is normal. Pathogenesis, differential diagnosis, and treatment of this condition are discussed in Chapter 4.

SEVENTH-NERVE NEUROPATHY (BELL'S PALSY). The majority of instances of peripheral facial paralysis are classified as idiopathic and are called Bell's palsy. The picture of Bell's palsy is one of acute, complete or partial unilateral facial weakness without involvement of other cranial nerves or of the CNS and no sensory abnormalities. There is no evidence of ipsilateral ear disease, although pain behind the ear is often present at the onset. If the lesion of the facial nerve is proximal to the origin of the chorda tympani, taste may be impaired on the ipsilateral side of the tongue. An accurate diagnosis can usually be established by routine clinical examination alone. Electrodiagnostic tests are sometimes helpful in questionable cases and may help prognosticate recovery in severe cases, but they are rarely essential for diagnosis and management. Recovery may be rapid and complete within from 2 to 6 weeks, or it may be delayed and incomplete with eventual signs of aberrant reinnervation. About 50% of patients have complete spontaneous recovery. Factors associated with incomplete recovery include complete facial paralysis, nonear pain, and hypertension. When there are no contraindications, short-term treatment with prednisone (60 mg daily in divided doses for 4 days) may enhance recovery. The dosage is subsequently tapered and discontinued over 6 days. Treatment should be initiated as early as possible following onset of the facial paralysis. In some instances, it may be necessary to close the eyelid with tape at night and to use artificial tears to prevent drying of the cornea. There is no good evidence that either surgical decompression of the facial nerve or galvanic stimulation of paralyzed facial muscles results in better recovery.

Other Mononeuropathies

HERPES ZOSTER NEUROPATHY. Infection of the sensory nerve ganglion by the varicella zoster virus produces an acute painful vesicular eruption of the skin (shingles), which is typically confined to a unilateral dermatomal or cranial nerve distribution. The acute picture occurs in adults and is thought to be due to reactivation of dormant virus by a variety of factors—including trauma, advancing age, cancer, and immunosuppressive therapy. Pain usually precedes the appearance of cutaneous lesions and may persist as postherpetic neuralgia after the lesions have disappeared. If the disorder involves lower cervical or lumbosacral nerve roots or the facial nerve, muscle weakness may also be present. The cutaneous lesions heal, and the pain resolves in most cases within several weeks. Treatment of this uncomplicated course is directed at relief of pain with analgesics, drying of vesicles with calamine or other topical drying agents, and appropriate systemic antibiotic therapy of secondary bacterial infections. Acyclovir (800 mg 5 times daily for 7 days) appears to result in fewer new lesions, more rapid crusting of lesions already present, and reduced severity and duration of severe pain. The effect of this treatment on postherpetic neuralgia is uncertain. The addition of steroids is not indicated. Whenever there is evidence of involvement of the ophthalmic division of the trigeminal nerve, an ophthalmologist should be consulted promptly because of the possibility of keratitis, uveitis, and acute glaucoma with resultant blindness. Sometimes, particularly in older patients, neuralgia persists after the disappearance of the cutaneous lesions. This pain may gradually subside over months or may persist indefinitely. Treatment of postherpetic neuralgia is best accomplished by combination therapy with amitriptyline (25 mg at night, increasing by 25 mg every 3 to 4 days to a total dose of 150 mg) and fluphenazine (1 mg 3 times a day). In some patients, additional 1 mg doses may be given as necessary for pain. On occasion, because of concern about side effects of fluphenazine, treatment with amitriptyline alone is first tried. If the patient does not have significant relief with this, the combination regimen is then used. Treatment should be discontinued if there is no alleviation of symptoms after 14 days at the maximum dosage levels.

TRAUMATIC MONONEUROPATHY. Many cases of mononeuropathy are caused by blunt trauma to the nerve or by direct penetration of the nerve. These include patients with perioperative neuropathies, who will complain of some combination of pain, sensory abnormality, and weakness in the distribution of the affected nerve. Clinical and electrophysiological examinations will confirm the presence of the lesion and will often identify the location of the lesion along the course of the nerve. The prognosis and treatment of the traumatic mononeuropathy will depend on whether or not the lesion is incomplete. If the lesion is incomplete, there will be evidence of some preservation of function on clinical or electrophysiological examinations. In this case, the nerve and nerve sheath are at least partially intact. Any part of the nerve that has been permanently damaged will generally die back to the anterior horn cell and/or sensory root ganglion and then regrow along the nerve sheath if that is not damaged. The prognosis will then be good for partial or complete recovery. Nerve fibers grow at a rate of about 1 inch per month. In the meantime, supportive therapies such as physical therapy, braces, and splints are employed. If the nerve injury is complete and the nerve sheath is disrupted, the nerve will have no well-defined course to follow when it attempts to regrow, and recovery will be poor. For this reason, the patient with a complete lesion and a history suggesting that the nerve sheath may not be intact should have surgical exploration at the site of the lesion with the intent of repairing the injury to the nerve sheath. Persistent pain at the site of a nerve injury may be an indication for exploration to look for either an irritating foreign body, such as a suture, or a posttraumatic neuroma.

Reflex sympathetic dystrophy (RSD) is a poorly understood syndrome that develops several weeks after a precipitating event, most commonly trauma to the wrist, hand, or foot. Many other conditions, ranging from bruises to spinal cord trauma to stroke, have been reported to precipitate this syndrome. Neurologically, there is no sign of nerve injury. When a patient develops a similar syndrome after peripheral nerve damage, the condition is called causalgia. The primary clinical features of RSD are burning pain, hyperesthesia, allodynia, shiny skin, excessive sweating, trophic changes in skin and nails, and osteoporosis. The pain and other symptoms are almost always located distally in the hand or foot. The pain is often quite severe, continuous, poorly localized, and frequently aggravated by movement and contact with the involved body part. Early in the development of this condition there is edema, erythema, and hyperhydrosis. This stage is followed by pallor and atrophy of skin and nails. The outcome is variable. Some patients recover completely in a few years, while many end up with a useless, pale, atrophic hand or foot. Patients with RSD often have an associated dystonia involving the painful extremity. The diagnosis is principally a clinical one. If a plain x-ray or bone scan does not show localized osteopenia, this does not rule out the condition. Tests for autonomic dysfunction are nonspecific and are not a guide for therapy. Thermography usually shows a cold extremity, which is already known clinically. For a variety of reasons, response to sympathetic block may give false positive and false negative results. Treatment in general is rather unsatisfactory. Treatment modalities include physiotherapy, nerve stimulators, sympathetic blockade, regional intravenous sympatholytic infusions, corticosteroids, propranolol, phenoxybenzamine, tricyclic antidepressants, calcium channel blockers, Dilantin, Tegretol, and narcotics.

Multiple Mononeuropathies

The category of multiple mononeuropathy implies discrete lesions of several individual peripheral nerves. The causes of multiple mononeuropathies are listed in Table 11–2. The collagen vascular diseases, including periarteritis nodosa, rheumatoid arthritis, systemic lupus erythematosus, and Strauss syndrome may cause multiple mononeuropathies as a result of a disruption of the vascular supply to peripheral nerves. The nerve damage typically occurs in association with systemic activity of the disease, although multiple mononeuropathy may be the presenting complaint in periarteritis nodosa. A series of acute-onset mononeuropathies manifested as pain and sensory symptoms, followed by weakness in the distribution of the affected nerves, is the typical picture. The mononeuropathies should be treated symptomatically and appropriate therapy given for the underlying disease.

Diabetes may produce a multiple mononeuropathy secondary to small-vessel vasculopathy. Cranial or peripheral nerves may be involved, and the clinical presentation is one of a series of sometimes painful, acute-onset mononeuropathies. An unrelated diabetic multiple mononeuropathy, which predominantly involves proximal mid-lumber roots, has been termed diabetic polyradiculopathy, diabetic plexopathy, and diabetic femoral neuropathy. Typically, middle-aged or elderly diabetics experience the acute onset of unilateral severe thigh pain that is rapidly followed by weakness and atrophy of the anterior thigh muscles and loss of the knee reflex. Other muscles in the leg may occasionally be involved, and the condition sometimes occurs in the other leg after a period of weeks or months, or at the same time. The pain usually subsides over several weeks to months, and in many patients there is a tendency for complete or incomplete recovery of strength over a period of months. The neuropathies are treated symptomatically. Analgesics should be used liberally. Vigorous efforts to control blood sugar are also considered helpful in the treatment of this disorder. Not infrequently, the diagnosis of diabetes mellitus is made when the patient presents with this neuropathy.

Less common causes of multiple mononeuropathy include sarcoidosis, Wegener's granulomatosis, lymphomatoid granulomatosis, postinfectious or dysimmune multiple mononeuropathy, tumors (neurofibromatosis), and leprosy.

POLYNEUROPATHIES

A polyneuropathy is produced by a pathologic process that affects all the peripheral nerves in a relatively symmetrical fashion. Most polyneuropathies have a distal, symmetrical distribution, and the deficit is frequently more severe in the legs than in the arms. Occasionally, a polyneuropathy may be predominantly proximal. The time course may be acute, subacute, chronic or relapsing; and the predominant neurologic involvement may be motor, sensory, sensorimotor, or autonomic. The likely etiology can often be inferred from the pattern of neurologic involvement and the time course. Table 11–3 groups the more common causes of polyneuropathy by mode of clinical presentation. Laboratory investigation to discover the etiology of a polyneuropathy should be based on the clinical impression and is detailed in Table 11–4. It must be emphasized that examination of family members is the single procedure most likely to show that an unexplained chronic polyneuropathy is hereditary.

GUILLAIN-BARRÉ SYNDROME. Guillain-Barré syndrome (GBS), or acute inflammatory polyneuropathy, is the most commonly encountered acute polyneuropathy. Its incidence is about 1.5 cases per 100,000 per year in the United States. The syndrome may follow infections of various kinds, immunizations, and surgery; or it may occur spontaneously. A viral syndrome, occurring approximately 1 to 3 weeks prior to onset of symptoms of polyneuropathy, is seen in 50% to 60% of patients. Swine flu vaccine, used in 1976, and rabies vaccine are the only vaccines ever shown to be causally related to GBS. Chance associations of GBS and other vaccines occur predictably, but no causal relationship has ever been proven. A much-cited case report from Australia in 1976

TABLE 11-3. Common Causes of Polyneuropathy

Predominantly motor
  Guillain-Barré syndrome
  Porphyria
  Diphtheria
  Lead
  Hereditary sensorimotor neuropathy, types I and II
  Paraneoplastic neuropathy
Predominantly sensory
  Diabetes
  Amyloidosis
  Leprosy
  Lyme disease
  Paraneoplastic neuropathy
  Vitamin B^{12} deficiency
  Hereditary sensory neuropathy, types I–IV
Predominantly autonomic
  Diabetes
  Amyloidosis
  Alcoholic neuropathy
  Familial dysautonomias
Mixed sensorimotor
  Systemic diseases
    Renal failure, hypothyroidism, acromegaly, rheumatoid arthritis, periarteritis nodosa, systemic lupus erythematosus, multiple myeloma, macroglobulinemia, remote effect of malignancy
  Medications
    Isoniazid, nitrofurantoin, ethambutal, chloramphenicol, chloroquine, vincristine, vinblastine, dapsone, disulfiram, diphenylhydantoin, cisplatin, l-tryptophan
  Environmental toxins
    N-hexane, methyl n-butyl ketone, acrylamide, carbon disulfide, carbon monoxide, hexachlorophene, organophosphates
  Deficiency disorders
    Malabsorption, alcoholism, vitamin B^1 deficiency, Refsum's disease, metachromatic leukodystrophy

describes a unique patient who developed three episodes of GBS in close temporal relationship to the administration of tetanus toxoid. That this individual is unique is supported by the fact that after publication of the report, the patient suffered several additional attacks of GBS unrelated to any vaccination. An immunopathologic mechanism is thought to be involved in the pathogenesis of the disorder.

Prodromal symptoms, often consisting of malaise and nonspecific aches and pains, are followed by progressive weakness of the extremities that may be associated with complaints of distal numbness and tingling. The illness usually progresses for 7 to 10 days, plateaus for 1 to 2 weeks, and is then followed by a period of slow, complete or partial recovery, which may take many months. Initially, the weakness may be predominantly proximal or distal. Approximately 10% of patients may

TABLE 11-4. Laboratory Tests in the Evaluation of Polyneuropathy*

Blood and urine tests
  Blood count, fasting blood sugar, glycosylated hemoglobin, glucose tolerance test, urea, creatinine, free T4, TSH, ESR, ANA, other tests for collagen vascular disease, hepatitis B surface antigen, serum protein electrophoresis, quantitative immunoglobulins, Bence Jones proteins, folate and vitamin B^{12} levels, toxicology screen, lipoprotein electrophoresis, urinalysis
Other tests
  Nerve conduction studies and needle EMG
  Spinal fluid examination (cell count, glucose, protein, VDRL, cytology)
  Evaluation for occult malignancy
  Sural nerve biopsy

* Which of these tests are done, and in which order, will depend on the clinical setting.

have a recurrent, independent episode, often many years after the first attack. Weakness is the predominant finding on examination, and sensory impairment is often relatively minor. The muscle stretch reflexes are diffusely diminished or absent. Involvement of the cranial nerves may produce peripheral-type facial weakness, abnormalities of ocular motility, or other cranial nerve dysfunction. After several days of illness, the total protein of the CSF is elevated in the majority of cases, and the cell count is normal. Electrophysiological evaluation may show diffuse slowing of motor and sensory nerve conduction velocities, absence or delay of F-wave responses, and evidence of acute lower motor neuron dysfunction.

Although most cases of GBS are classified as idiopathic, the same clinical picture can be seen in association with viral hepatitis, infectious mononucleosis, and AIDS. Therefore, these infections should be routinely excluded by appropriate laboratory tests. Furthermore, porphyria, diphtheria, and tick paralysis must be considered in the differential diagnosis, because they also produce an acute, predominantly motor polyneuropathy that may closely resemble GBS.

Patients who are initially suspected to have acute inflammatory polyneuropathy should be admitted to the hospital for observation, since respiratory insufficiency may develop precipitously during the progressive phase of the illness. Respiratory function should be monitored carefully in a controlled environment until the patient's clinical status has stabilized or begun to improve. If sequential respiratory tests indicate a decline in function to a critical level, tracheotomy to permit mechanical ventilation, or endotracheal intubation followed by tracheotomy, should be carried out prior to the appearance of frank respiratory failure. Episodes of severe automatic dysfunction with cardiac arrhythmias and lability of blood pressure may present life-threatening problems that require treatment in an intensive care setting. Dysphagia is common, and feeding by nasogastric tube may be necessary. Paralyzed patients require passive range of motion of the extremities and alert nursing care to prevent complications of immobility, such as superimposed compression neuropathies of the ulnar and peroneal nerves. Plasma exchange has conclusively been shown to reduce the period of hospitalization, time required for mechanical ventilation, and length of time before the patient walks again. This therapy should be started within 2 weeks of the onset of the disease. Four to 6 treatments usually suffice. Recently, intravenous immunoglobulin (0.4 g per kg of body weight per day for 5 consecutive days) has been shown to be as effective as plasmapheresis. Prednisone has not been shown to be of any benefit.

The prognosis for spontaneous recovery is excellent in the majority of patients. Only a few patients will be left with significant residual neurologic deficits. The prognosis is worse in elderly individuals. Mortality in the acute phase of the illness and with optimal management should be less than 3%. Even though muscular strength may recover completely, the muscle stretch reflexes often remain permanently depressed or absent.

CHRONIC INFLAMMATORY DEMYELINATING POLYNEUROPATHY. Chronic inflammatory demyelinating polyneuropathy (CIDP) is thought to be distinctly different from GBS, and its incidence is much lower. The diagnosis is made on the basis of a pattern of clinical symptoms and signs, electrodiagnostic studies, CSF examination, and other laboratory tests. The clinical course is characterized by progressive or relapsing motor and sensory (rarely motor *or* sensory) dysfunction in more than one limb of a peripheral nerve nature, developing over at least 2 months. Muscle stretch reflexes will be decreased or absent, usually in arms and legs. Nerve conduction studies show reduction in conduction velocity in two or more nerves, partial conduction block, prolonged distal latencies, and absent F waves. The cerebrospinal protein is usually elevated without a pleocytosis. Most cases are idiopathic, but systemic lupus erythematosus, HIV infection, monoclonal or biclonal gammopathy, Castelman disease, diabetes, and CNS demyelinating disease may be present concurrently. Patients with CIDP have a protracted course over many years; treatment with plasmapheresis or intravenous immunoglobulin has been shown to be effective in some patients.

DIABETIC POLYNEUROPATHY. The reported incidence of polyneuropathy in diabetic patients varies from 10% to 50%. It may be seen as a complication of both insulin and noninsulin-dependent diabetes, although it is uncommon in diabetic children. The polyneuropathy in diabetes is typically symmetrical, distal, and predominantly sensory in nature. Symptoms are frequently mild and, early in the course, examination may show only decreased vibratory perception in the toes and feet and depression or loss of the ankle jerks. Symptoms are worse in the legs than in the arms and may be described as an unpleasant burning, numbness, or tingling in the feet, along with aching pain of the legs. Rarely, ulceration of the feet may develop in association with a severe sensory neuropathy. Muscular weakness and atrophy are usually not very prominent and, when present, tend to involve distal musculature. Disturbances of autonomic function are frequent with diabetic polyneuropathy. Autonomic abnormalities include Argyll Robertson–type pupils (small pupils that react not to light but to accommodation), postural hypotension due to vasomotor instability, anhidrosis, atonic dilation of the stomach, nocturnal diarrhea, atonic neurogenic bladder, and sexual dysfunction in males.

The pathogenesis of diabetic polyneuropathy is unclear. Recent evidence suggests that all forms of diabetic neuropathy might have a vascular component. In clinical practice there is considerable uncertainty about the relationship of the development of polyneuropathy to the degree of hyperglycemia. In rare instances, polyneuropathy may be the presenting symptom of noninsulin-dependent diabetes, in which the diagnosis of diabetes is confirmed only after a glucose tolerance test. On the other hand, the more severe cases of peripheral neuropathy tend to occur in poorly controlled diabetics who have chronic hyperglycemia.

An EMG and nerve conduction studies are usually abnormal in diabetic polyneuropathy. Abnormalities of sensory conduction are especially prominent, and sensory and motor nerve conduction studies correlate with the degree of pathologic involvement of the nerves.

No current therapy will effectively arrest or reverse the progression of diabetic neuropathy. Nevertheless, there is a general consensus that efforts to avoid chronic hyperglycemia are worthwhile, as long as such control is not obtained at the expense of hypoglycemia. Symptomatic treatment of painful sensory complaints is difficult. Carbamazepine or diphenylhydantoin as prescribed for trigeminal neuralgia or amitriptyline and fluphenazine as prescribed for postherpetic neuralgia are sometimes helpful. Proper foot care is of utmost importance in the diabetic who has lost pain sensation in the feet.

UREMIC POLYNEUROPATHY. Uremic neuropathy became a significant clinical problem when the introduction of long-term hemodialysis and renal transplantation led to long-term survival of patients with renal failure. Chronic renal failure is the common denominator of this neuropathy. Uremic neuropathy is typically a mixed motor and sensory polyneuropathy with a distal, symmetrical pattern of involvement of the extremities that is most prominent in the legs. Restless legs and leg cramps, which occur frequently, are thought to be caused by the underlying neuropathy rather than by a metabolic consequence of renal failure. Dysesthesias and painful, burning sensations of the feet are also common. Absence of the ankle jerks is seen early. Distal weakness and atrophy may follow. Uremic neuropathy is usually slowly progressive over a span of months. The diagnosis of uremic neuropathy is based on the presence of symptoms and signs of diffuse neuropathy in the setting of chronic renal failure, with significant uremia of at least several months' duration. Conditions that may produce kidney and nerve damage—such as neurotoxic agents, collagen vascular disease, multiple myeloma, or diabetes—must be ruled out. Electrophysiological studies of patients with uremic neuropathy show slowing of conduction velocities that correlates with the severity of the neuropathy. Serial measurements of the motor nerve conduction velocity have been used to gauge the adequacy of dialysis.

Uremic polyneuropathy responds favorably to treatment of the underlying uremia. Most patients experience stabilization or improvement of their neuropathy if treated by adequate long-term peritoneal dialysis. Hemodialysis is not as successful in improving the neuropathy. Successful renal transplantation is generally followed by resolution, or at least by significant improvement, of the polyneuropathy. Thus, in the patient with chronic renal failure, evidence of progression of neuropathy is a signal to intensify efforts at dialysis or to consider transplant surgery.

ALCOHOLIC POLYNEUROPATHY. The relation of alcoholism to peripheral neuropathy has been recognized since the nineteenth century. The incidence of neuropathy in chronic alcoholics is variable, although it was approximately 10% in a series of consecutive hospital admissions at a Boston hospital. Most series have reported a somewhat higher incidence of neuropathy in alcoholic women than in men. Long-standing alcohol abuse and dietary deficiency, resulting in a chronic state of semistarvation, are uniformly present in association with the development of alcoholic neuropathy. The alcoholic diet is low in vitamins and consists mainly of carbohydrates; this provides an ideal setting for the development of thiamine deficiency, since this vitamin is consumed during carbohydrate metabolism. There is a strong clinical and pathologic similarity between the neuropathy of alcoholism and the neuropathy of beriberi, which is due to a specific deficiency of thiamine. For this reason, deficiency of B vitamins in general and of thiamine in particular are suspected to play a role in the pathogenesis of alcoholic neuropathy.

Evidence of mild peripheral neuropathy with loss or depression of ankle jerks and distal sensory impairment may be found in asymptomatic alcoholics. Those who develop symptoms usually complain of distal paresthesias, distressing burning sensation of the feet, and weakness. The rate of progression is typically slow and gradual. Examination may reveal sensory, motor, and reflex impairment that is distal and symmetrical in location. Foot drop may be apparent in advanced cases, and the muscles of the feet and legs may be tender to palpation. Electrophysiological studies show findings consistent with mixed motor and sensory polyneuropathy. Typically, there is a mild to moderate slowing of nerve conduction velocities, with EMG evidence of a variable degree of denervation in the distal extremity muscles.

Efforts to treat alcoholic neuropathy are often frustrated by the patient's tendency to continue abusing alcohol. Nevertheless, it is reasonable to offer supplementation with B-complex vitamins in the hope of preventing further neuropathic damage due to nutritional deficiency. Alcoholics with neuropathy who stop drinking permanently may experience partial improvement of symptoms.

POLYNEUROPATHY DUE TO DRUGS AND TOXINS. The polyneuropathies caused by medications or toxic agents are an important etiologic category, since discontinuation of the use of the responsible neuropathic agent may lead to stabilization or improvement. Vincristine, if given in adequate doses and for sufficient duration, will invariably produce a mixed motor and sensory polyneuropathy with loss or depression of reflexes. Weakness is a prominent feature, and an unusual predilection for the extensor muscles of the fingers and wrist has been reported. Vincristine neuropathy typically improves when treatment is stopped or if the dosage is reduced. Consequently, the beneficial effects of cancer chemotherapy with vincristine must be carefully balanced against neurotoxic side effects. Isoniazid has been found to produce a deficiency of vitamin B^6 in some patients, thereby producing a peripheral neuropathy. Prophylactic supplementation with vitamin B^6 during isoniazid therapy will prevent development of this undesired side effect. Therapy with nitrofurantoin, which is used for the treatment of urinary tract infections, may be associated with a severe and rapidly developing sensory and motor polyneuropathy. Renal failure appears to be a predisposing factor, and the higher blood levels of nitrofurantoin found in this setting may enhance the neurotoxic potential of the drug. For this reason, it is probably inadvisable to use nitrofurantoin for the treatment of urinary tract infections in patients with renal failure. Diphenylhydantoin is used extensively and effectively as a long-term maintenance therapy for epilepsy. Evidence of peripheral neuropathy, usually mild, has been reported in up to half of patients on treatment for more than 15 years. Loss or depression of lower limb reflexes and impairment of vibratory sensation are the most frequent findings. It is suspected that this neuropathy may be caused by a diphenylhydantoin-induced folate deficiency. Supplementation with folate usually corrects the neuropathy, and diphenylhydantoin may be continued. Disulfiram is used in the treatment of alcoholism, a disorder in which polyneuropathy is fairly common. Nevertheless, instances have been reported in which the appearance of a polyneuropathy has been linked to disulfiram. This possibility, therefore, should be considered in an alcoholic patient who develops neuropathy or experiences progression of a preexistent neuropathy while under therapy with disulfiram. Recently, peripheral neuropathy associated with the eosinophilia-myalgia syndrome has been reported in individuals who have chronically used large amounts of l-tryptophan. It is believed that a contaminant was responsible for the development of this syndrome.

Intoxication with a variety of metals may produce polyneuropathy. These include arsenic, lead, mercury, thallium, antimony, and zinc. Arsenic intoxication may be the result of deliberate poisoning or of exposure to certain pesticides. It is typically associated with gastrointestinal complaints and prominent sensory symptoms in the extremities. The presence of light-colored transverse bands (Mee's lines) in the fingernails may be a clue to the diagnosis. Thallium intoxication is usually accompanied by severe hair loss. Polyneuropathy due to lead and mercury is usually due to industrial or environmental exposure. In contrast to the sensory-motor neuropathy of arsenic poisoning, lead neuropathy is a predominantly motor neuropathy. The diagnosis of intoxication with lead, mercury, or arsenic may be confirmed by quantitative laboratory analysis of hair, fingernail clippings, or urine. Removal from exposure to the offending metal is the first step in therapy. Chelation therapy with British anti-Lewisite (BAL) or D-penicillamine (for arsenic, lead, and mercury) and calcium disodium edetate (for lead) are usually reserved for patients with disabling symptoms.

A variety of nonmetallic neurotoxic substances in widespread use in industry and agriculture may all produce peripheral neuropathy. These include n-hexane glue, trichlorethylene, carbon monoxide, carbon disulfide, methyl butyl ketone, hexachlorophene, triorthocresol phosphate, gasoline, and acrylamide.

POLYNEUROPATHY AS A REMOTE COMPLICATION OF MALIGNANCY. The incidence of polyneuropathy in association with carcinoma in general is about 5%, although it is somewhat higher in carcinoma of the lung and stomach. Symptoms and signs may be present months before a malignancy is found. The neuropathy is often painful. It is typically sensorimotor but it may be predominantly sensory *or* motor and often follows a chronic progressive course, although acute and relapsing-remitting courses may occur. The cause of the neuropathy is unknown; it is clearly not related to the presence of direct metastasis into peripheral nerves. Cases have been reported in which the neuropathy regressed following removal of the primary carcinoma, which suggests the possibility of an unidentified toxic factor in the circulation. Peripheral neuropathy also occurs in association with lymphoma, multiple myeloma, and Waldenstrom's macroglobulinemia.

Hereditary Neuropathies

A large number of hereditary neuropathies have been identified. It is beyond the scope of this book to address these interesting disorders in any detail, and the reader is referred to specialized texts. One of the more common hereditary neuropathies will be dealt with briefly below.

CHARCOT-MARIE-TOOTH DISEASE. The peroneal-type progressive muscular atrophy, or Charcot-Marie-Tooth disease, is the most common hereditary neuropathy. The disease is autosomal dominant and is characterized by much variability in the degree of expression among individual family members. Some individuals do not know that they have the disease until abnormalities are detected on neurologic examination or by electrophysiological testing. The onset of symptoms is generally in the second to fourth decades, at which time gait difficulty due to weakness of the distal extremity muscles and foot deformity are often first noticed. In contrast to many of the acquired chronic polyneuropathies, sensory symptoms are not a prominent part of the typical clinical picture. High arched feet and hammertoe deformities are common. A distal and symmetrical distribution of weakness and atrophy, greater in the legs, is usually present, and bilateral foot drop is present in more advanced cases. Reflexes are depressed or absent, especially in the legs, and sensory abnormalities are mild or absent on routine examination. Peripheral nerves may be palpably enlarged. Nerve conduction studies show diffuse slowing of conduction velocities, and chronic denervation is observed on needle examination of affected muscles. The rate of progression is indolent in most patients, and the outlook is favorable for a full life span with mild to moderate ultimate disability.

Although there is no specific treatment that will alter the natural course of events, the physician has much to offer in terms of supportive therapy and genetic counseling. Foot braces and special shoes may be beneficial for certain patients with foot drop, foot deformity, and gait difficulty. Consultation with specialists in orthopedics and rehabilitation medicine is often helpful in this regard. Other aids to ambulation may be required later in the course of the disease. The physician may be asked to give advice about the prognosis and risk of transmission of the disease to future offspring. In this case it is important to review and examine all available relatives in order to establish the pattern of transmission, rate of progression, and the degree of expression present in a particular family.

REFERENCES

Pollard JD: Relapsing neuropathy due to tetanus toxoid. J Neurol Sci 1978; 37: 113–125.

Heiman-Patterson TD, Bird SJ, Parry GJ, Varga J, Shy ME, Culligan NW, Edelsohn L, Tatarian GT, Heyes MP, Garcia CA, Tahmoush AJ: Peripheral neuropathy associated with eosinophilia-myalgia syndrome. Ann Neurol 1990; 28:522–528.

Ad hoc subcommittee of the American Academy of Neurology AIDS task force: Research criteria for diagnosis of chronic inflammatory demyelinating polyneuropathy (CIDP). Neurology 1991; 41:617–618.

Van Doorn PA, Brand A, Strengers PFW, Meulstee J, Vermeulen M: High-dose intravenous immunoglobulin treatment in chronic inflammatory demyelinating polyneuropathy: A double-blind, placebo-controlled, crossover study. Neurology 1990; 40:209–212.

Working group of the American Academy of Neurology AIDS task force: Nomenclature and research case definitions for neurologic manifestations of human immunodeficiency virus-type 1 (HIV-1) infection. Neurology 1991; 41: 778–785.

Lange DJ, Trojaborg W, Latov N, Hays AP, Younger DS, Uncini A, Blake DM, Hirano M, Burns SM, Lovelace RE, Rowland LP: Multifocal motor neuropathy with conduction block: Is it a distinct clinical entity? Neurology 1992; 42:497–505.

Ropper A: The Guillain-Barré Syndrome. N Engl J Med 1992; 326:1130–1136.

Dyck PJ, Dyck PJB, Chalk CH: The 10 P's: A mnemonic helpful in characterization and differential diagnosis of peripheral neuropathy. Neurology 1992; 42: 14–18.

Schaumburg H, Berger A, Thomas P: Disorders of Peripheral Nerves. Philadelphia, FA Davis, 1992.

Logigian EL, Steere AC: Clinical and electrophysiologic findings in chronic neuropathy of Lyme disease. Neurology 1992; 42:303–311.

Nobile-Orazio E, Meucci N, Barbieri S, Carpo M, Scarlato G: High-dose intravenous immunoglobulin therapy in multifocal motor neuropathy. Neurology 1993; 43:537–544.

Thornton CA, Ballow M: Safety of intravenous immunoglobulin. Arch Neurol 1993; 50(2):135–136.

Suarez GA, Kelly JJJ: Polyneuropathy associated with monoclonal gammopathy of undetermined significance: Further evidence that IgM-MGUS neuropathies are different than IgG-MGUS. Neurology 1993; 43:1304–1308.

Dyck PJ, Thomas PK, Griffin JW, Low PA, Poduslo JF (ed): Peripheral Neuropathy, 3rd ed, vols I and II. Philadelphia, WB Saunders, 1993.

Simmons Z, Albers JW, Bromberg MB, Feldman EL: Presentation and initial clinical course in patients with chronic inflammatory demyelinating polyradiculoneuropathy: Comparison of patients without and with monoclonal gammopathy. Neurology 1993; 43:2202–2209.

Wood MJ, Johnson RW, McKendrick MW, Taylor J, Mandal BK, Crooks J: A randomized trial of acyclovir for 7 days or 21 days with and without prednisone for treatment of acute herpes zoster. N Engl J Med 1994; 330(13):896–900.

Chad DA: The evaluation and diagnosis of peripheral neuropathy. Neurology Chronicle 1994; 4(1):1–8.

12
Radiculopathies

ANATOMY, PATHOPHYSIOLOGY, ETIOLOGY, AND CLINICAL PRESENTATION

The vertebral column is made up of 33 vertebrae, arranged as follows: 7 cervical, 12 thoracic, 5 lumbar, 5 sacral, and 4 coccygeal. Each vertebra is composed of a body that permits weight bearing and a vertebral arch that surrounds the spinal cord. Immediately behind the attachment of the arch to the vertebral body, the arch is notched above and below. Together, the two vertebral notches constitute the intervertebral foramen. It is through this foramen that the ventral and dorsal roots of the corresponding spinal cord segment exit as the spinal nerve. There are 8 cervical, 12 thoracic, 5 lumbar, 5 sacral, and 1 coccygeal root.

A radiculopathy is the clinical syndrome produced by damage to a dorsal or ventral nerve root or both. Since the roots do not join until quite close to the neural foramen, lesions may affect primarily sensory fibers, primarily motor fibers, or both. Thus, it is possible to have in a radiculopathy almost exclusively sensory symptoms (radicular pain or paresthesias); motor symptoms (painless weakness); or, more commonly, a combination of both. The ventral and dorsal roots and spinal nerve are subject to damage by a variety of etiologies, including vascular, inflammatory, congenital, neoplastic, and traumatic disorders. The anterior horn cell or dorsal root ganglion may be damaged by infectious agents, such as poliomyelitis virus in anterior horn cells and herpes zoster virus in sensory ganglia, which can lead to an inflammatory radiculitis. Rheumatoid disease of the spine, osteoarthritis, primary neoplasms of the bone, metastasis to the vertebral column from primary tumors—including breast, lung, and prostate—all may cause damage to the spinal roots or nerves and produce radicular symptoms and signs. However, by far the most common cause of a radiculopathy is compression of a root by a protruded intervertebral disc. In this condition, a portion of one or more intervertebral discs is displaced posteriorly into the spinal canal and exerts pressure on one or more roots and, occasionally, the spinal cord. The intervertebral disc that separates each vertebral body is contained by a hyalin cartilage plate over the surface of each vertebral body and within a fibrous ligament (the annulus fibrosis). Physical stress, strain, repeated minor trauma, or one major trauma may cause the disc to bulge into the canal through the annulus fibrosis. Disc protrusions usually occur in a posterolateral direction and affect nerve roots without involving the spinal cord. However, should the disc protrusion be midline or large (above the L2–L3 level), the spinal cord may be damaged.

Disc protrusions can occur at any level but are most commonly seen at the cervical and lumbosacral levels. This distribution may be due to the fact that these segments of the vertebral column are subject to the most movement in daily activities. In the cervical region, disc protrusions at the fifth and sixth cervical interspace, with damage to the C6 root, and at the sixth and seventh cervical interspace, with damage to the C7 root, are the most common. In the lumbosacral region, disc protrusions at the fourth and fifth lumbar interspace, with damage to the L5 root, or disc protrusions at the fifth lumbar and first sacral interspace, with damage to the S1 root, are most common. In both areas, these protrusions represent more than 90% of all disc syndromes. Disc protrusions in the thoracic area are quite uncommon. They are usually located in the lower portion of the thoracic spine. Compression of the spinal cord is common with intervertebral thoracic disc protrusions because of the narrowness of the spinal canal in this region.

Clinical Presentation

An intervertebral disc protrusion should be suspected if a patient complains of sudden onset of neck or back pain with radicular symptoms and/or signs. A patient may complain of local neck or back pain that radiates to the shoulder or buttock, or to a limb. Such pain may be accompanied by paresthesias in a dermatomal distribution. Both the pain and paresthesias are commonly aggravated by coughing, sneezing, or spine movements. It is often possible to identify the affected spinal root from the patient's description of the distribution of the pain and paresthesias combined with documentation of muscle weakness, sensory loss, and changes in muscle stretch reflexes in a radicular pattern. Common radicular syndromes due to cervical and lumbar disc disease are detailed in Tables 12–1 and 12–2.

TABLE 12-1. Distribution of Symptoms and Signs of Cervical Root Damage

Root	Pain	Paresthesias	Weakness	Depressed reflexes
C5	Neck, shoulder, lateral arm (distal to elbow)	Shoulder	Deltoid, infraspinatus	Biceps, brachioradialis
C6	Neck, shoulder, scapula, thumb, radial forearm	Thumb	Biceps, brachioradialis, wrist extensors	Biceps, brachioradialis
C7	Neck, shoulder, dorsal or volar forearm	Middle finger	Triceps	Triceps
C8	Neck, shoulder, ulnar forearm	Little finger	Intrinsic hand muscles	Triceps or none

Clinical Examination

In the evaluation of patients with radiculopathies it is important to observe the patient's behavior. A patient with cervical radiculopathy tends to hold the head in a slightly flexed position and avoids any head movement because it aggravates the pain. Similarly, the patient with a lumbosacral radiculopathy stands in a slightly stooped position and walks stiffly to avoid excessive motion in the lumbar area. Changes in position are accomplished with great difficulty, and getting up may be a major chore. Both in cervical and lumbar radiculopathies, one of the earliest signs is loss of the normal lordosis. Movements in the affected areas are

TABLE 12-2. Distribution of Symptoms and Signs of Lumbosacral Root Damage

Root	Pain	Paresthesias	Weakness	Depressed reflexes
L4	Posterolateral hip, anterior thigh	Anterior thigh, anterolateral leg	Quadriceps	Quadriceps
L5	Posterolateral thigh, leg, dorsum of foot	Lateral calf, dorsum of foot	Tibialis anterior, tibialis posterior, gastrocnemius	Hamstrings (internal)
S1	Posterior thigh, leg, heel	Posterior calf, lateral and plantar foot	Foot muscles, hamstrings, gastrocnemius	Hamstrings (external) Gastrocnemius-soleus

usually severely restricted, and the paraspinal muscles are contracted. Tenderness to palpation and/or percussion is frequently present. Each patient with a radiculopathy requires a thorough neurologic examination. In cervical disease the spinal cord may be compressed. Specific inquiry into problems with gait, urination, and defecation are important, as is an examination of the lower extremities. An evaluation of a patient with low back problems always requires specific examination of the perineal area, elicitation of the anal reflex, and a rectal examination. Patients with L5–S1 midline disc protrusion may compress only the S2–S3 roots, which may lead to sensory loss in the perineal areas and absent anal reflex, decreased anal sphincter tone, and bladder dysfunction without any other neurologic abnormalities.

In addition to the standard neurologic examination with particular emphasis on the areas affected, some specific maneuvers help to delineate the patient's problem and to follow a patient's clinical course.

CERVICAL FORAMINAL COMPRESSION TEST. Narrowing of the cervical foramina is achieved by pressure on the vertex of the head while the neck is hyperextended, laterally flexed, and rotated. The test is considered positive if it produces or aggravates radicular pain and/or paresthesias.

MANUAL CERVICAL TRACTION TEST. Widening of the cervical neural foramina is achieved by manual traction. With the patient sitting and the head slightly flexed, the examiner holds the patient's head laterally with both hands and pulls up. The test is considered positive if the patient's radicular pain and/or paresthesias are transiently relieved.

CHIN-CHEST MANEUVER. This maneuver causes the spinal cord to ascend in the spinal canal and places the spinal nerve roots under tension. If a nerve root is trapped by a protruded disc, radicular pain may be induced or aggravated.

STRAIGHT-LEG RAISING TEST. This maneuver places the fifth lumbar and first sacral roots and the sciatic nerve under tension. The test is best performed when the patient is supine and relaxed, with the head supported by a pillow. The extended leg is passively raised by the examiner. To eliminate hamstring tightness, the leg is slightly rotated internally and adducted as it is raised. The test is considered positive if it produces or aggravates pain in the back or leg at an angle of less than 70 degrees. Raising of the contralateral leg may also produce or aggravate pain on the affected side. To eliminate the possibility that the pain produced is related to pathology of the hip or knee joint, the hip and knee should be flexed and the hip rotated externally, a maneuver that does not stretch the sciatic nerve but does move both hip and knee joints. Because most patients today are quite familiar with the straight-leg raising test, the results are often unreliable. A good alternative is to accomplish the same, that is stretching of roots, when the patient does not expect it. With the patient sitting, the leg is extended and strength of the quadriceps muscle is tested. In this position the extended leg is at a right-angle to the spine, and considerable stretch is placed on a trapped lumbosacral root. If a patient does not report any pain in this position, then any pain reported when doing the straight-leg raising test in the classic manner is of dubious value.

FEMORAL NERVE STRETCH TEST. This maneuver places the second, third, and fourth lumbar roots and the femoral nerve under tension. The test is best performed with the patient resting in the prone position. The leg is flexed at the knee and slowly hyperextended at the hip. The test is positive if the maneuver produces or aggravates the patient's radicular pain.

Other Examinations

Plain radiographs of the spine are of value in excluding bony destructive lesions, spondylosis, and spondylolisthesis. In most disc protrusions, radiographs are either normal or show a narrowed disc space corresponding to the presumed level of disc protrusion. Loss of lordosis is often present and best seen on lateral films. An MR scan of the spine can provide direct documentation of a disc protrusion without the need for more invasive procedures. A major advantage of MRI is that it provides information not only about discs but also about spinal cord, roots, subarachnoid space, and extradural space. Where the procedure is available, MRI has also eliminated the need for myelography. An EMG and nerve conduction studies are usually not required in the initial phases of management unless one is quite uncertain regarding the clinical diagnosis of radiculopathy.

Treatment

Patients with suspected cervical, thoracic, or lumbosacral disc protrusions and root compression should be treated with bed rest, moist cold followed by moist heat, and analgesics. Initially, the patient should be placed on bed rest to reduce movement of the painful area. If the pain is in the neck, sandbags should be positioned on both sides of the head to limit neck and head motion. If the pain is in the thoracic or lumbosacral region, the patient should assume a comfortable reclining position. Although in many cases the patient chooses the modified Trendelenburg position with the back slightly elevated and the knees slightly flexed, in some cases the patient may find that lying in the lateral decubitus position is more comfortable. Generally, it is best to permit the patient to use the bathroom, since this is less stressful than attempting to use a bedpan. Patients with lumbosacral disc protrusions should use crutches or a walker for support when up. During the first day after the onset of the pain, moist cold should be applied directly to the painful area. A moist towel containing crushed ice should be applied for a period of 10 to 20 minutes 4 to 5 times a day while the patient is awake. After the first day, if muscle spasms, percussion tenderness, and limitation of spine movements persist, then moist heat (hot towels) should be applied in a similar fashion. If the patient insists on remaining ambulatory because the symptoms are mild, relative immobilization of the neck may be achieved by using a soft cervical collar or dry towel folded lengthwise and wrapped around the neck. The widest or highest part of the collar should be on the back of the neck to produce slight flexion of the head. Corsets are rarely useful. Adequate analgesia is essential. Aspirin or acetaminophen should be given every 3 to 4 hours and supplemented with codeine (30–60 mg) as needed while the patient is awake. Overuse of analgesics should be avoided if the patient insists on remaining ambulatory. If patients are anxious, mild sedation with Valium during the day and a short-acting sleeping pill at night are indicated. The bedridden patient may also benefit from a stool softener. After the initial discomfort has largely subsided, one may start a program of graded exercises to assist in strengthening extensor and flexor muscles of the spine, as well as to increase the range of motion. This recommendation is analogous to the range-of-motion exercises encouraged in patients with inflammatory disorders of other joints to prevent fibrosis and subsequent painful limitation of motion. Whether or not strengthening exercises are of any help is doubtful, except in a patient with overtly weak abdominal muscles.

Cervical traction for cervical disc protrusion is often beneficial. It should be applied for 5 to 10 minutes 3 to 4 times a day, starting with 2 to 3 lbs. Slight flexion of the head during traction is essential, because other head positions may aggravate the patient's condition. Cervical traction can readily be done at home after proper instruction by a physiotherapist. Traction has no place in the management of thoracic or lumbosacral disc protrusion.

When symptoms have persisted for 2 to 3 weeks, an EMG is often valuable in confirming the presence of the site of motor root damage, especially if one includes needle examination of the paraspinal muscles. The latter both increases the diagnostic yield of the test and helps exclude a plexus lesion.

Resolution of a soft disc protrusion with relief of root irritation is manifested by a reduction in the severity and frequency of pain and paresthesias, as well as by improvement of strength and reduced reflexes. If the patient shows signs of improvement over a week, it is reasonable to continue with the program. The majority of patients respond quite well to conservative therapy. Surgical intervention should be considered urgently in the following situations: (1) when signs or symptoms suggestive of cord (spastic paresis, bladder incontinence, transverse sensory level) or cauda equina compression (flaccid paralysis, bladder incontinence) develop; (2) when there is progression of a motor deficit within a few days; and (3) when, over a period of weeks, there is persistence or worsening of radicular pain.

An MR scan prior to a surgical procedure is an important step for several reasons. First, although it is frequently possible to identify the site of cervical disc protrusion from the neurologic signs and symptoms, it is not possible to do so reliably in the lumbosacral area. Cervical nerve roots exit the spinal canal almost at their level of origin in the spinal cord. In the lumbosacral area, because the spinal cord ends at the upper border of the L2 vertebra, some roots exit at a considerable distance from their origin. Thus, an L5–S1 disc protrusion may (and frequently does) cause neurologic signs and symptoms in the distribution of the first sacral root, although this nerve root exists below the disc by the full height of a vertebral body. The second reason for performing an MR scan is that radicular signs and symptoms may be caused by intraspinal lesions other than disc protrusion, including primary neoplasms of nerve or leptomeningeal origin, as well as arteriovenous malformations. It is important to identify both the cause of the root damage and its location as accurately as possible prior to surgical exploration so that the appropriate surgical approach may be planned. LP is not recommended prior to surgery in a suspected disc protrusion, because if incomplete or complete block of CSF flow is present, worsening of the neurologic condition may follow removal of CSF. Myelography or CT myelography are still procedures of choice prior to surgery in areas where MR scanning is not available. Myelography should be done only if a surgeon familiar with the patient is available to intervene should the patient's condition worsen because of the myelogram.

If radiographic or magnetic studies confirm the presence of root and/or spinal cord compression due to a soft disc protrusion, surgical therapy is based on laminectomy and foraminotomy, with removal of the protruded soft disc fragment as well as the remaining disc material to prevent recurrence. Morbidity has been drastically reduced by modern surgical techniques. Results of surgery are quite favorable if surgical intervention is based on good indications as outlined above.

REFERENCES

Haymaker W, Woodhall B: Peripheral Nerve Injuries. Philadelphia: WB Saunders, 1953, pp 3-37.

Mayo Clinic and Mayo Foundation: Clinical Examination in Neurology. Philadelphia, WB Saunders, 1976; pp 7-11.

Mulder D, Dale A: Spinal cord tumors and discs. *In* Baker AB, Baker LH (eds), Clinical Neurology, chapter 33. New York, Harper, 1980.

Keim HA, Kirkaldy-Willis WH: Low back pain. Clinical symposia, Ciba, Summit, 1980.

Deyo RA: Conservative therapy for low back pain: Distinguishing the useful from the useless therapy. JAMA 1983;250:1057-1062.

Borenstein DG, Wiesel SW: Low Back Pain: Medical Diagnosis and Comprehensive Management. Philadelphia, WB Saunders, 1989.

13
Seizure Disorders

A seizure is a brief paroxysmal clinical event characterized by loss of consciousness, an altered state of consciousness, cessation of motor activity, abnormal motor activity, abnormal sensory perceptions, and loss of bladder and bowel control. Each manifestation may occur alone or in combination with any or all of the others. During a seizure the EEG almost always shows epileptiform activity. When seizures are recurrent, the condition is referred to as a seizure disorder or epilepsy. The occurrence of seizures is not rare. Approximately 1% of children under the age of 5 years will have at least one seizure. Most of these are associated with high fever and are not recurrent. The incidence of recurrent seizures is approximately 0.5% of the population. Seventy-five percent of seizure disorders begin before the age of 20 years; 30% by the age of 4. Less than 2% of seizure disorders have an onset after 50 years of age. There is an overall male predominance.

CAUSES OF SEIZURES

A seizure disorder is a manifestation of underlying brain dysfunction, not a disease entity. Thus, any person with a seizure requires a careful diagnostic evaluation to determine the etiology. A specific cause can be found in approximately 50% of both adult-onset and childhood-onset seizures. When no specific cause can be found, the patient is usually said to have an idiopathic seizure disorder. This implies that the structural or metabolic abnormality responsible for the seizure disorder cannot be detected with currently available clinical or laboratory tests.

PERINATAL INSULTS. Toxic ischemic damage to the brain can occur during labor or delivery for a variety of reasons, including tight nuchal umbilical cord, meconium aspiration, and respiratory depression. Cerebral contusion or infarction can develop during difficult deliveries. Intraventricular hemorrhage is a major problem in premature infants. All of these can result in cerebral damage that may predispose to seizures either immediately or later in infancy or childhood.

HEREDOFAMILIAL CONDITIONS. A large variety of familial disorders are associated with epilepsy. The neurocutaneous syndromes, especially tuberous sclerosis and Sturge-Weber syndrome, are associated with seizures in a high percentage of cases. Children with inherited metabolic disorder such as Tay-Sachs disease may also develop seizures. Petit mal epilepsy is familial, with an autosomal dominant pattern of inheritance. At least two forms of familial myoclonic epilepsy have been described. Benign febrile convulsions are familial in a majority of cases. In the last few years probable chromosomal loci for the genes of benign familial neonatal convulsions and juvenile myoclonic epilepsy have been determined. Furthermore, genes have been identified for several neurodegenerative disorders associated with prominent seizures and myoclonus (juvenile ceroid lipofuscinosis, juvenile Gaucher's disease, cherry-red spot myoclonus, and Unverricht-Lundborg progressive myoclonic epilepsy). The inherited epileptic syndromes have been thought to present with generalized seizures, but recently an autosomal dominant inheritance has been demonstrated in partial seizures of frontal lobe origin.

TRAUMA. At any age, significant head trauma with loss of consciousness may result in either immediate or delayed seizures. Most posttraumatic seizures occur within 1 year after the injury. Head injury may cause contusions or infarctions. Neck trauma can result in carotid artery dissection with occlusion and cerebral infarction. Nonaccidental trauma, for example child abuse, can result in significant brain injury with predisposition to recurrent seizures.

ANOXIA. Anoxic brain damage at any age can lead to residual seizure disorders. In addition to generalized tonic-clonic seizures, a particular susceptibility to action myoclonus occurs after anoxia.

INFECTIONS. Seizures may occur as a sequel to viral encephalitis, bacterial and fungal meningitis, brain abscess, and parasitic infestations of the brain (e.g., cysticercosis). Seizures may be the presenting symptom in any type of CNS infection or may occur as a result of brain damage during the course of the acute infectious process. Several infectious agents that invade the fetus in utero can produce seizure disorders during infancy (cytomegalovirus, toxoplasma, rubella, syphilis, and herpes virus).

METABOLIC DISORDERS. Numerous metabolic derangements produce seizures. Electrolyte imbalances are common causes of seizures, especially in infants and children. Hypoglycemia can produce seizures at any age. Infants of diabetic mothers and infants who were small for their age throughout gestation are particularly prone to hypoglycemia and hypocalcemia in the neonatal period. Metabolic encephalopathies due to end-organ failure (e.g., hepatic and uremic encephalopathies) are often accompanied by seizure activity. Inborn errors of metabolism (e.g., phenylketonuria, maple syrup urine disease, galactosemia), as well as acquired metabolic encephalopathies of childhood (e.g., Reye's syndrome), are marked by epileptic activity.

TOXINS. Many toxic ingestions, both acute and chronic, are accompanied by seizure activity. Toxic substances that may be ingested include lead, atropine, diphenhydramine, scopolamine, tricyclic antidepressants, camphor, chloroquine, and ethanol. Seizures are also precipitated by sudden withdrawal of drugs such as ethanol or barbiturates.

DEGENERATIVE DISEASES OF THE CNS. Tay-Sachs disease, subacute necrotizing encephalomyelopathy (Leigh's syndrome), and occasionally the leukodystrophies may give rise to seizures in children. In adults, Alzheimer's disease, Pick's disease, and MS may occasionally produce seizures.

TUMORS. Seizures are the initial manifestation in approximately 15% of patients with primary and metastatic brain tumors. Slowly growing lesions and those involving the cerebral hemispheres are most likely to produce seizures. In general, tumors are more likely to cause focal seizures, focal changes on the EEG, and focal abnormalities on the neurologic examination. Any or all of these problems should lead to the suspicion of a mass lesion. However, generalized seizures may also result from mass lesions.

VASCULAR DISORDERS. Cerebral infarcts, arteriovenous malforma-tions, bleeding aneurysms, and cerebral arteritis may cause focal and sometimes generalized or multifocal seizures. In the older age group, most seizures are due to strokes from atherosclerotic cerebrovascular disease.

CLASSIFICATIONS OF SEIZURES

Terms such as grand mal and petit mal are no longer considered sufficient to describe the numerous varieties of seizures known. Table 13–1 shows a general classification of seizure types.

TABLE 13–1. Classification of Seizures

Generalized (bilaterally symmetrical and without focal onset)
  Tonic
  Clonic
  Tonic-clonic
  Absence
  Infantile spasms
  Myoclonus
  Akinetic
  Atonic
Partial seizures (seizures beginning focally)
  Partial with secondary generalization
  Partial elementary (without impairment of consciousness)
    With motor symptoms
    With somatosensory symptoms
    With autonomic symptoms
    Compound forms
  Partial complex (with alteration of consciousness)
    With affective disturbances
    With cognitive disturbances
    With complex motor behavior
    With subjective visceral or sensory symptoms
Unilateral seizures
Miscellaneous
  Reflex seizures (stimulus-induced; e.g., pattern or photic-induced, musicogenic)

Generalized Seizures

Primary generalized seizures are bilateral, symmetrical, and without focal onset. These usually result from conditions that affect the brain bilaterally, such as genetic, metabolic, and anoxic etiologies.

TONIC-CLONIC SEIZURES. This type of seizure occurs without warning and consists of sudden loss of consciousness, and tonic (stiffening) contractions of all muscles followed by clonic jerking. During the tonic phase all of the muscles contract, including muscles of respiration, and apnea and cyanosis are commonly observed. The patient falls at the onset of the tonic phase and may suffer injuries due to the fall. During the clonic phase the patient may bite his tongue. Jerking may be so intense that bones can be broken if the extremities are tightly restrained. Urinary and fecal incontinence are common. Following the clonic phase the patient lapses into an unresponsive state and muscles become flaccid. After the seizure activity subsides, there is usually a postictal confusional period followed by sleep for several hours. There is total amnesia concerning the ictal events. Other seizure manifestations include only tonic or only clonic phases. Tonic seizures are particularly common in children. During a seizure, the EEG typically shows continuous generalized spike-and-wave discharges. The interictal EEG pattern in generalized seizure disorders varies form normal to generalized epileptiform discharges, usually on a background of normal rhythms. Several anticonvulsant medications are effective in preventing this type of seizure. They include phenobarbital, phenytoin, valproic acid, carbamazepine and primidone.

INFANTILE SPASMS. Infantile spasms typically occur in infants between 4 and 18 months of age. They are usually the result of severe brain injury and are found in infants with anoxic brain damage, tuberous sclerosis, untreated phenylketonuria, and Tay-Sachs disease. The prognosis is poor for children who develop infantile spasms; approximately 80% will be mentally retarded. There is recent evidence suggesting that the prognosis is improved if the infantile spasms are successfully treated within the first month of onset. The clinical pattern of infantile spasms consists of multiple daily episodes of sudden brief flexion movements of the neck, trunk, and limbs. Crying may accompany each spasm, and the eyes may roll back, have a blank stare, or appear frightened. As many as 20 to 40 spasms may come in rapid succession, and multiple flurries occur each day. Often the flurries will occur on awakening or when the infant is drowsy. By 2 to 3 years of age, the seizure pattern changes from infantile spasms to generalized or partial complex seizures, and often to a mixed seizure disorder. The EEG pattern typically seen with infantile spasms is hypsarrhythmia. This is an extremely disorganized pattern of multifocal spikes, multispikes, and slow wave activity, with virtually no normal background activity. Infantile spasms are difficult to treat. They respond best to adrenocorticotropic hormone (ACTH) gel (40 units per day by intramuscular injection for 6 weeks). Less consistently, valproic acid or clonazepam may control the seizures.

TYPICAL ABSENCE (PETIT MAL EPILEPSY). Typical absence occurs almost exclusively in childhood between the ages of 3 to 12 years and is familial, with a probable autosomal dominant pattern of inheritance. The seizures consist of brief (less than 15 seconds) episodes of altered states of consciousness without changes in muscle tone, during which the child has a vacant stare and, at times, eyelid blinking at a rate of 3 per second. Automatisms such as lip smacking and picking movements of the fingers are not part of typical absence seizures but are found in atypical absence. After the seizure the child goes on with normal activities, having no recollection of the seizure. There is no postictal drowsiness and no incontinence. Multiple petit mal attacks may occur daily. Because the seizures are subtle, there is often a delay in diagnosis. The child may exhibit poor school performance because of frequent lapses of awareness. The EEG is characteristic of this type of seizure. It contains frequent generalized spike-and-slow-wave discharges at a rate of

3 per second. Both the seizures and the EEG abnormalities can often be elicited by having the child hyperventilate for 3 minutes. By adolescence the seizure pattern changes to one of generalized convulsive or partial complex seizures. This change is more likely if the absence attacks remain untreated. The prognosis for seizure control is very good if begun early. Ethosuximide is the anticonvulsant of choice for petit mal seizures. Valproic acid or clonazepam may be substituted if an allergic reaction to ethosuximide develops.

ATYPICAL ABSENCE. This seizure type can occur at any age and is often mistaken for petit mal epilepsy. There are some important differences, however. Atypical absence is usually the result of a temporal lobe focus and responds to different medications from those effective in petit mal epilepsy. The seizures are characterized by brief altered states of consciousness, with staring and eyelid blinking. They tend to last longer (15 to 30 seconds) and to be associated with automatisms such as lip smacking and picking at clothes. The EEG ranges form normal to atypical spike-and-wave discharges (epileptiform discharges may be faster or slower than in typical petit mal). Ethosuximide is usually ineffective. Carbamazepine, diphenylhydantoin, primidone, and valproic acid are all effective for this type of seizure.

AKINETIC SEIZURES. An akinetic seizure is manifested by a sudden fall to the ground. The episode is often so violent that observers describe the patient as being thrown to the ground. The patient then arises and goes about normal activity with no postictal drowsiness. Each seizure is extremely brief, but significant injuries can occur during the fall. Akinetic seizures most often occur between the ages of 2 and 8 years, and rarely in adolescence. The EEG is most often markedly abnormal, with generalized or multifocal epileptiform discharges. This type of seizure is difficult to treat. Some patients respond to valproic acid or clonazepam. Patients with akinetic seizures have been treated most successfully with the medium chain triglyceride (MCT) variant of the ketogenic diet.

Partial Seizures

PARTIAL SEIZURES WITH SECONDARY GENERALIZATION. Seizures may begin focally and then generalize. This type of seizure may begin with an aura (a brief stereotyped episode), which may be olfactory, gustatory, or a vague feeling of abdominal discomfort. The aura is actually the beginning of the seizure, commonly reflecting the focal nature of the epileptic discharge at its onset. Patients may be aware of what is happening during the aura but later not remember anything because of retrograde amnesia. Any partial seizure may secondarily generalize, but some are more likely to do so than others. Since the beginning of the seizure is not dramatic and the patient frequently does not remember the initial symptomatology, it is important to obtain information about this initial period from those who have witnessed the seizure.

PARTIAL ELEMENTARY SEIZURES (NOT ASSOCIATED WITH ALTERATIONS IN CONSCIOUSNESS)

Partial Elementary Seizures with Motor Symptoms. This type of seizure consists of sudden onset of tonic and/or clonic movements of one or more muscles on one side of the body (e.g., unilateral face, hand, and arm twitching). The clonic movements may begin in one muscle group (usually distal) and progress more proximally, at times eventually involving the entire side of the body. This spread of seizure activity is known as Jacksonian march. Adversive seizures are a form of partial seizure in which the head and eyes involuntarily deviate to one side. Although fully conscious, the patient cannot control these body movements (this is true for all partial elementary seizures). Another form of partial elementary seizure consists of speech arrest. Usually these types of seizure are brief, lasting seconds to at most a few minutes. There may be a postictal Todd's paralysis on the affected side lasting as long as 24 hours. Seizure activity may persist unabated or with only brief periods of abatement over many hours (epilepsia partialis continua). The EEG may show focal spike discharges arising from the affected hemisphere.

Partial Elementary Seizures with Somatosensory Symptoms. Sudden onset of sensory disturbances over one part of the body may occur as a seizure manifestation. Sensory changes include feelings of numbness, tingling, and temperature changes. Seizures may be confined to a small area (e.g., one hand), may spread proximally, or may involve the entire half of the body. As with partial elementary seizures with motor manifestations, partial elementary seizures with somatosensory symptoms may be prolonged and result in epilepsia partialis continua.

PARTIAL COMPLEX SEIZURES (ASSOCIATED WITH ALTERED STATES OF CONSCIOUSNESS). This group of disturbances has been combined in the past under the heading psychomotor seizures. Many of them originate in the temporal lobe. They are usually classified according to the initial symptom of the seizure, which indicates the focal nature at the onset. Partial complex seizures may at times become generalized, with loss of consciousness and tonic-clonic activity. There are almost as many types of partial complex seizure as there are patients with epilepsy. Only a few general types will be described.

Partial Complex Seizures with Disturbance of Thinking. These patients report hallucinatory experiences, déjà vu, a dreamlike state, compulsive thoughts, and feelings of unreality (e.g., being "outside one's body"). Sensory illusions (e.g., objects changing shape, appearing smaller or larger than they really are, sounds becoming louder or quieter) are also common symptoms of this seizure type.

Partial Complex Seizures with Speech Disturbance. Aphasia and speech automatisms (forced repetitions of syllables or phrases) are encountered with partial complex seizures of this type.

Partial Complex Seizures with Complex Motor Behavior. Numerous stereotyped motor behaviors are associated with partial complex seizures. These include, among many others, picking at clothes, wandering around the room, uncontrollable running, rearranging furniture, lip smacking, and eye blinking. For an individual patient, the same type of automatism usually heralds the onset of each seizure.

Partial Complex Seizures with Affective Symptomatology. Intense fear is the most common affective disturbance reported. Others include sadness and less commonly, pleasurable feelings.

Partial Complex Seizures with Sensory Symptomatology. Some patients complain of intense olfactory hallucinations that in most cases are unpleasant (e.g., a smell of rotten eggs or burnt toast). Other patients describe a sudden onset of an intensely bitter taste in the mouth. Unusual abdominal sensations are a relatively common manifestation of psychomotor seizures. They may include epigastric pain, a queasy epigastric feeling described as "butterflies," and other similar visceral sensations. When the visceral complaint is severe, it may lead to the erroneous conclusion that the patient has a gastrointestinal disorder. Prominent visceral symptomatology has led to the diagnosis of abdominal epilepsy.

The EEG in all types of partial seizures may demonstrate focal or generalized epileptiform discharges. However, it is often normal interictally, especially with seizure disorders that arise in the temporal lobe.

Anticonvulsant medications that are successful in treating partial seizures, with and without secondary generalization, include carbamazepine, phenytoin, valproic acid, primidone, and gabapentin.

Benign Febrile Convulsions

This entity occurs with a strong familial predisposition in children between the ages of 6 months and 4 years. If all characteristics are present (see Table 13–2) and there is only a single febrile seizure, the prognosis is excellent that the child will not develop recurrent seizures. Repeated febrile seizures, however, may be associated with later development of partial complex seizures. Thus, after two or more febrile seizures, the child should be treated with anticonvulsant medication for 2 years or until he or she reaches 4 years of age. Phenobarbital is the drug of choice. Febrile seizures should not be confused with seizures provoked by fever.

TABLE 13-2. Characteristics of Benign Febrile Convulsions

Age	6 months to 4 years
Temperature	>38.9 °C
Duration of convulsion	<15 minutes
Type of convulsion	Generalized without focal features
Interictal EEG	Normal
Family history	Positive in 50% of patients

The latter refers to a condition suffered by a person of any age in which seizures are triggered by fever. Many other types of stress may trigger seizures in susceptible individuals (Table 13-3). Seizures with focal onset, prolonged ictus (greater than 15 minutes), or abnormal interictal EEGs should not be considered in the category of benign febrile convulsions but should be treated as any other seizure disorder would be.

DIFFERENTIAL DIAGNOSIS OF SEIZURES

The cause of paroxysmal loss of consciousness or unusual motor or sensory symptoms can be difficult to delineate (Table 13-4). Syncope is a brief loss of consciousness usually preceded by a feeling of dizziness or light-headedness. It always occurs in the standing or sitting position unless precipitated by a cardiac arrhythmia. There may be one or two limb twitches during the syncopal episode. Loss of consciousness lasts 1 to 2 minutes, after which the patient may feel tired but is oriented and can clearly relate the events leading up to the time when consciousness was lost. There is no tongue biting, and only rarely is there incontinence. Causes of syncope include vasovagal syncope, orthostatic hypotension, Stokes-Adams attacks, carotid sinus hypersensitivity, micturition, and coughing. Rarely, a patient may suffer a generalized seizure when syn-

TABLE 13-3. Events That May Trigger Seizures

Fever
Intercurrent infection
Lack of sleep
Lack of food
Psychological stress
Drugs that lower seizure threshold (e.g., phenothiazines, tricyclic antidepressants, theophylline)
Alcohol
Puberty

TABLE 13–4. Differential Diagnosis of Seizures

Syncope
Breath-holding spells
Hyperventilation
TIAs
Complicated migraine
Hypoglycemia
Sleep myoclonus
Drug intoxication
Decerebrate-decorticate posturing
Clonus
Pseudoseizure

cope is prolonged. This does not indicate that the patient has a seizure disorder, because the seizure is secondary to cerebral hypoxia.

Migraine headaches, especially basilar migraine, are occasionally associated with a brief loss of consciousness. The patient usually complains of a throbbing occipital headache, often with visual prodromes (e.g., scintillating scotomata), and then a brief loss of consciousness without tonic or clonic activity. On awakening, the symptoms are similar to those in patients with syncope. In older patients with cerebral atherosclerotic disease, hyperextension of the neck may produce vertebral basilar insufficiency with a brief loss of consciousness. The patient may be aware of other symptoms of vertebral basilar insufficiency prior to the loss of consciousness (for example, weakness of the legs, loss of vision, or vertigo). Cerebral vascular disease involving the carotid distribution may produce TIAs, brief episodes of hemiparesis, hemisensory symptoms, or aphasia. These episodes may last anywhere from a few minutes to several hours and may be difficult to differentiate from seizures. It is likely that an elderly patient with atherosclerotic disease who complains of these symptoms has TIAs. TIAs usually last longer (10 to 30 minutes) than seizures.

Prolonged hypoglycemia can produce seizures, especially in children. However, reactive hypoglycemia that is relatively mild in degree more likely produces dizziness or syncope. These episodes usually occur at times that correlate with the time of the patient's meals.

Infants and young children may have breath-holding spells in which they cry, suddenly stop breathing, then turn blue, and finally lose consciousness. They may have stiffening of the body or arching of the back during loss of consciousness. The episode is brief, and when they awaken there is no postictal drowsiness or confusion. The key factor in differentiating breath-holding spells from seizures is that the former usually occur when the infant has had some sudden fright or shock (for example, after falling and hitting the head). Also, breath-holding spells always begin with infants holding their breath, whereas apnea associated with seizure activity occurs after the onset of tonic movements. In older children and adults, sustained hyperventilation may produce a brief syncopal episode. There are usually other accompanying symptoms (for example, carpal pedal spasms and perioral tingling).

Sleep myoclonus is a normal phenomenon. This is not usually mistaken for seizure activity, although it may be in a situation in which the person does have a genuine seizure disorder. Sustained clonus, particularly in a young infant, may be mistaken for partial elementary seizures with motor symptoms. Clonus is generally induced and can be inhibited by holding the extremity involved. In a comatose patient, decorticate or decerebrate posturing may be mistaken for seizure activity. Finally, many psychotropic drugs may produce bizarre psychomotor symptomatology that can be confused with seizure activity. The patient may be disoriented and confused, with visual or auditory hallucinations. There are usually no motor components to this type of activity. However, ingestion of phenothiazines may produce dystonic posturing that may resemble tonic seizure activity.

Pseudoseizures, also referred to as psychogenic seizures, are episodic patterns of behavior that are interpreted by patients, family, and medical personnel as due to epilepsy. Pseudoseizures are well recognized among certain religious sects. Pseudoseizures and real seizures may coexist. The clinical manifestations may be difficult to differentiate from real seizures. Side-to-side head movements, pelvic thrusting, directed violence (e.g., biting, and unintelligible talking) are often manifestations of pseudoseizures. Urinary or bowel incontinence, while it may occur, is rare. Hyperventilation is often a precipitating event; every patient suspected of pseudoseizures should therefore be hyperventilated for 4 to 5 minutes. Pseudoseizures should be suspected in patients who carry the diagnosis of epilepsy and do not respond at all to optimal management with anticonvulsants. In most patients the diagnosis of pseudoseizures can be made with certainty only after prolonged EEG and video monitoring of attacks. The EEG is extremely unlikely to be normal during a genuine seizure. Some patients will cease having pseudoseizures once the diagnosis is established and has been explained, but most will require psychiatric care.

EVALUATION OF PATIENTS WITH SEIZURES

Any evaluation of a patient with seizures should begin with a thorough history, physical examination, and comprehensive neurologic examination. The most important task initially is to decide whether or not the patient suffered from a primary generalized seizure or from a partial seizure with or without secondary generalization. Primarily generalized seizures are caused by substrate deprivation (e.g. hypoxia, hypoglycemia), withdrawal states (e.g., sedatives, alcohol), toxic-metabolic disturbances, or one of the inherited seizure disorders. Partial seizures with or without secondary generalization are due to focal brain disease, which in most instances is not detectable clinically or by laboratory examinations. Secondary generalization may be so brief as to be unrecognizable clinically. The diagnostic evaluation should include blood tests for glucose, calcium, magnesium, electrolytes, renal and liver function tests, VDRL, complete blood count, and ethanol level. A urine specimen should be collected for a toxicology screen in adults and for an amino acid screen in infants and children.

The EEG is a useful diagnostic tool in the evaluation of patients with seizures. The sooner after a seizure an EEG is obtained, the greater is the likelihood that it will show a specific abnormality. The EEG can be helpful in establishing whether a seizure disorder is of the primary generalized type or of the focal type. Persistent obtundation or persistent abnormal behavior may suggest focal seizure status, and an EEG may be extremely helpful in diagnosing this condition.

A CT or MR scan should be performed on all patients presenting with a new seizure disorder. Even in the absence of focal neurologic or EEG abnormalities, structural abnormalities may be detected by these procedures.

Whenever an infectious etiology, particularly fungal and parasitic, is suspected, an LP should be performed and CSF examined for cell count, protein, glucose, and bacterial and fungal cultures. Antibody titers should be determined both in CSF and blood.

THE EEG IN SEIZURE DISORDERS

The EEG is performed with scalp electrodes recording electrical activity from the superficial cerebral cortex. It may show normal background activity, with or without focal or generalized abnormalities. These abnormalities may include slowing of background rhythms or epileptiform activity suggestive of an irritative focus. However, in as many as 40% of seizure disorders the EEG is normal. Thus, the EEG cannot be used to exclude the diagnosis of epilepsy. It also cannot be used to diagnose epilepsy in a patient who has never had seizures but has epileptiform activity on the EEG, since a small percentage of patients who have never had a clinical seizure will have an abnormal EEG. The following steps can, however, maximize the usefulness of the EEG:

1. Obtain the EEG during waking and sleep. Sleep may bring out epileptiform discharges that are not present during wakefulness.
2. Stress the patient. Sleep deprivation or a 12- to 24-hour fast may unmask abnormalities not present on a routine examination.
3. Repeat the EEG. The EEG is recording only a small temporal window of brain electrical activity. Repeated EEGs are more likely to detect intermittent paroxysmal abnormalities than a single recording.
4. Hyperventilate the patient for 3 minutes during each EEG recording. Hyperventilation will almost always trigger petit mal seizures. Likewise, photic stimulation should be performed during all EEG recordings and may be helpful in eliciting a photoconvulsive response. If the patient is aware of any specific stimulus that triggers the seizures, such as a certain piece of music, this stimulus should be applied during the EEG.
5. Place sphenoidal electrodes to help detect electrical abnormalities not recorded from standard surface electrodes.

In summary, the EEG is useful in the evaluation of the patient with a seizure disorder because it can delineate an area of focal pathology in the brain and in some situations (e.g., petit mal epilepsy) may be quite specific. However, the EEG must be correlated with the clinical situation. It cannot be used as the sole criterion to make a diagnosis of epilepsy.

TREATMENT OF SEIZURES

The primary goal of therapy is to prevent any further seizures from occurring whenever possible. In almost all patients this goal implies that some anticonvulsant medication must be taken daily. Patients who suffer seizures as a result of toxic-metabolic disturbances may require anticonvulsant medication acutely, but if the underlying condition can be adequately treated, they do not need to be on chronic medication. All anticonvulsant medications have unpleasant side effects, idiosyncratic reactions, and potentially serious complications from prolonged use. Therefore, it is essential that anyone prescribing these medications do so judiciously and with an awareness of the problems that can arise. In some patients the risks associated with taking anticonvulsant drugs may far outweigh the risk of doing nothing. For example, a patient who averages one seizure a year during sleep is not a candidate for drug therapy.

One of the most important rules is to begin with one medication only. There are several reasons for this. Many patients will require only one drug. Thus, side effects are minimized, no drug interactions can occur, and compliance is better. Furthermore, an allergic reaction to a given drug requires stopping that medication. If a patient is on more than one medication, it will be impossible to know which one is responsible for the allergic reaction, and all will have to be discontinued. The physician will then be denied the opportunity of using any of these drugs on the same patient in the future. Some patients certainly will require several drugs to control their seizures. Unfortunately, less than one quarter of patients uncontrolled with monotherapy will achieve better seizure control with the addition of a second drug.

Once a single medication has been initiated, the dosage should be increased until seizures are controlled. It takes five half-lives of a given anticonvulsant before an increase becomes therapeutically effective. If seizures are not completely controlled and side effects prevent further dosage increase of one anticonvulsant, then a second medication can be added. A minimum of 2 weeks' trial on therapeutic levels of one anticonvulsant should be given before a second one is added. If an anticonvulsant drug is totally ineffective, there is no logical reason to continue with it and add a second drug. In this situation the ineffective drug should be stopped and another one started. Finally, the dosage schedule should be kept as simple as possible. For example, if the medication being used has a long half-life, it can be given once a day rather than in divided doses. A simple dosage schedule will greatly increase compliance. Once a patient is seizure-free, anticonvulsant medications should be continued daily for a minimum of 2 years. Medications should never be stopped abruptly but should be tapered slowly over 1 to 2 months. In patients whose seizures are caused by structural lesions (e.g., unresectable brain tumors or arteriovenous malformation), the irritative focus causing the seizures will persist; in these cases, the patient may require anticonvulsant medications for life.

The choice of medication depends on seizure type, pharmacologic properties of the drug, potential side effects, age and sex of patient, and cost. Common anticonvulsant medications and their indications for use by seizure type are listed in Table 13–5. Several drugs may effectively control a certain seizure type, in which case other factors will dictate which drug to use. The lowest incidence of side effects is seen with valproic acid and carbamazepine. Certain aspects of drug metabolism are age-related. During the first weeks of life drug metabolism is slow, but children aged between 1 and 10 years have a higher metabolic rate than do older children and adults. In patients over 65, sedative and cognitive side effects may be much more prominent. In this older age group it is advisable to start anticonvulsants at a low dose and increase very gradually, unless seizures have to be controlled urgently. Diphenylhydantoin has nonlinear kinetics, and a small increase in dosage may be followed by a dramatic increase in side effects not seen at lower daily doses.

Furthermore there is great variability in individual responses, not only to this drug but to most anticonvulsants. Because of its side effects of hirsutism and acne, diphenylhydantoin is not the drug of first choice in women. On the other hand, because of its long half-life, diphenylhydantoin need be taken only once a day, resulting in improved compliance. Carbamazepine leads to autoinduction of its own metabolism, often resulting in a decrease of blood levels as the dose is increased. Valproic acid blood levels correlate poorly with clinical effectiveness, and its pharmacologic activity may persist for weeks after it is cleared from serum. Fatal hepatotoxicity of valproic acid is rare and occurs predominantly when the drug is used in conjunction with another anticonvulsant in children under age 2. The hyperammonemia seen in about 50% of patients on valproic acid is separate and is almost always asymptomatic. Gabapentin, a new anticonvulsant, is not protein-bound, is not metabolized, does not induce hepatic microsomal enzymes, does not inhibit metabolism of other anticonvulsant drugs, and is excreted unchanged in urine. Because of its pharmacologic and metabolic properties, the drug appears to be particularly useful for patients requiring multiple anti-epileptic drugs. Its efficacy as a single drug also appears promising.

All anticonvulsants increase the risk of congenital malformations when taken during the first trimester of gestation. Monotherapy and use of the lowest possible dose probably reduce this risk somewhat. Valproic acid and possibly carbamazepine increase the risk of spina bifida, and amniocentesis and alpha-fetoprotein determination are advisable.

Benzodiazepines are mostly used to control seizures acutely. Occasionally, patients uncontrolled on other anticonvulsants may benefit from long-term use of this class of drugs. One major obstacle is the frequent development of tolerance and breakthrough seizures.

Anticonvulsant blood levels are only a guide to therapy and constitute a statistical abstract that may be meaningless in a given patient. Some patients may be well controlled even though their blood anticonvulsant level is below the empirically derived therapeutic range. Other patients' blood levels may be well above it without any side effects. The primary goal of treatment of epileptic patients is to make them seizure-free with the least amount of medication and no or tolerable side effects. If that goal is achieved, blood anticonvulsant levels are irrelevant. Serum anticonvulsants can be expressed as either total levels or nonprotein-bound free levels. When seizures are uncontrolled and when drug toxicity is a problem, determination of serum anticon-

TABLE 15-5. Commonly Used Anticonvulsants

Drug	Total daily dose	Half-life (hours)	Doses per day	Seizure type for which most effective	Common side effects	Idiosyncratic reactions	Laboratory studies
Phenobarbital	Child 4–5 mg/kg Adult 100–300 mg	50–150	1–2	Major motor, partial motor, febrile convulsions	Drowsiness, hyperactivity, personality changes	Rash, Stevens-Johnson syndrome	Annual blood count
Diphenylhydantoin	Child 5–7 mg/kg Adult 300–500 mg	10–40	1–2	Major motor, focal motor, partial complex	Ataxia, nystagmus, dysarthria, gingival hyperplasia, hirsutism, acne	Rash, Stevens-Johnson syndrome, liver toxicity, fever, lymphadenopathy	SGOT, blood count every 6 months
Carbamazepine	Child 15–20 mg/kg Adult 600–1200 mg	12–35	2–3	Partial complex, major motor, focal motor	Drowsiness, ataxia, hallucinations	Rash, Stevens-Johnson syndrome, liver toxicity, bone marrow depression	CBC, SGOT monthly for 3 months, then every 2 months
Valproic acid	Child 15–16 mg/kg Adult 1000–2000 mg	8–12	2–4	Petit mal, major motor, infantile spasms	Nausea, vomiting, anorexia, hair loss	Fatal hepatic necrosis, thrombocytopenia, hyperammonemia	CBC, platelets, SGOT every month for 6 months, then every 2 months

Drug	Dose	Half-life (hr)	Dosing (per day)	Indication	Side effects	Toxicity	Monitoring
Gabapentin	Child not approved Adult 900–1800 mg	5–9	3	Partial simple and complex	Somnolence, dizziness, ataxia, fatigue, nystagmus	Rash	CBC, urea, creatinine every 2–3 months
Clonazepam	Child 0.03–0.2 mg/kg Adult 1.5–20 mg	22–33	3–4	Petit mal, myoclonic, akinetic, infantile spasms, partial complex	Lethargy, ataxia, dysarthria	Liver toxicity	SGOT, CBC every 2–3 months
Primidone	Child 10–25 mg/kg Adult 500–2000 mg	6–18	2–4	Major motor, focal motor, partial complex	Drowsiness, ataxia, personality changes	Rash, megaloblastic anemia	CBC every 3 months
Ethosuximide	Child 15–30 mg/kg Adult 750–2000 mg	20–60	3–4	Typical absence	Nausea, drowsiness, headache	Rash, bone marrow depression, liver toxicity	SGOT, CBC every 3 months
ACTH gel (IM)	Infant 20–80 units for 6–8 weeks		1	Infantile spasms	Weight gain, hypertension, hyperglycemia, hirsutism, acne		Serum glucose every 3–4 weeks

vulsant levels is helpful in comatose patients whose drug history is unknown, in patients on multiple anticonvulsant drugs, and in those taking other medications.

Anticonvulsant monitoring includes certain blood tests (see Table 13–5). The value of such monitoring is uncertain in predicting rare and serious complications. Normal tests at one point may provide false reassurance. Mild leukopenia, mild thrombocytopenia, and asymptomatic mild elevation of liver enzymes may cause undue alarm. The suggested frequency of monitoring is rather arbitrary. The best approach is to conduct baseline studies prior to instituting anticonvulsant drug therapy and to advise patients to seek prompt medical attention for unexpected and unusual symptoms and signs.

A difficult question is whether or not to institute chronic preventive drug therapy in a patient with a single seizure. Should another seizure occur, it commonly does so within 6 months of the initial event. The risk of another seizure is somewhere between 40% and 70%. Patients without any risk factors have a recurrence rate of about 20% within 3 years. Patients with risk factors—focal seizure, family history of seizures, abnormalities on neurologic examination, abnormal EEG, known neurologic injury, and transient paralysis after the first seizure—have a 50% chance of having another seizure within 3 years. It is probably prudent to treat patients who have a risk factor for recurrent seizures.

Another difficult question is whether or not to give anticonvulsant drugs routinely to a patient with a head injury to prevent the development of posttraumatic epilepsy, which is estimated to occur in approximately 7% to 60% of patients. The higher likelihood is seen in patients with severe head injuries, including posttraumatic amnesia of 24 hours or longer, depressed skull fracture, dural penetration, intracranial hematoma, and seizures within the first week after head trauma. An immediate seizure does not necessarily correlate with the later development of posttraumatic epilepsy. Severe head injury is probably an indication for instituting prophylactic treatment immediately after the incident and continuing for about 1 year.

Of the approximately 2 million persons with epilepsy in the United States, about 40% receive regular medical care for their seizures. The majority of these do well on a single anticonvulsant, about 10% to 15% require multiple drugs, and another group no longer needs medication or finds the treatment worse than the disorder. When should anticonvulsants be discontinued? Except in the most refractory patients, an attempt should be made to achieve monotherapy with one of the nonsedative drugs (diphenylhydantoin, carbamazepine, valproic acid, or ethosuximide). There are no clear-cut guidelines for discontinuing anticonvulsant drugs altogether. Gradual withdrawal of a single anticonvulsant is suggested for a patient who has been seizure-free for 2 years, had a low frequency of seizures prior to seizure control, has a normal or only mildly abnormal EEG, and has a normal neurologic examination. Estimates of seizure recurrence after complete drug withdrawal are highly variable but range around 50%. Withdrawal should be over a prolonged period of many weeks to minimize the possibility of drug withdrawal seizures. Patients who are withdrawing should be advised not to drive for several months.

Hormonal changes during puberty are a stress to the nervous system and may precipitate seizures in susceptible individuals. New seizure disorders frequently begin at this time of life. For this reason, it is generally unwise to taper and discontinue anticonvulsant medication in a youngster, even if he or she has been seizure-free for several years. The more prudent choice is to wait until the major growth spurt and other pubertal changes have occurred and at that point to taper or discontinue medication, provided seizures are controlled.

Laws pertaining to driving by epileptic individuals differ from state to state, and it behooves the treating physician to be familiar with these laws.

Other modalities of treatment that have been and are being advocated, e.g., acupuncture and biofeedback, do not appear to have any promise. In selected patients, surgery has become safer and more successful. Patients with medically intractable seizures and a single, resectable focus should be considered for surgery.

Treatment of Generalized Status Epilepticus

Generalized status eplepticus is defined as a single seizure lasting for 20 minutes or longer or recurrent generalized seizures with no regaining of consciousness in between each seizure episode. Generalized status is a life-threatening medical emergency and requires prompt and intensive therapy. The treatment of status epilepticus is outlined in Table 13–6. The goals in the treatment of status epilepticus are to protect the patient and to stop seizure activity. The patient should not be tightly restrained but minimally restrained only, to ensure protection from hitting sharp objects or falling to the floor. Any tight clothing should be removed. There is no place for intramuscular administration of anticonvulsants in the treatment of status epilepticus. Absorption is erratic in some cases, lengthy in others, and will complicate management as well as increase the risk of complications. It is best to use only one medication to obtain seizure control, since significant additive effects on respiratory depression can occur (for example, with concomitant use of Valium and phenobarbital). The most significant drawback to the use of large doses of phenobarbital in treating status epilepticus is that since the patient is likely to remain extremely sedated for many

TABLE 13-6. Outline of Treatment of Generalized Status Epilepticus

1. Admit to an intensive care unit.
2. Do not use tight restraints.
3. Remove constricting clothing (necktie, scarf).
4. Establish airway. Intubate if proper ventilation is impaired.
5. Maintain adequate blood pressure.
6. Draw blood for CBC, differential, glucose, calcium, magnesium, electrolytes, blood urea nitrogen (BUN), liver function tests, ethanol level, and toxicology screen. Obtain arterial blood for pH, pO^2, and pCO^2.
7. Begin intravenous (IV) drip and administer 50 ml 50% glucose (in children, 25% glucose) and 100 mg thiamine.
8. If seizures persist, give IV diazepam 10 mg slowly over 5–10 minutes (for children, 0.1–0.3 mg/kg to maximum of 10 mg). This dose may be repeated four times if necessary. Be prepared to ventilate the patient, since diazepam may cause respiratory depression.
9. If seizures recur after one dose of Valium, one of the following medications should be given:
    IV diphenylhydantoin 500–1000 mg at rate of 40 mg/min (child: 15 mg/kg to maximum of 500 mg) with ECG recorded continuously (since this medication may cause complete heart block). Infusion should be discontinued if prolonged P–R or Q–T intervals are observed or if T waves become depressed.
    IV phenobarbital 200 mg over 10 minutes (child: 5–10 mg/kg to maximum of 200 mg). This dose may be repeated every 20 minutes 4 times if necessary but may cause respiratory arrest.
    Rectal paraldehyde 10 ml (child: 0.3 ml/kg to maximum of 6 ml) mixed with equal amount of mineral oil and injected through glass syringe.
10. If seizures cannot be stopped within 30 to 60 minutes, the patient should be paralyzed and ventilated, preferably with continuous EEG monitoring.

hours, an adequate determination of mental status and neurologic evaluation cannot be performed during this time. This drawback is particularly crucial in patients for whom the cause of the status epilepticus is unknown.

If generalized status epilepticus cannot be controlled, such patients should be intubated, paralyzed, and ventilated. The EEG needs to be monitored, and additional amounts of anticonvulsant medication should be given. If 1000 mg of diphenylhydantoin was given, another 500 to 1000 mg should be administered. In extreme cases, generalized anesthesia may be required.

REFERENCES

Commission on classification and terminology of the International League against Epilepsy: Proposal for revised clinical and electroencephalographic classification of epileptic seizures. Epilepsia 1981; 22:489–501.

Wiederholt WC: Seizure Rx: How to select and use anticonvulsants. Modern Medicine Oct. 1983;135–158.

Fenichel GM, Greene HL: Valproate hepatotoxicity: Two new cases, a summary of others, and recommendations. Pediat Neurol 1985; 1:109–113.

Lockman LA: Management of generalized seizures in childhood. Pediat Neurol 1985; 1:265–273.

Porter RJ, Morselli PL (eds): The Epilepsies. London, UK, Butterworth, 1985.

Trauner DA: Medium-chain triglyceride (MCT) diet in intractable seizure disorders. Neurology 1985; 35:237–238.

Mattson RH, Cramer JA, Collins JF, Smith DB, Delgado-Escueta AV, Browne TR, Williamson PD, Treiman DM, McNamara JO, McCutcheon CB, Homan RW, Crill WE, Lubozynski MF, Rosenthal NP, Mayersdorf A: Comparison of carbamazepine, phenobarbital, phenytoin, and primidone in partial and secondary generalized tonic-clonic seizures. N Engl J Med 1985; 313:145–151.

Callaghan N, Garrett A, Goggin T. Withdrawal of anticonvulsant drugs in patients free of seizures for two years. N Engl J Med 1988; 318:942–946.

Niedermeyer E: The Epilepsies, Diagnosis and Management. Baltimore, Urban and Schwarzenberg, 1990.

Shen W, Bowman ES, Markand ON: Presenting the diagnosis of pseudoseizure. Neurology 1990; 40:756–759.

Pellock JM, Willmore LJ: A rational guide to routine blood monitoring in patients receiving antiepileptic drugs. Neurology 1991; 41:961–964.

Gabapentin—a new anticonvulsant: Med Lett Drug Ther 1994; 36:39–40.

Mattson RH: Current challenges in the treatment of epilepsy: Neurology 1994; 44:Suppl 5:S4–S9.

Scheffer I, Bhatia KP, Lopes-Cendes I, Fish DR, Marsden CD, Andermann F, Andermann E, Desbiens R, Cendes F, Manson JI, Berkovic SF: Autosomal dominant frontal epilepsy misdiagnosed as sleep disorder. Lancet 1994; 343:515–517.

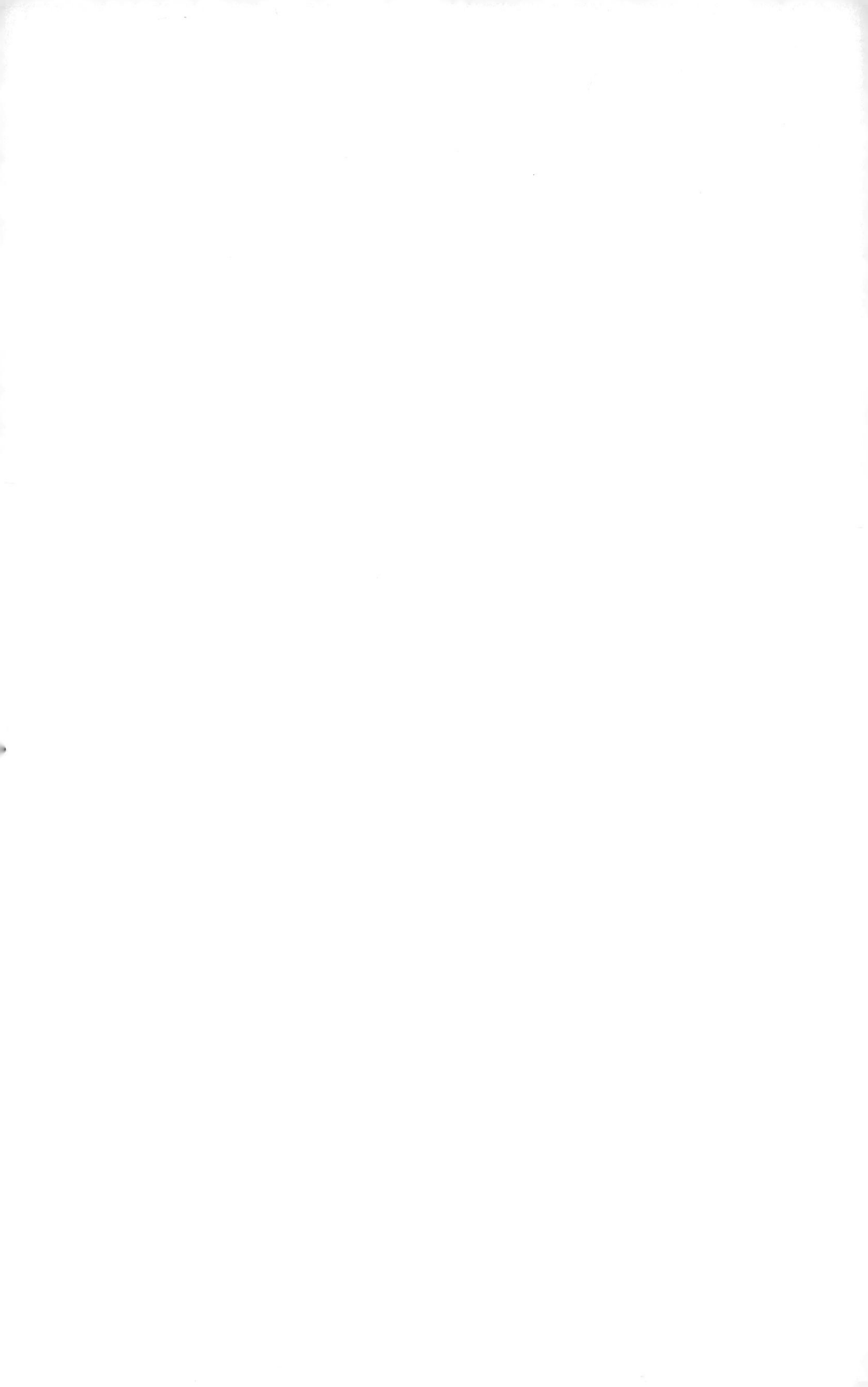

14

Parkinson's Disease and Other Movement Disorders

Under this heading are included neurologic disorders that produce abnormalities of muscle tone, abnormal posturing, and tremors. In most instances the pathology is in the basal ganglia, brainstem, and cerebellum. They also represent a group of disorders in which neurotransmitter function has been demonstrated to be abnormal or is postulated to be so. In this chapter certain abnormalities of tone and movement and certain tremors will be described, and specific diseases will then be discussed.

Spasticity is seen in patients with disorders of the pyramidal and extrapyramidal system. It is tested by passively moving a patient's extremity. Typically, resistance increases rapidly but is followed by instantaneous total relaxation (clasp-knife phenomenon or lengthening reaction). Rigidity, a classic sign of disorders of the basal ganglia, is characterized by different degrees of resistance to passive movement that remain about the same throughout the entire range of motion. In dystonia, another classic sign of basal ganglia disorders, the patient may assume bizarre postures. When extremities are moved passively, resistance increases progressively, but there is no giving as in spasticity. When the extremity being moved is released, it will fly back into a flexed position as if attached to a spring. Choreiform movements, also associated with basal ganglia disorders, are characterized by quick, purposeless, small-amplitude movements usually involving predominantly distal parts of the extremities but also involving the tongue and lips. Athetosis refers to rather slow writhing movements, which may involve all parts of the body. The extreme positions in athetosis of the upper extremities are adduction and flexion of the arm, supination of the hand with the fingers usually tightly flexed, and the opposite of these positions (arm abducted and extended, hand pronated, and fingers hyperextended). The upper extremity moves slowly between these two postures. These movements are thought by some to be the forerunner of dystonic posturing, which usually consists of tight flexion of both upper and lower extremities. Damage to the subthalamic nucleus produces hemiballismus, which consists of violent, gross movements of the arm and leg opposite to the side of the lesion. Paratonia consists of a rather subtle resistance to passive movement of the extremities and is usually seen in patients with frontal lobe damage. This abnormality in tone may be difficult to distinguish from the resistance to passive movement seen in anxious patients. Myoclonus is present in a variety of disorders with lesions from the cortex to the brainstem and cerebellum. It consists of abrupt gross movements involving proximal muscles and is frequently aggravated by intentional or passive movements of the extremity. Palatal myoclonus is a rapid oscillation of the soft palate that at times includes the musculature of the pharynx, the larynx, and even the diaphragm. The lesion responsible is in one of the following structures: inferior olive; projections of the inferior olive to the cerebellum; outflow from the cerebellum to the red nucleus; or central tegmental tract, which connects the red nucleus and the inferior olive. This movement disorder is the only one that persists during sleep.

Tremor is defined as a regular involuntary oscillation. In that sense, the so-called cerebellar tremor is not a true tremor, because it is characteristically irregular in rate and amplitude. The classic Parkinsonian tremor has a rate of oscillation of approximately 4 to 6 cps and consists of regular contractions of agonist and antagonist muscles. It is most commonly seen in the fingers and hands but may involve the entire arm, the lower extremity, and facial musculature. The tremor disappears with complete relaxation and very often is reduced during voluntary movements. Rubral tremor is a somewhat irregular oscillation involving proximal and distal muscles. The diagnosis of this tremor cannot be made with any degree of certainty unless there is a coexisting third-nerve paresis. Essential or familial tremor is most commonly seen in the fingers and hands, has a low to medium amplitude, has a frequency of 6 to 7 cps and is aggravated during volitional movements. When muscles of the neck are involved, oscillations of the head are seen. Involvement of tongue, vocal cords, and diaphragm produces a characteristic tremulousness of the voice. In so-called cerebellar tremor, the movement is in the horizontal plane and is strikingly accentuated when the extremity reaches the intended target. This manifestation simply reflects the fact that the movement has to be much more precise close to the target than far away from the target, and the movement abnormality consequently will be more obvious. Tardive dyskinesias are the result of treatment with phenothiazines and butyrophenones. They are characterized by rather bizarre facial and oral movements consisting of incessant tongue protrusion and/or twisting, licking of the lips, puckering and smacking of the lips, grimacing of the face, and similar bizarre movements of the extremities. Patients with tardive dyskinesia may also show incessant movements of their feet.

PARKINSON'S SYNDROME

A large number of patients with a movement disorder have Parkinson's disease. It is rather common in middle and old age, usually beginning between 40 and 70 years of age. The peak of onset is in the sixth decade. Incidence is lower among African Americans and Asians. Familial cases are rare. Approximately 40,000 to 50,000 new cases are diagnosed in the United States every year, and the incidence is about 150 individuals per 100,000. There are several conditions that may produce the clinical picture of Parkinson's disease. The most common is the idiopathic form in which the etiology is unknown. Pathologically, the disorder is characterized by the presence of cytoplasmic inclusions (Lewy bodies) and progressive loss of dopamine-synthesizing neurons in the zona compacta of the substantia nigra that project to the caudate and putamen. As a consequence, dopamine is depleted in the neostriatum. The next most common Parkinsonian-type syndrome is that secondary to therapy with chlorpromazine, prochlorperazine, trifluoperazine, and perphenazine. The symptoms and signs are dose-related and will disappear when the drug dosage is lowered or the drug is withdrawn. Symptoms and signs are also sometimes markedly ameliorated by the concurrent use of anticholinergic drugs. Postencephalitic Parkinsonism usually occurs at an earlier age than the idiopathic form. Oculogyric crises, though uncommon, distinguish this disorder from the idiopathic variety. In oculogyric crisis, the patient's eyes repeatedly turn extremely upwards and remain fixed in this position for minutes to hours. Manganese poisoning produces a picture similar to Parkinson's disease and is usually accompanied by dementia. In idiopathic orthostatic hypotension (primary dysautonomia or Shy-Drager syndrome), patients present with orthostatic hypotension, bladder dysfunction, and Parkinsonian features. In progressive supranuclear palsy, in addition to certain features of Parkinsonism, the typical findings are progressive restriction of voluntary eye movements. Initially, downward gaze is preferentially impaired and oculocephalic reflexes are preserved. The etiology of this disorder is unknown. It progresses relentlessly, with the patient ultimately showing no voluntary or spontaneous eye movement, marked generalized rigidity, and dementia. Levodopa (l-dopa) therapy is rarely of any help. Even though most textbooks discuss a subgroup classified as arteriosclerotic Parkinsonism, there is no convincing evidence that such an entity exists. It is of more than passing interest that in opiate addicts and monkeys, MPTP (a neurotoxin) can produce irreversible signs of Parkinson's with selective destruction of neurons in the substantia nigra. In striatonigral degeneration there is extensive loss of putaminal and nigral neurons but no Lewy bodies in the substantia nigra. The patient presents with typical Parkinsonian features but tremor is usually absent. It often occurs with olivopontocerebellar degeneration. Because of loss of striatal neurons, dopaminergic receptors are markedly diminished or absent, and response to l-dopa is minimal or absent.

Idiopathic Parkinson's Disease

The cardinal manifestations of Parkinson's disease are expressionless face, infrequent blinking, typical tremor (seen best with the extremity partly relaxed), rigidity (often detected earliest in the neck muscles), bradykinesia (slowness of movements), and disturbances of gait and station. A careful history will frequently reveal that the rate at which patients perform their daily routine has markedly slowed, tremor may or may not have developed, gait has become shuffling, and patients may fall for no apparent reason. Other symptoms include a soft voice, which in some patients may become inaudible, dysphagia, drooling, seborrhea of the face, and progressive difficulty with writing, which is very often extremely small. Constipation is common, but impairment of bladder function is not. On clinical examination, patients may or may not have the typical tremor. The absence of tremor does not exclude the diagnosis of Parkinsonism. Blinking is usually decreased in frequency, and patients often have an expressionless face with a general lack of normal spontaneous small movements of the face and the rest of the body. There are variable degrees of rigidity. Bradykinesia may be present, and in some patients any voluntary act is performed at such a slow rate that it is painful simply to watch. Speech may or may not be impaired, but if it is, it is characterized by its low volume and monotony of pitch. Patients often have great difficulty rising from a sitting position and also are extremely slow when trying to turn from one side to the other in the recumbent position. It is this latter feature that very often interferes with the patient's sleep. In fact, as an early indication of response to medication, many patients will report improved sleep. Patients will stand in a slightly stooped fashion with the arms flexed. When pushed they will be easily toppled, particularly when pushed backward. The ability to maintain balance while standing on one foot is often impaired. When attempting to walk, patients may have great difficulty getting started. When they finally succeed, steps are short; arm swing is decreased or absent; and when turning, the normal fluid movements become replaced by turning in one block. When patients are asked to stop walking, they may have difficulty stopping immediately and may take several extra steps. Subtle early gait abnormalities not readily apparent when the patient walks forward may be clearly visible when the patient walks backward. Early manifestations may be unilateral, but ultimately both sides are involved. Most patients with Parkinson's will have glabellar, pouting, and sucking reflexes.

Dementia is present in 8% to 30% of patients. Whether or not this is due to coexisting Alzheimer's disease is difficult to determine. There are some patients who are demented and do not show the typical Alzheimer pathologic changes. In others the pathology is characterized by widespread distribution of Lewy bodies (Lewy body disease). In this latter group dementia may precede the onset of Parkinsonian symptoms. Depression is a not uncommon feature in Parkinson's disease.

Therapy

The introduction of l-dopa has revolutionized the treatment of patients with Parkinson's disease, although not all patients with Parkinson's disease respond dramatically to this new form of therapy, as was initially hoped. Nevertheless, compared with previously available treatment modalities, the management of patients with Parkinson's disease has markedly improved. About 50% to 75% of patients significantly improve on l-dopa therapy. All major manifestations improve, although tremor usually takes longer to respond than other manifestations. Speech disturbances are least helped. Bradykinesia, akinesia, and postural instability may also respond poorly. Early institution of l-dopa therapy may prolong the patient's life. Because of unpleasant peripheral side effects of l-dopa, sinemet, a combination of l-dopa and carbidopa, was introduced. Carbidopa inhibits peripheral dopa decarboxylase but does not pass the blood-brain barrier. Consequently, side effects, particularly gastrointestinal disturbances, are reduced; and the total amount of l-dopa needed to achieve a therapeutic effect can be reduced to about one fourth of that used without carbidopa. Either l-dopa or sinemet should be gradually increased over a period of 2 to 3 months to a dose equivalent to approximately 3 to 4 gm of l-dopa per day, which is equal to 3 to 4 tablets of sinemet 25/250 per day (the first number refers to mg of carbidopa and the second to mg of l-dopa). In some patients a higher dose of 5 gm per day may be beneficial, but after 1 year of therapy most patients will achieve maximum benefit at a dosage of 3 gm of l-dopa per day. To reduce gastric irritation, medication should preferably be taken at mealtimes or with some food between meals. It is very often advantageous to let the patient determine optimal scheduling of the drug. Blood levels of l-dopa peak 1 to 3 hours after ingestion, which is also true for sinemet; but the half-life of sinemet is substantially longer than for plain l-dopa. Therefore, a longer-lasting response can be expected with the latter medication. Levodopa is available in 100 mg, 250 mg, and 500 mg tablets, sinemet in 10/100, 25/250 and 25/100 tablets. When treating with l-dopa, it is important for patients not to ingest more than 5 to 10 mg of pyridoxine (vitamin B^6) per day, because it increases the activity of dopa decarboxylase, directly counteracting the intended therapeutic effect. A controlled-release sinemet (sinemet CR; 200 mg l-dopa; 50 mg carbidopa) has become available and may be used advantageously in some patients. The combination of sinemet CR with regular sinemet may be optimal in other patients.

Selegeline (Deprenyl), a selective inhibitor of monoamine oxidase, has been reported to be neuroprotective, but its effect may not last longer than 1 year. The daily recommended dose is 5 mg with breakfast and lunch. Deprenyl can increase the efficacy of l-dopa, but it may also exacerbate side effects, and it can produce insomnia.

While a patient is taking l-dopa, monoamine oxydase inhibitors (MAOI) should not be given, because concurrent use may precipitate a hypertensive crisis. Phenothiazines and butyrophenones should be used only for essential indications, because they may aggravate the clinical manifestations of Parkinson's disease. Patients with narrow-angle glaucoma and those known to be hypersensitive to dopamine should not receive l-dopa. Nausea, vomiting, and anorexia—common side effects when plain l-dopa is given—are rare when sinemet is used. Orthostatic hypotension is a common early complication. In most patients, orthostatic hypotension does not persist, but if it does and patients are symptomatic, liberalized salt intake and elastic support stockings may be helpful. In some instances where these measures do not produce a desirable effect, fluorocortisone (0.1–0.3 mg per day) may be tried. In a small number of patients, acute psychotic behavior may develop during the institution of l-dopa therapy. In such cases it is best to withdraw the drug completely and start again with very small amounts that are increased very gradually.

The vast majority of patients who have been on l-dopa therapy for a year will develop choreiform movements that may involve the face, upper extremities, and diaphragm. Reduction in dosage will usually alleviate these symptoms, but many patients prefer these movements to the greater disability that may develop when the drug dosage is reduced. In some patients on l-dopa therapy, there may be periods of total akinesia. These akinetic periods may occur many times per day and vary in duration from a few minutes to as long as an hour. This on-off effect is less often seen when sinemet is used. sinemet CR may be beneficial in patients with fluctuations of motility on regular sinemet. In some patients motor fluctuations correlate with delayed gastric emptying, preventing absorption of the drug from the intestine. In this situation the drug is best taken as a powder mixed with water or some carbonated beverage on an empty stomach. Furthermore, patients should move about and not lie down, and they should avoid taking drugs that increase delayed gastric emptying, e.g., anticholinergic drugs. Patients taking l-dopa may experience deterioration of motor functions following a heavy protein meal and will benefit from eating frequent snacks during the day and reserving the major protein intake for the evening. After patients have been treated for a number of years with l-dopa, some will become nonresponsive to any drug therapy.

In some patients, adding anticholinergic drugs or amantadine to the treatment with l-dopa may be beneficial. The recommended daily dose of amantadine is 200 mg. The recommended daily dose for trihexyphenidyl (Artane) ranges from 1.5 to 15 mg and for benztropine mesylate (Cogentin) from 0.5 to 6 mg per day. Dopamine receptor agonists currently available include bromocryptine and pergolide. There do not appear to be significant differences among these agonists. Dopamine agonists are usually not as beneficial as l-dopa, but their action is longer and they cause less dyskinesia. Bromocryptine mesylate may be used as the initial drug of choice, and some authors have suggested that it is more effective than l-dopa in long-term treatment. Patients unresponsive to l-dopa therapy are poor candidates for this therapy. As adjunctive treatment to l-dopa, bromocryptine therapy may provide additional benefits in those patients maintained on optimal dosages of l-dopa and in those who are beginning to deteriorate. The use of bromocryptine may permit a reduction of the maintenance dose of l-dopa and thus may reduce the frequency and severity of the on-off phenomenon and dyskinesias. Patients treated with bromocryptine have significantly more adverse reactions—including nausea, hypotension, confusion, and hallucinations—than patients treated with l-dopa. Therapy with bromocryptine is started at a low dose and increased very slowly. Initially, patients should be maintained on their daily l-dopa dosage and bromocryptine should be given as one-half tablet (one tablet = 2.5 mg) twice a day with meals. If necessary, the dosage may be increased every 2 to 4 weeks by 2.5 mg per day with meals. The overall goal is to use the smallest dose of l-dopa and bromocryptine that produces optimal benefits with the least side effects. Pergolide offers no advantage over bromocryptine but is less expensive.

There is no agreement on when and how best to treat a patient with pharmacotherapy. Most physicians probably start patients on deprenyl plus sinemet or sinemet CR and use other drugs when the response is unsatisfactory. The way in which patients respond to pharmacotherapy is variable, and the optimal therapy is the one that works best for an individual patient. Unfortunately, none of the drugs currently in use has any effect on the dementia when present. In addition to drug therapy, maintenance of optimal health, including treatment for depression, is important. Even though they may respond quite adequately to therapy, patients with Parkinson's disease very often severely limit their daily activities. Continuous encouragement, gentle prodding, and establishment of a regular exercise schedule are beneficial in attempting to keep the patient mobile. Physical therapy may be helpful in achieving these goals.

Stereotactic surgery may still be indicated in an occasional patient who has a severe unilateral tremor and does not respond to drug therapy. Parkinson's disease is an excellent candidate for consideration of treatment by transplantation of neural tissue. Results of implantation of fetal adrenal medullary tissue and fetal nigral cells have been mixed, but investigations continue.

ESSENTIAL TREMOR

Essential tremor is probably the most common movement abnormality encountered in clinical practice. Other names applied to it are benign essential tremor, familial tremor, senile tremor, and intention tremor. In 50% of patients, other members of the family have a similar tremor. The tremor is not accompanied by any other neurologic abnormalities but may occasionally be present in patients with other neurologic disorders such as Parkinson's disease. It may start at any age, but most commonly patients will seek help in their thirties and forties. In some patients, the onset is not until senescence. The etiology is unknown, except that it appears to be inherited in about 50% of patients. There is no known pathology. The tremor is most prominent during volitional movements, particularly skilled movements such as writing, and is aggravated when the patient is tense or after caffeine use. It is absent at rest. Tremor of the head and voice is common and is often confused with the tremor of Parkinson's disease. Essential tremor is faster (6–7 Hz versus 4–5 Hz), is not present during rest, and is not accompanied by other neurologic symptoms or signs.

Frequently, simple reassurance is all that is needed. Most patients will have discovered on their own that alcohol in any form will significantly reduce the tremor. Phenobarbital and diazepam are quite effective in suppressing the tremor temporarily, and many patients may take an occasional 5 mg or 10 mg diazepam tablet when they know they will be in social situations in which their tremor is embarrassing. For long-term control of the tremor, propranolol is probably the drug of choice. This drug diminishes the amplitude of the tremor but does not alter its frequency. The tremor is rarely totally abolished, but the amount of reduction is usually sufficient to be of significant benefit to the patient. It is unknown if the site of action that reduces the tremor is peripheral or central. Treatment may be started with propranolol (10 mg t.i.d.) and increased by 10 to 30 mg per day at 4- to 5-day intervals. In most patients, a dosage of between 200 and 240 mg per day is sufficient. An occasional patient, however, may require much higher dosages. While on propranolol therapy, the pulse rate should remain above 50 per minute and systolic blood pressure above 110 mm Hg. If the drug is to be discontinued, it should be tapered off gradually; abrupt withdrawal may lead to myocardial infarction. Because most patients with essential tremor are not significantly incapacitated, treatment with propranolol is rarely justified. In some patients small doses of mysoline (50 mg 3 times per day) may substantially reduce the tremor. Unlike propranolol and sedative drugs, which only reduce the increase in tremor by anxiety or stimulant use and have no effect on the baseline tremor, mysoline reduces the baseline tremor. Unfortunately, the drug is ineffective in the majority of patients.

DYSTONIA

The characteristic features of dystonia consist of slow involuntary movements as described. Voluntary movements may precipitate dystonic postures. In severe cases or cases at the end stage of the disease, severe postural deformities and fixed contractions result. Dystonic movements and dystonic posturing may involve all extremities but may be confined to only one part of the body. In some patients, the dystonia is secondary to encephalitis, degenerative basal ganglia diseases, trauma, or intoxication. In the majority of patients, the cause is unknown. Although onset frequently occurs during childhood, the disease may begin at all ages. Progression is usually slow and may even cease after a number of years. Dystonia that has its onset in childhood is accompanied by dysarthria in 50% of patients and dysphagia in approximately 20%. These symptoms occur less frequently when the onset is later in life. The disorder is usually associated with normal intelligence.

In young children an autosomal recessive form occurs, which progresses slowly. A dominantly inherited form has its onset in later childhood, is milder in its manifestations, and progresses more slowly than does the recessive form. One rare form of childhood dystonia responds to l-dopa therapy. In adulthood most cases are sporadic, often involve only one extremity or one side of the body, and are characterized by very slow progression. Isolated writer's cramp, bleopharospasm, and spastic dysphonia are probably restricted forms of dystonia. These disorders are also referred to as segmental dystonias.

A great number of drugs have been tried, but none has emerged as predictably beneficial. Haloperidol and high doses of artane may be helpful in some patients. Patients severely disabled by the dystonia can be considered for stereotactic lesions of the thalamus. In recent years, local injections of botulinum toxin have been shown to be very helpful in the restricted forms of dystonia. The duration of the therapeutic effect is usually 3 to 4 weeks, and repeated injections have to be given.

SPASMODIC TORTICOLLIS

In this disorder, which can be considered a restricted form of dystonia, contraction of neck muscles leads to turning of the head, usually to one side, and hyperextension of the head. Typically, the patient may move the head back to the midline position by just gently touching that side of the face to which the head is rotated. The frequency of these movements varies from moment to moment. They are usually more prominent during periods of tension and anxiety. Even though torticollis may appear superficially to be a minor disorder, many patients are totally and permanently disabled and frequently withdraw from all job-related and social contacts. Patients with torticollis are at increased risk for suicide. In some patients, neuronal degeneration has been observed in the basal ganglia. An occasional patient with torticollis will develop generalized dystonia. This disorder is notoriously resistant to all forms of therapy. In some patients, haloperidol may be of some benefit. Destructive surgical treatment of neck muscles, extensively used in the past, has not been shown to be effective. Many patients who suffer from this disorder for many years will develop significant cervical osteoarthritis that, when symptomatic, can be managed with physiotherapy and analgesics. Local injections of botulinum toxin have been shown to be of great benefit to these unfortunate patients.

CHOREA

A number of neurologic disorders have chorea as a common feature. They also share pathologic changes in the caudate and putamen. These disorders include Huntington's chorea, Sydenham's chorea, familial chorea (which may be episodic), chorea gravidarum, and drug-induced chorea. Sydenham's chorea, a manifestation of rheumatic fever, and chorea gravidarum are self-limited entities.

Huntington's Disease

This is a dominantly inherited disorder that affects the basal ganglia and cerebral cortex. The gene abnormality is on the short arm of chromosome 4. The disease presents with progressive dementia and chorea. One or the other may be the initial manifestation, but eventually both are present. Tragically, the illness does not usually manifest itself until the third and fourth decades of life, well into the child-bearing years. In some families, the disease begins in the mid- or late teens, and the earliest manifestation is usually rigidity. The estimated prevalence of the disease is 5 to 10 cases per 100,000 population. Pathologically, there is loss of neurons and proliferation of astrocytes in the corpus striatum and less severe neuronal loss in the cortex. Grossly, there is striking shrinkage of the head of the caudate and the putamen. The caudate shrinkage is readily evident on CT or MR scan of the brain. There is reduction of gamma-aminobutyric acid (GABA), glutamic acid decarboxylase, choline acetyltransferase, cholinergic receptors, serotonergic receptors, and substance P.

Initially, the choreiform movements are subtle and are very often interpreted as fidgetiness or restlessness. At this stage, mental changes are subtle and may consist of lability of mood, difficulties in interacting with other people, withdrawal, heightened anxiety, and problems in maintaining adequate performance at work. The abnormal movements are inappropriate, but many patients quickly learn to convert them into seemingly appropriate movements. As the disease progresses, the movements become more obvious and more abundant, and the patient may appear to be dancing. Later, athetoid movements and dystonic posturing develop. Mental changes progress, and most patients die within 15 to 20 years. Suicide early in the course of the illness in not uncommon.

There is no known therapy for the progressive dementia. Early in the course of the illness, psychiatric manifestations may predominate and are difficult to manage. When depression is severe, tricyclic antidepressants are helpful. Monoamine oxidase inhibitors should not be used, because they may aggravate the abnormal movements. The most commonly used form of therapy for the movement disorder is haloperidol. This drug may be started at 1 mg q.i.d. and increased to the point of tolerance and optimal control of abnormal movements. In patients who present with the rigid form, l-dopa may occasionally be of some temporary benefit. Genetic counseling is of the utmost importance. Even in the best of situations, the impact of genetic counseling is very often quite disappointing. This is largely due to the fact that in most patients the onset of the disease is past the child-bearing age. Patients should be seen at reasonable intervals so that the physician may determine how to adjust daily activities as the disease progresses. Ultimately, all patients will be totally dependent and will need institutional care.

MYOCLONUS

Myoclonus may be seen as a manifestation of a variety of different disorders without a consistent pathologic process. Myoclonus may be a manifestation of epilepsy, and in some instances, such as infantile myoclonic epilepsy, may dominate the clinical picture. In this disorder, myoclonic seizures eventually cease, but they are frequently replaced by other types of seizures. Children suffering infantile myoclonic epilepsy are almost always retarded. Early treatment with adrenocorticotropic hormone (ACTH) appears to provide some benefit. Myoclonus is also seen in a number of familial degenerative disorders, including Lafora body disease, heredofamilial ataxias, leukodystrophies, and lipidosis. Furthermore, myoclonus is frequently observed in patients with Jakob-Creutzfeldt disease, subacute sclerosing panencephalitis, and epidemic encephalitis.

Severe hypoxia of the brain, frequently secondary to cardiopulmonary arrest or drug overdose, may lead to posthypoxic intention myoclonus. In this entity, voluntary or passive limb movements precipitate trains of myoclonic jerks that cease when the extremity comes to rest. A number of pharmacologic agents are currently under investigation for use in myoclonus. Unfortunately, no single agent or combinations of different agents have proven to be consistently effective. Presently, two drugs approved by the Federal Food and Drug Administration may provide some benefit. These are clonazepam, which may be started at 1 mg per day and gradually increased to 7 to 12 mg per day, and valproic acid.

HEMIBALLISMUS

The pathology in this disorder consists of infarction or hemorrhage in the subthalamic nucleus on the side opposite the extremities showing the violent, purposeless movements. Care should be taken to protect the patient from self-injury. Fortunately, the disease is self-limited from a few days to several months in almost all patients. Haloperidol in doses of 2 to 8 mg per day has been reported to be beneficial, but no treatment at all appears to be just as effective.

ATHETOSIS

This disorder is usually the result of perinatal brain injury to the fetus during prolonged, difficult labor. The basal ganglia show a marbled appearance. In kernicterus, the globus pallidus is predominantly involved.

The disease rarely occurs in adult life but may be seen in posthypoxic encephalopathy. No effective therapy is known.

GILLES DE LA TOURETTE SYNDROME

This disorder usually has its onset between the ages of 2 and 15. It is characterized by stereotyped repetitive movements (tics), compulsive uttering of inarticulate sounds, and coprolalia. The tics involve the eyelids, head, and face. Patients may blink, grimace, twitch the head, shrug the shoulders, and jerk the arms. More complex movements such as skipping, hopping, squatting, and pelvic thrusting and tilting may be seen. In about 50% of these patients, there may be a history of hyperactivity, and subtle neurological abnormalities may be found. The incidence of left-handedness is increased in these patients. Additional family members, parents as well as children, are affected in approximately 35% of patients. No pathologic lesion has been identified. Patients with this syndrome have a normal distribution of intelligence. Chronically administered haloperidol is the drug of choice for treatment of this condition.

TARDIVE DYSKINESIAS

The term tardive dyskinesia is derived from the observation that these abnormal movements were first observed after prolonged, high-dose treatment with antipsychotic drugs. Once established, withdrawal of the offending agent will in most instances not reverse the condition. The prognosis for these abnormal movements to cease is much more favorable when they occur after short-term therapy of several weeks' or months' duration. The subacute development of Parkinsonian-type abnormalities with antipsychotic treatment is invariably reversible. Not only psychotic patients are at risk of developing tardive dyskinesias but also those who receive antipsychotic medications for treatment of nausea or chronic anxiety. In addition to the duration of treatment and total amount of drug given, sex and age are important factors. The elderly and women are more prone to develop tardive dyskinesia. No specific neuropathologic changes have been reported. It has been postulated that chronic striatal dopamine receptor blockade by these drugs results in hypersensitivity of the chemically denervated receptors.

It is rather disappointing that no effective therapy has been introduced. When tardive dyskinesias develop subacutely, the offending agent or agents should be markedly reduced or withdrawn. Antipsychotic agents, particularly in the elderly, should be used for long-term therapy only if absolutely necessary. Whether or not periodic withdrawal decreases the incidence of tardive dyskinesias is unknown. When Parkinsonian-type symptoms and signs appear, anticholinergic drugs or l-dopa will effectively counteract these dyskinesias but may worsen tardive dyskinesia. It has been observed that increasing the daily dosage of the antipsychotic drug will frequently control the dyskinesias, but this benefit is only short term, sooner or later the same symptoms will reemerge.

REFERENCES

Lance JW Adams RD: The syndrome of intention or action myoclonus as a sequel of hypoxic encephalopathy. Brain 1963; 86:111–136.

Hoehn MM, Yahr MD: Parkinsonism: Onset, progression, and mortality. Neurology 1967; 17:427–442.

Johnson WG, Fahn S: Treatment of vascular hemiballism and hemichorea. Neurology 1977; 27:634–636.

Kobayashi RM: Drug therapy of tardive dyskinesia. N Engl J Med 1977; 296:257–260.

McAllister RG, Markesberry, WR, Ware RW, Howell SM: Suppression of essential tremor by propranolol: Correlation of effect with drug plasma levels and intensity of beta-adrenergic blockade. Ann Neurol 1977; 1:160–166.

Duvoisin R: Parkinson's Disease: A Guide for Patient and Family. New York, Raven Press, 1978.

Joseph C, Chassan JB, Kock ML: Levodopa in Parkinson's disease: A long-term appraisal of mortality. Ann Neurol 1978; 3:116–118.

Shoulson I, Fahn S: Huntington's disease: Clinical care and evaluation. Neurology, 1979; 29:1–3.

Jankovic J: Progressive supranuclear palsy: Clinical and pharmacologic update. Neurol Clin 1984; 2:573–586.

Stoessl AJ: Managing the refractory Parkinsonian patient. In Hachinski VC (ed), Challenges in Neurology. Philadelphia, FA Davis, 1992, pp 195–212.

Comella CL, Buchman AS, Tanner CM, Brown-Toms NC, Goetz CG: Botulinum toxin injection for spasmodic torticollis: Increased magnitude of benefit with electromyographic assistance. Neurology 1992; 42:878–882.

Markham CH, Diamond SG: Clinical overview of Parkinson's disease. Clin Neuroscience 1993; 1(1):5–11.

Nutt JG: Pharmacotherapy of Parkinson's disease. Clin Neuroscience 1993; 1(1):64–68.

Drugs for Parkinson's disease: Med Lett Drugs Ther 1993; 35:31–34.

Surgical treatment of Parkinson's disease: Med Lett Drugs Ther 1993; 35:103–104.

Calne DB: Initiating treatment for idiopathic Parkinsonism. Neurology 1994; 44 (Suppl 6):S19–S22.

Koller WC, Pahwa R: Treating motor fluctuations with controlled-release levodopa preparations. Neurology 1994; 44(suppl 6):S23–S28.

Olanow CW, Fahn S, Muenter M, Klawans H, Hurtig H, Stern M, Shoulson I, Kurlan R, Grimes JD, Jankovic J, Hoehn M, Markham CH, Duvoisin R, Reinmuth O, Leonard HA, Ahlskog E, Feldman R, Hershey L, Yahr MD: A multicenter double-blind placebo-controlled trial of pergolide as an adjunct to sinemet in Parkinson's disease. Movement Disorders 1994; 9(1): 40–47.

Tolosa ES, Valldeoriola F, Marti MJ: New and emerging strategies for improving levodopa treatment. Neurology 1994; 44(suppl 6):S35–S44.

15

Infections of the Nervous System

Prevalence of pathogens in bacterial meningitis varies with age. In neonates group B streptococcus, Escherichia coli (E coli), and other gram-negative enteric organisms are most common. In infants the most frequent organisms are Haemophilus influenzae type b, Neisseria meningitidis, and Streptococcus pneumoniae. In adults the most common organisms are Streptococcus pneumoniae and Neisseria meningitidis.

The CNS is subject to infection by a wide variety of viruses, bacteria, fungi, and other organisms. Most often, infections are diffusely distributed but may have a predilection for the meninges (meningitis), the cerebral cortex and subcortical white matter (encephalitis), or both (meningoencephalitis). Less commonly, infections localize in a specific area of the nervous system (cerebritis, abscess). In addition, infections may cause secondary nervous system dysfunction because of mass effect or hydrocephalus. Cerebral infarction or damage to cranial or spinal nerves may also occur. Because the morbidity and mortality of many CNS infections, particularly bacterial ones, increases when the onset of treatment is delayed by days or even hours, every effort must be made to make a prompt diagnosis and to begin appropriate therapy immediately.

This chapter will generally recommend one specific drug treatment for each CNS infection discussed. Alternative drugs for patients who are allergic to the recommended drug will be given for the most commonly encountered situations. The references contain other suggested therapies, complete information about alternative treatments for drug-allergic patients, and pediatric doses of the drugs used in the treatment of CNS infections. Because of the frequent introduction of new antimicrobial drugs, as well as changes in drug sensitivities of organisms, infectious disease specialists should frequently be consulted to provide optimal management of the patient with a CNS infection.

VIRAL INFECTIONS

In dealing with viral infections of the CNS it is helpful to take into account that some are more prevalent in certain seasons. In summer and fall St. Louis encephalitis, California encephalitis, Western equine encephalitis, Eastern equine encephalitis, and enterovirus meningoencephalitis are common. In fall and winter lymphocytic choriomeningitis occurs often. In winter and spring the mumps virus has to be considered in the differential diagnosis. Viruses that cause encephalitis year-round are herpes virus, Epstein-Barr virus, and cytomegalovirus (CMV). Epidemiological information from local health departments and the Centers for Disease Control in Atlanta, Georgia, is often helpful in determining the causative agent.

Acute Meningitis

Acute viral meningitis commonly presents as the syndrome of aseptic meningitis, namely fever, headache, photophobia, stiff neck, and predominantly mononuclear pleocytosis with elevated CSF protein and normal CSF glucose. At the beginning of the illness, there may be a predominance of polymorphonuclear cells in the CSF. Many viruses produce this syndrome, and these can often be identified by culture or antibody titers. While patients may be quite ill at the onset, viral meningitis generally has a self-limited, benign course; the approach to the patient should be an expectant, supportive one. The differential diagnosis of viral meningitis includes partially treated bacterial meningitis, bacterial parameningeal infection, syphilitic meningitis, tuberculous meningitis, cryptococcal meningitis, carcinomatous meningitis, lymphomatous meningitis, and Behçet's disease. Thus, the patient should be examined carefully for sinusitis, mastoiditis, or brain or other abscess. Appropriate diagnostic tests should be done if necessary. Moreover, the spinal fluid of the patient with aseptic meningitis should be sent for VDRL, TB stain and culture, fungal stain and culture, and cytology, to avoid delaying the diagnosis of a treatable disease.

Acute Encephalitis

The patient with acute encephalitis or meningoencephalitis has fever, headache, and stiff neck, together with symptoms and signs of direct brain involvement. These include some combination of altered level of consciousness (delirium, stupor, or coma), seizures (focal or generalized), and focal neurologic signs (hemiparesis, aphasia, amnesia, movement disorder, ataxia, or myoclonic jerks). A number of organisms may produce viral encephalitis, including the arthropod-borne viruses, herpes simplex, and rabies. CSF exam is generally necessary to confirm the diagnosis. Spinal fluid shows the picture of aseptic meningitis, and the organism may be identified by virus antibody titer, culture, or fluorescent antibody study. Patients with suspected encephalitis should generally have a CT head scan prior to LP to exclude the possibility of a mass lesion. If encephalitis is present, the scan may be normal or may show evidence of focal or diffuse brain inflammation. EEG often shows focal and/or diffuse slowing and may show epileptiform activity. The morbidity and mortality of encephalitis depend on the infectious agent, being quite high for herpes simplex and intermediate for the arthropod-borne viruses. Except for the patient with herpes simplex infection, treatment of the patient with acute encephalitis is supportive. Increased intracranial pressure should be controlled, and seizures should be treated.

Herpes simplex encephalitis (HSE) is the most common cause of nonepidemic encephalitis. It is almost always caused by the HSV-1. Type 2 virus may also cause encephalitis, usually in the neonatal period. It may also cause aseptic meningitis, myelitis, and—rarely—a polyradiculitis. The HSV-1 infection is characterized, in its severest form, by the evolution over several days of fever, headache, seizures, confusion, stupor, and coma. Personality change, Wernicke's aphasia, and hallucinations are frequently seen. The CSF is often under increased pressure and shows a lymphocytic pleocytosis (usually 50 to 100 cells), elevated protein, and on occasion a low glucose. Rarely there may also be xanthochromia and an increased number of red cells. The CSF is normal in 10% of cases on initial LP. Because herpes simplex is an intracellular virus, for all practical purposes the virus cannot be grown from CSF. An EEG showing periodic high-voltage sharp waves over one or both temporal lobes is highly suggestive of the diagnosis. CT may show low-density areas, particularly in the temporal lobes. MRI is also helpful in the diagnosis. There may be associated hemorrhagic areas or mass effect. Definitive diagnosis depends upon cerebral biopsy of an infected area. Intranuclear inclusions in neurons suggest virus infection, and a fluorescent antibody study can identify the virus. Virus particles may sometimes be seen on electron microscopy. The virus can be grown from the tissue specimen in 24 to 72 hours.

Intravenous acyclovir (10 mg/kg over 1 hour every 8 hours for 14 to 21 days) is the treatment of choice. Corticosteroids for short periods may be helpful in controlling brain edema and prevent herniation. As necessary, patients should be treated medically for seizures. Untreated HSE has a 70% mortality, with most survivors having significant neurologic disability, including dementia, amnesia, aphasia and seizures. The prognosis is better in treated cases, particularly for those who are younger and have milder symptoms at the time the antiviral drug is started. There is no agreement on whether or not brain biopsy should precede treatment with acyclovir. It appears prudent to start patients suspected of having HSE on acyclovir immediately and then proceed with brain biopsy. The drug should be discontinued if another diagnosis is discovered or if the viral culture of brain tissue is negative after 5 days. About 25% of biopsy-negative patients have another treatable disease.

Poliomyelitis

In this country the polio patient—a rare phenomenon—is often an unvaccinated person who has been exposed to someone recently vaccinated with live attenuated virus. A generally benign syndrome similar to poliomyelitis can be caused by Coxsackie viruses A and B and echoviruses. The patient with acute poliomyelitis develops an aseptic meningitis together with painful, flaccid weakness of voluntary muscles. The weakness usually progresses over 2 to 5 days; typically involves the extremities asymmetrically; and may affect facial, pharyngeal, and respiratory muscles. The spinal fluid picture is that of an aseptic meningitis. Electrophysiological examination of nerves and muscles confirms the presence of acute anterior horn cell disease. Viral cultures and titers may establish the diagnosis with certainty. The patient with suspected polio should be isolated and treated supportively with analgesics and physical therapy. Respiratory status should be followed carefully; mechanical ventilation may be required. In the 90% to 95% of patients who survive, there is considerable recovery of function during the first 4 months after infection. Respiration and swallowing generally recover completely, and extremity weakness may also improve considerably. Physical therapy and/or orthopedic evaluation may help the patient achieve maximal recovery of function. (See Chapter 8 for a discussion of postpolio syndrome).

Herpes Zoster

Herpes zoster is responsible for the painful cutaneous vesicular eruption in a dermatome distribution generally known as shingles. The incidence is 3 to 5 cases per 1000 per year. The varicella-zoster (chicken pox) virus infects the host at a young age and persists in sensory ganglion cells. Advancing age or immunoincompetence are risk factors for reactivation of the virus. While most patients have involvement of only one dermatome, the disease may disseminate, particularly in immunocompromised hosts. The proportion of patients with zoster who are found to have a concurrent malignancy is 5%, which is twice the expected incidence. The patient with herpes zoster should be isolated from anyone who has not had chicken pox. Specific treatment is described in Chapter 11.

Subacute, Chronic, and Slow Virus Infections

A number of viruses produce neurologic symptoms and signs that progress gradually over weeks to months. Because fever, leukocytosis, and CSF pleocytosis are generally absent, these conditions simulate CNS degenerative diseases. No specific treatments are available, and the patients must be treated supportively. Subacute sclerosing panencephalitis (SSPE) generally begins several years after a measles infection, presenting as progressive personality change, dementia, seizures, and myoclonus in a child or adolescent. The EEG often shows characteristic periodic discharges, and the CSF has greatly elevated gamma globulin and measles-antibody titers. Almost all patients die within 1 to 3 years. Remissions are rare but do occur. No effective therapy exists. Progressive multifocal leukoencephalopathy (PML), caused by a polyoma virus often occurs in an immunosuppressed patient. Hemiparesis, quadriparesis, visual field deficits, aphasia, dementia, and ataxia may be present. CSF is normal, and CT brain scan often shows multifocal white matter lesions. The course of this disease is usually 3 to 6 months. Jakob-Creutzfeldt disease (JC), caused by an unusual viruslike agent, generally presents as rapidly progressive dementia and myoclonus in a middle-aged or elderly adult. Signs of pyramidal or extrapyramidal involvement may also be seen, and there may be prominent ataxia or cortical blindness. CT scan is usually normal, and CSF may have elevated protein. The EEG may show characteristic periodic discharges that strongly suggest the diagnosis, but only a brain biopsy can confirm the diagnosis. Cerebral and cerebellar cortices are principally affected with loss of neurons, gliosis, and prominent vacuolation without inflammatory changes. The patient usually dies within a year. Great care must be taken in handling cerebral and other tissue because of the possibility of transmitting the infection. Any patient with possible JC (this includes all patients with dementia of unknown etiology) must not be a tissue donor during life or at the time of death. Any reusable instruments that may have been exposed to the virus should be treated by autoclaving at 121 degrees C and 20 psi for 1 hour or by immersion in 5% sodium hypochlorite (household bleach).

Acquired Immunodeficiency Syndrome (AIDS)

AIDS dementia ("subacute encephalitis") may present before or after the appearance of other manifestations of AIDS. Direct brain infection by the HIV-1 virus that causes AIDS is the likely etiology. The clinical picture is generally one of insidious onset and gradual progression of forgetfulness, poor concentration, mental slowing, and apathy. Leg weakness and gait unsteadiness may also occur early in the course. Three months after onset more than 50% of patients have moderate to severe global dementia and psychomotor slowing. At this stage there may also be severe ataxia, spastic weakness, and incontinence of bladder and bowels. Tremor, myoclonus, or seizures may be present. HTLV-III serology is positive in almost all patients. CT brain scan may show atrophy, and MRI brain scan may show abnormalities in the central white matter. EEG and CSF exam show only nonspecific abnormalities. Although there is currently no treatment for AIDS dementia, it is important to rule out depression, treatable brain infection, or tumor in the AIDS patient with new cerebral dysfunction.

HIV-1–associated progressive encephalopathy of childhood may start as early as 2 months of age. Usually children fail to acquire developmental milestones or lose those already reached. In older children decreasing school performance is usually an indicator of cognitive impairment. Eventually the disease progresses to severe mental impairment and spastic quadriparesis. CT and MRI often show cerebral atrophy and, in young children, bilateral basal ganglia calcifications. HIV-1 infection may be associated with a great number of primary neurologic and opportunistic infections and neoplasms (Table 15–1). All disorders require laboratory confirmation of systemic HIV-1 infection. There is no specific therapy for primary HIV-1–associated disorders. Specific therapies, if available, are used for secondary infections and neoplasms.

Tropical Spastic Paraparesis

This disorder, caused by the human T lymphotrophic virus type 1 (HTLV-1), is endemic in many tropical and subtropical areas but also occurs sporadically in western countries. Slowly progressing spastic paraparesis, loss of sphincter control, and variable sensory abnormalities characterize the clinical picture. The CSF usually shows a pleocytosis of 10 to 50 mononuclear cells. Protein and glucose are normal, but IgG is elevated and antibodies to HTLV-1 are present.

Parainfectious Encephalitis

Up to 20% of apparent encephalitis cases may actually be due to a delayed hypersensitivity reaction to a viral infection or vaccination. Nonspecific upper respiratory infection is associated with 70% of cases. Varicella and measles infections, together with the smallpox and the old rabies vaccines, were previously the most common causes. The symp-

TABLE 15–1. HIV-1 Associated Central and Peripheral Nervous Sytem Disorders

Primary CNS infections
  Dementia complex
  Acute encephalitis
  Meningitis
  Progressive encephalopathy of childhood
  Vacuolar myelopathy
Secondary CNS infections
  Predominantly diffuse
    Herpes simplex encephalitis
    Cytomegalovirus encephalitis
    Cryptococcal, tuberculous, syphilitic meningitis
  Predominantly focal
    Cryptococcosis
    Toxoplasmosis
    Herpes zoster
    Tuberculous abscess
    Meningovascular syphilis
    Progressive multifocal leukoencephalopathy
    Herpes zoster and herpes simplex myelitis
Secondary CNS tumor
  Predominantly diffuse
    Metastatic lymphomatous meningitis
  Predominantly focal
    Primary CNS lymphoma
Primary peripheral nervous system and muscle
  Acute inflammatory demyelinating polyradiculoneuropathy
  Chronic inflammatory demyelinating polyradiculoneuropathy
  Mononeuritis multiplex
  Predominantly sensory polyneuropathy
  Distal painful sensory polyneuritis
  Myopathy
Secondary peripheral nervous sytem
  Herpes zoster radiculitis
  Cytomegalovirus polyradiculoneuritis

toms usually begin abruptly 4 to 14 days after a nonspecific upper respiratory infection, and the clinical picture is identical to that of an acute viral encephalitis. Mortality varies from 5% (for varicella) to 25% (for measles). Permanent neurologic sequelae are uncommon except when the disorder is due to measles.

BACTERIAL INFECTIONS

Bacterial meningitis

The clinical features of bacterial meningitis in the adult and older child include fever, headache, and stiff neck. Seizures, cranial neuropathies, and focal neurologic signs are occasionally present. The level of consciousness may be depressed, and signs of meningeal irritation may be absent in the very young and in those patients who are deeply stuporous or comatose. There is often a history of antecedent upper respiratory symptoms. Patients usually deteriorate rapidly. Symptoms and signs often have been present for less than 24 hours at the time of diagnosis. In contrast to adults, the infant or newborn with bacterial meningitis may have only nonspecific signs of an infection or a systemic illness.

The likely etiology of bacterial meningitis can often be predicted from the patient's age and the presence of other risk factors. E coli and group B streptococcus are the predominant pathogens in neonates. In patients older than 2 months, Haemophilus influenzae, Neisseria meningitidis (meningococcus), and Streptococcus pneumoniae (pneumococcus) account for 80% to 90% of cases. Listeria monocytogenes is the fourth most common cause. Pneumococcus should be suspected in alcoholics, splenectomized patients, those with sickle cell anemia, and those with basilar skull fracture. Infections with staphylococcus, group A streptococcus, E coli, Proteus, Klebsiella, and Pseudomonas are the most common causes of bacterial meningitis in the neurosurgical patient or the patient with penetrating head injury.

A CSF examination must be done to diagnose bacterial meningitis. A CT scan must be done first only if a cerebral mass lesion is suspected. The spinal fluid is almost always under increased pressure. There is usually a pleocytosis of 1000 to 10,000 white blood cells with 90% to 95% neutrophils. Sometimes there is a normal or near normal cell count in the first hours of meningitis, and on occasion there may be a mononuclear predominance to the pleocytosis. Protein is generally 100 to 500 mg/dl and sugar is typically low, (less than 40 mg/dl). Organisms are seen on gram stain of centrifuged CSF in 80% to 90% of patients who have a positive bacterial culture. Counter immunoelectrophoresis and latex agglutination tests are useful for detection of bacterial antigens in partially treated meningitis due to some strains of haemophilus, meningococcus, and pneumococcus. Cultures are positive in 70% to 90% of cases of bacterial meningitis. Bacterial sensitivity to antimicrobial drugs should always be determined.

Blood leukocyte count is usually elevated, with an associated shift to the left. Blood cultures are positive in 40% to 60% of individuals with meningitis due to haemophilus, meningococcus, or pneumococcus. Cultures of the nasopharynx generally show haemophilus or meningococcus when these organisms are responsible for meningitis. X-rays of the chest may show an associated pneumonia. Skull and sinus films may demonstrate underlying sinusitis, mastoiditis, or skull infection. A CT head scan should be obtained if there is an abnormal level of consciousness that might be due to hydrocephalus or if focal neurologic signs are present that could be caused by subdural empyema, abscess, or stroke.

In cases of suspected bacterial meningitis prompt treatment with antibiotics is essential and should start immediately after a CSF sample has been obtained from the patient. Initial antibiotic therapy for the patient without an identifiable bacterial organism depends on which organism is most likely to be present. Organisms commonly responsible for meningitis are Streptococcus pneumoniae, Neisseria meningitides, and (in children) Haemophilus influenzae type b. In newborns meningitis is often caused by group B or other streptococci, gram-negative enteric organisms, or Listeria monocytogenes. Pending results of cultures, most infectious disease specialists recommend cefotaxime or ceftriaxone in adults and children more than 3 months old, and ampicillin plus cefotaxime with or without gentamicin in newborns. Once an organism has been identified and sensitivities established, adjustments in antibiotic therapy may be necessary. Drugs of first choice and alternative drugs for meningitis are listed in Table 15–2. For exact dosages for adults, children, and infants, drug inserts and other appropriate references have to be consulted. The treatment of choice for many of the enteric gram-negative bacteria is a third-generation cephalosporin such as cefotaxime. When treating a staphylococcal meningitis, the choice of drug depends on whether the organism is nonpenicillinase-producing, penicillinase-producing, or methicillin-resistant. In penicillin-allergic patients, cefotaxime or ceftriaxone are sometimes used, but such patients may also be allergic to cephalosporins. In this situation chloramphenicol may be used for initial treatment, but it may not be effective against enteric gram-negative bacilli or resistant pneumococci. Vancomycin plus rifampin can be used to treat pneumococcal or staphylococcal meningitis. When a patient with Listeria meningitis is allergic to penicillin, trimethoprim-sulfamethoxazole is the drug of choice. Antibiotics are generally given for 10 to 14 days, or for 10 days after the culture is sterile in gram-negative meningitis.

Appropriate therapy for associated infections or for complications of meningitis must also be given. In children, the early use of dexamethasone has been shown to decrease the incidence of hearing loss and other neurologic complications. Prolonged or recurrent fever in the patient who is receiving the correct antibiotic suggests subdural effusion, intercurrent hospital-acquired infection, or drug fever. Less commonly, it may signify the development of venous sinus thrombosis or brain abscess.

Household contacts of patients with Haemophilus influenzae or meningococcal meningitis should be treated with 4 days of rifampin (600 mg daily for adults and 20 mg/kg—maximum 600 mg—daily for children). Haemophilus influenzae type b vaccine, which should be ad-

TABLE 15–2. Treatment of Bacterial Meningitis

Infecting organism	Drug of first choice	Alternative drugs
Unknown (adults and children > 3 months old)	Cefotaxime or ceftriaxome	
Unknown (infants < 3 months old)	Ampicillin and cefotaxime with or without gentamicin	
Streptococcus pneumoniae	Penicillin G or V	An erythromycin, a cephalosporin, vancomycin, rifampin, trimethoprim-sulfamethoxazole, azithromycin, clarithromycin, clindamycin, chloramphenicol
Neisseria meningitidis	Penicillin G	Cefotaxime, ceftizoxime, ceftriaxone, chloramphenicol, a sulfonamide
Haemophilus influenzae	Cefotaxime or ceftriaxone	Chloramphenicol
Pseudomonas	Ceftazidime and an aminoglycoside (tobramycin, gentamicin, amikacin)	Imipenem, a fluoroquinolone
Listeria monocytogenes	Ampicillin with or without gentamicin	Trimethoprim-sulfamethoxazole
Staphylococcus aureus or epidermidis	Penicillin G or V	A cephalosporin, vancomycin, imipenem, clindamycin, a fluoroquinolone

ministered to children at the age of 2 years, will greatly reduce the risk of subsequent meningitis due to this organism. The vaccine should also be given to children 18 to 23 months old who are at increased risk of exposure to Haemophilus influenzae, including any child who attends a day-care center. Similarly, pneumococcal vaccine should be given to any patient at increased risk for pneumococcal infection and to all patients over 65 years who have chronic pulmonary or cardiac disease.

The course of untreated bacterial meningitis is one that invariably leads to death or severe, permanent neurologic sequelae. Even with treatment, the mortality of bacterial meningitis is 5% to 10% for haemophilus, 10% to 30% for meningococcus, and 20% to 40% for pneumococcus. The highest fatality rates are in very young and very old persons and in those infected with less common organisms. Among survivors, 5% to 30% have permanent neurologic residua—including sensorineural hearing loss, mental retardation, seizures, focal neurologic deficits, and hydrocephalus.

Brain Abscess

Most brain abscesses are due to spread of disease from paranasal sinuses, mastoid or middle ear; hematogenous spread from infection in the lungs or pleura; acute bacterial endocarditis; congenital heart disease with right-to-left shunt; or traumatic or neurosurgical penetrating wounds. Bacterial meningitis is only very rarely a cause of brain abscess. In about 20% of cases, the cause of brain abscess cannot be determined. The common organisms responsible for brain abscesses are anaerobic streptococci, bacteroides species, E coli, and proteus species. Generally, multiple organisms can be cultured. Staphylococcus aureus is usually the responsible organism following penetrating head injuries.

The patient with brain abscess may present with headache, drowsiness or confusion, focal or generalized seizures, or focal neurologic deficits. Although fever, signs of systemic infection, and leukocytosis may be present in the early cerebritis stage, these symptoms are often absent once a well-encapsulated abscess is formed. Intracranial pressure is often elevated, and there is a particular danger of cerebral herniation when LP is performed on a patient with brain abscess. Diagnosis is usually based on the appropriate clinical setting, together with CT evidence of a lucent lesion showing enhancement in a ringlike pattern after contrast injection. Abscesses are usually solitary but may be multiple.

The treatment of brain abscess due to unknown organisms is penicillin G (4 million units every 4 hours intravenously) and chloramphenicol (1.5 gm every 6 hours intravenously for at least 4 to 6 weeks). Antibiotics are adjusted accordingly if the organisms are known, or if there is a reason to suspect Staphylococcus aureus or some other organism not covered by this regimen. The patient is followed closely with serial neurologic examinations and serial CT head scans. If there is clinical deterioration or significant worsening of the CT picture, then surgical intervention will probably be required.

Immediate surgery, with pre- and postoperative antibiotics, is generally indicated for the patient with a large, easily accessible abscess; an abscess that is located where it may suddenly rupture into a ventricle; an impending herniation; or a mass effect sufficient to produce stupor or coma. In all patients, increased intracranial pressure should be treated, if present, and prophylactic anticonvulsant therapy (phenytoin) should be administered. Untreated brain abscess is almost always fatal. The mortality in patients with treated brain abscess is about 10%. Seizure disorders and focal neurologic deficits are found in about 30% of survivors.

Subdural Empyema

A subdural empyema is a collection of pus in the subdural space on one side, usually secondary to spread from sinus, mastoid, or middle ear infection. It is one fifth as common as brain abscess. The clinical presentation is one of headache and fever, progressing to decreasing level of consciousness and focal neurologic signs. Skull films typically show sinus or mastoid infection and may show osteomyelitis. CT head scan shows the empyema, and rules out brain abscess. The patient must have immediate surgical drainage. Penicillin G (4 million units every 5 hours intravenously) and chloramphenicol (1.5 gm every 6 hours intravenously) are started after pus is obtained. The therapy may be changed when the organism is identified and its sensitivities to antibiotics are determined. Many patients who are promptly treated have significant recovery of neurologic function.

Spinal Epidural Abscess

Spinal epidural abscess often presents as back or leg pain together with fever and malaise. Signs of meningeal irritation follow, and there is progressive spinal cord compression. The source of infection may not be obvious, although there may have been an infection of the skin or another part of the body days or weeks previously. The patient should have immediate myelography and spinal fluid examination to confirm the diagnosis and to rule out multiple sclerosis or transverse myelitis. Prompt surgical drainage combined with antibiotic therapy will maximize the recovery of spinal cord function.

Cerebral Thrombophlebitis (Septic Venous Sinus Thrombosis)

Thrombophlebitis of the large dural sinuses is generally due to extension from a local infection. Patients have headache and fever, together with symptoms and signs of systemic infection. Increased intracranial pressure may be present. Lateral sinus thrombophlebitis is associated with middle ear or mastoid infection and presents as headache and papilledema. Cavernous sinus thrombophlebitis is often associated with infection of either ethmoid, sphenoid, or maxillary sinuses or of the skin around the eyes or nose. The patient has orbital edema, chemosis, and ophthalmoplegia on the infected side. The signs often become bilateral as the infection spreads to the other cavernous sinus. Superior sagittal sinus thrombophlebitis presents as unilateral hemiparesis and focal seizures. Other focal signs may be present, and signs may become bilateral. Jugular venography or cerebral angiography are necessary for diagnosis of lateral or superior sagittal sinus thrombophlebitis, while the diagnosis of cavernous sinus thrombophlebitis is usually made clinically. The therapy of septic thrombophlebitis includes antibiotics effective against Staphylococcus aureus and gram-negative rods. Associated meningitis, brain abscess, or subdural empyema must be diagnosed and treated.

OTHER INFECTIONS OF THE NERVOUS SYSTEM

Tuberculosis

Tuberculous (TB) meningitis occurs in patients of all ages. Untreated, it is invariably fatal. Headache, malaise, drowsiness or confusion, and fever with stiff neck evolve over a week or longer. Cranial nerve palsies, signs of focal cerebral involvement or increased intracranial pressure, or seizures may become apparent. The tuberculin test may be negative, the CBC is often normal, and erythrocyte sedimentation rate may be unremarkable. The classic CSF findings are elevated opening pressure, lymphocytic pleocytosis (generally 100 to 500 cells), elevated protein (generally 100 to 500 mg/dl), and depressed glucose (less than 45 mg/dl). There may be a polymorphonuclear predominance early in the course, and CSF glucose may be normal. Acid fast bacilli (AFB) may be visible on the stained CSF sediment, particularly if CSF from four consecutive spinal taps is examined. Centrifuged sediment from at least 10 ml of CSF should be used for the AFB stain. CSF culture for TB is positive in about 80% of cases. CT brain scan is positive in about 80% of cases and may show basilar meningitis, secondary hydrocephalus, infarct, or tuberculomas.

The differential diagnosis of TB meningitis includes other infectious and noninfectious causes of the syndrome of chronic meningitis (fever, headache, stiff neck, confusion, altered level of consciousness, seizures, focal neurologic signs, and CSF abnormalities, developing in a subacute or chronic fashion and persisting for at least 4 weeks). Fungal meningitis, neurosyphilis, Lyme disease, toxoplasmosis, cysticercosis, carcinomatous meningitis, sarcoidosis, and vasculitis can all present in this fashion.

Therapy should be initiated as soon as the presumptive diagnosis of TB meningitis is made. Waiting 4 to 6 weeks for confirmation by culture may lead to irreversible neurologic abnormalities. The adult patient should be treated orally with 3 drugs for 9 months and 6 months after culture conversion. Isoniazid (300 mg per day), rifampin (600 mg per day), and ethambutol (15 mg/kg per day) are recommended. Pyridoxine (50 mg per day) should be administered in conjunction with INH. Tuberculomas generally respond well to this antituberculous therapy but may require surgical intervention. The recent rising incidence of drug resistance, which is often due to poor compliance, has led to the suggestion that patients take their medication under direct observation.

Hydrocephalus often requires shunt placement. Seizures need to be treated with anticonvulsants. Corticosteroids (prednisone, 60 mg per day) should probably be given in conjunction with antituberculous therapy in cases with impending subarachnoid block or cerebral edema.

The mortality and morbidity of TB meningitis are greatest in very young and very old patients, in patients with longer duration of illness and more prominent neurologic signs at the time of treatment initiation, and in those with severe basilar meningitis on CT scan. Thus, as for bacterial meningitis, therapy is most likely to be successful if instituted early.

Cryptococcosis

Cryptococcal meningitis most commonly presents as headache and stiff neck. Fever, changes in mental status, seizures, or ocular signs may be present. Rarely, the disease presents as dementia, hydrocephalus, or a focal neurologic deficit. It is generally slowly progressive over weeks. Cryptococcus may also produce single or multiple brain abscesses or granulomas, alone or in association with meningitis. About 50% of cases are associated with underlying disease, especially with disorders of the lymphoreticular system or AIDS. Many patients have antecedent or concurrent cryptococcal pulmonary infections. The CSF picture is similar to that seen in TB meningitis, and repeated LPs may be required to make the diagnosis. India ink stain demonstrates the organism about 60% of the time, and fungal cultures are positive in about 75% of cases. Spinal fluid cryptococcal antigen is positive in about 90% of cases. The treatment of cryptococcal meningitis is generally 6 weeks of amphotericin B, (0.3 to 0.5 mg/kg per day intravenously) together with 5-fluorocytosine (150 mg/kg per day orally in 4 divided doses). Over 50% of patients are cured or significantly improved with this regimen, although relapses have been a problem in AIDS patients.

Coccidioidomycosis

The patient with meningitis due to Coccidioides immitis usually has headache, stiff neck, and fever. Personality change and other mental status abnormalities may be present. There is generally a history of travel in an endemic area, and there may be evidence of infection of other organ systems. The spinal fluid picture is similar to that of the patient with TB meningitis. Complement-fixing antibody to Coccidiodes immitis is present in the spinal fluid in 95% of cases. CSF cultures are positive in one third of cases. This organism rarely produces mass lesions but may cause secondary hydrocephalus because of blockage of normal spinal fluid flow. Amphotericin B should be administered intravenously in doses increasing to 40 to 60 mg daily or every other day, depending on patient tolerance and renal function. Serum BUN, creatinine, and potassium levels must be followed closely. Additionally, amphotericin should be given intrathecally 3 times weekly in a dose gradually increased to 0.1 to 0.5 mg, depending on location of infection and patient tolerance of therapy. Intrathecal amphotericin is administered either by an Ommaya reservoir that has been inserted into a lateral ventricle, by LP with barbotage, or by repeated cisternal punctures. The initial course of intravenous therapy is generally to a total dose of 0.5 to 1 gram. The duration of intrathecal therapy is generally guided by the clinical and CSF picture, including cellular and serologic responses. The total intrathecal dose is often 20 to 25 mg. Hydrocortisone (25 mg intravenously) may be given simultaneously to prevent local adverse reactions. Coccidiodal meningitis is frequently fatal, and intermittent treatment must often be given for the lifetime of the patient. Recently oral fluconazole (400 mg once a day for up to 4 years) has been shown to be quite effective, eliminating the need for intrathecal therapy. Unfortunately, not all patients respond to this drug.

Other Fungal Infections

Numerous other fungal disease, including mucormycosis, candidiasis, aspergillosis, histoplasmosis, and blastomycosis may involve the CNS. Several of these are particularly common in immunocompromised patients. The clinical and CSF pictures may be similar to those of TB, cryptococcal, and coccidioidal brain infections. Diagnosis is usually made by CSF culture. Amphotericin B is the treatment of choice for these infections.

Neurosyphilis

There are five classic presentations of neurosyphilis. Except as noted, they all have the CSF picture of aseptic meningitis, a positive VDRL in serum and CSF, and a positive FTA antibody test (FTA-ABS) in blood. Asymptomatic neurosyphilis is associated with absent symptoms or signs, together with CSF pleocytosis and/or positive CSF VDRL. Meningeal syphilis usually occurs within 2 years of the initial infection. The presentation is of an afebrile patient with headache, stiff neck, and on occasion cranial neuropathies. Seizures, confusion, and signs of increased intracranial pressure may also occur. Meningovascular syphilis presents as a stroke, often in the territory of the middle cerebral artery. It generally occurs 7 years after the primary infection but may occur at any time. Tabes dorsalis usually presents 15 to 20 years after initial infection with lightning pains, particularly in the legs; visceral crises; areflexia and loss of position and vibration sense in the legs; sensory ataxia; urinary incontinence; and pupillary abnormalities, especially Argyll-Robertson pupils. CSF abnormalities may be minimal. General paresis generally occurs 10 to 15 years after the primary infection. It presents as a progressive dementia, often accompanied by significant psychiatric symptoms. Seizures occur in half of these patients.

Atypical forms of neurosyphilis have become increasingly common in recent years, probably because of inadequately treated primary infections. For this reason, it is suggested that the diagnosis of presumptive neurosyphilis be made in patients who meet any of the following criteria: (1) positive blood FTA-ABS and one of the classic clinical pictures of neurosyphilis; (2) positive blood FTA-ABS, any degree of CSF pleocytosis, and no evidence of other infectious cause of meningitis; and (3) positive blood FTA-ABS, unexplained progressive neurologic disease, and a clinical or CSF response to penicillin therapy.

The treatment of neurosyphilis is aqueous crystalline penicillin G (4 million units intravenously every 4 hours for 10 days) or a 10-day course of aqueous procaine penicillin G (2.4 million units intramuscularly daily) plus oral probenecid (500 mg 4 times daily). Both of these regimens should be followed by benzathine penicillin G (2.4 million units intramuscularly weekly for 3 doses). Tetracycline, (500 mg orally 4 times a day) should be administered for 30 days to penicillin-allergic patients. The CSF should be checked every 6 months until it is normal or there is only a mild elevation of protein. The patient should be retreated if pleocytosis persists at any of these spinal taps.

The chance of arresting the progression of neurosyphilis is best when the patient is treated early. Asymptomatic, meningeal, and meningovascular syphilis have the best prognosis for recovery. Tabes dorsalis and general paresis patients may improve with therapy but are more likely to have persistent or even progressive neurologic deficits.

Lyme Disease

Lyme disease, a multisystem infection, is transmitted by ixodid ticks and caused by a spirochete, Borrelia burgdorferi. Several different species of this spirochete have been identified, which probably explains why the disease is usually much milder in Europe. It occurs primarily in endemic areas. Transmission of infection is unlikely unless the tick attachment persists for 48 hours. The disease usually presents as rash (erythema chronicum migrans) and nonspecific influenzalike symptoms, followed in weeks to months by arthritis, cardiac disease, and/or nervous system disease. Lyme disease may present neurologically as meningoencephalitis, peripheral neuropathy, polymyositis, cranial neuropathy (almost always involving the seventh cranial nerve), MS-like disease, transverse myelitis, and psychiatric disease. In CNS infection the CSF usually contains a lymphocytic pleocytosis, mildly elevated protein, and normal glucose. Plasma cells may be present. It is almost impossible to culture the spirochete from the spinal fluid. The best chance of isolating the organism is from skin biopsy at the edge of the expanding primary skin lesion (erythema migrans). Serum antibody titers to the spirochete often confirm the diagnosis but are usually not detectable until 4 to 6 weeks after the infection. Seronegativity occurs in some patients with proven diagnosis. Patients with neurologic manifestations of Lyme disease should be treated with ceftriaxone (2 gm daily intravenously) or penicillin G (4 million units intravenously every 4 hours) for 10 days. Mild neurologic manifestations, such as Bell's palsy, may be treated with doxycycline (100 mg twice a day) or amoxicillin (250 to 500 mg by mouth 3 times a day) for 10 days.

A post-Lyme syndrome has been reported. It is unclear if this represents a persistent infection or a postinfectious, immune-mediated process. The diagnosis requires that symptoms are chronic or intermittent, that they started at the time of the primary disease, and that they persist even though antibiotic treatment was administered. The most common presentations are cognitive impairment (encephalopathy), fatigue and malaise, joint and muscle pains, and headache. The currently recommended treatment is with antibiotics for 10 to 14 days. It has not been established that this treatment is effective.

Toxoplasmosis

Acquired toxoplasmosis is especially common in immunosuppressed patients. The patient may present with confusion and depressed level of consciousness, sometimes with associated seizures; headache and stiff neck, sometimes with focal neurologic signs and seizures; or focal signs due to one or more intracerebral mass lesions. The spinal fluid can be normal but usually shows a lymphocytic pleocytosis with elevated protein and normal glucose. CT brain scan may show multiple ring-enhancing lesions. Serologic tests are frequently positive, and the organism is sometimes identified in spinal fluid. Brain biopsy to establish a diagnosis is generally required if the patient does not respond to therapy within 7 to 10 days. Patients with a definite or presumptive diagnosis of CNS toxoplasmosis should be treated for at least 4 weeks with sulfadiazine (2 to 6 gm daily) and pyrimethamine (25 mg daily). Leucovorin (10 mg daily) counteracts the hematologic toxicity of pyrimethamine. Relapses will occur in 30% of patients. The mortality of acquired CNS toxoplasmosis is 70%, primarily because of the severity of the underlying systemic diseases.

Cysticercosis

CNS infections with the larval form of the pork tapeworm are particularly common in persons from Latin America and Southeast Asia. Seizures, increased intracranial pressure, and stroke are the most frequently seen presentations. The CSF may be normal or may show lymphocytic pleocytosis, elevated protein, and depressed or normal glucose. Serologic tests of serum of CSF are helpful in establishing the diagnosis. The CT scan often shows multiple, nonenhancing intracerebral calcified and noncalcified lesions and/or cysts. Less frequently, contrast-enhancing lesions or evidence of hydrocephalus are found. Seizures are generally well controlled with anticonvulsant therapy, and hydrocephalus responds to ventricular shunting. Patients with CT scan showing only parenchymal calcifications and/or hydrocephalus due to meningeal fibrosis have inactive disease and require no further treatment except possibly shunting. Patients with evidence of arachnoiditis; hydrocephalus due to active meningeal inflammation, parenchymal, intraventricular or spinal cysts; stroke due to vasculitis; or mass effect have active disease. These patients should be treated with praziquantel (50 mg/kg daily in 3 divided doses for 2 weeks). Corticosteroids should be given for several days before and during this therapy. Most patients will have transient worsening of neurologic symptoms and signs at the onset of therapy, but a favorable response to the course of treatment is generally seen. Seizures present prior to treatment with praziquantel continue in many patients, requiring long-term anticonvulsant therapy.

The clinical presentation of CNS schistosomiasis is similar to that seen with cysticercosis. Rarely, the ova may cause necrotizing foci in the brain and spinal cord. Treatment is with praziquantel.

Leprosy

Leprosy is transmitted by intimate and prolonged direct contact. After an incubation period of many years, the patient develops skin lesions and multiple mononeuropathy. Nerves may be enlarged, and there may be attacks of neuralgic pain as a nerve becomes infected. There is a predilection for involvement of distal nerves, and the multiple mononeuropathies often become confluent. This may produce a clinical picture of distal, predominantly sensory polyneuropathy. Severe trophic changes occur, and there may be distal ulcers, infections, or loss of digits. The diagnosis is made clinically and is often confirmed by the demonstration of the acid fast bacilli in skin or peripheral nerve specimens. The nerve disease is often slowly progressive when untreated, and the clinical course may be significantly improved with therapy. The patient should be given dapsone (100 mg daily) for 4 or more years, together with rifampin (600 mg daily) for 6 months or longer. A third antileprosy drug is sometimes added to this regimen. The duration of treatment depends on the clinical form of the disease and on the response to therapy.

INFECTIONS IN IMMUNOCOMPROMISED PATIENTS

Patients with compromised immune systems have increased susceptibility to CNS infections and have poorer outcomes when they develop such infections. Four types of immune system defects predispose the patient to different CNS infections. Defective cell-mediated immunity occurs in patients with organ transplants, lymphomas, chronic corticosteroid therapy, and AIDS. These patients are particularly likely to develop meningitis due to listeria, tuberculosis, cryptococcus and coccidioides immitis; encephalitis or meningoencephalitis due to varicella-zoster virus, listeria, cryptococcus and toxoplasmosis; progressive multifocal leukoencephalopathy; or brain abscess due to listeria, cryptococcus, aspergillus, mucor, nocardia, and toxoplasmosis.

Defective humeral immunity is seen in patients with chronic lymphocytic leukemia, multiple myeloma, and Hodgkin's disease. These patients are particularly susceptible to bacterial meningitis caused by pneumococcus, haemophilus, and menigococcus and to chronic meningoencephalitis from enterovirus infection. Patients with decreased numbers of neutrophils due to acute leukemia, aplastic anemia, or cytotoxic chemotherapy are susceptible to meningitis or meningoencephalitis caused by Pseudomonas, E coli, klebsiella, proteus, and candida; and to brain abscess produced by aspergillus, mucor, and candida. In general, the increased risk of infection is present with neutrophil counts below 1000 cells per cubic mm and is greatest with counts below 100 cells per cubic mm. Patients with defective splenic function caused by surgery, disease, or radiotherapy have an increased risk of developing meningitis due to pneumococcus, haemophilus, and meningococcus.

The immunocompromised patient with a CNS infection may initially show little clinical indication of an inflammatory response. Moreover, serologic tests that detect host antibodies to infecting organisms are often negative, and CSF and CT brain scan abnormalities may be delayed in their appearance. For this reason, immunocompromised patients with unexplained headache, fever, meningeal signs, decreased level of consciousness, or focal neurologic deficit must be immediately evaluated. If there is any possibility of CNS infection, a CT brain scan and CSF exam must be performed. When the diagnosis of presumed

CNS infection is made, treatment must begin promptly in order to offer the patient the best chance of significant recovery.

REFERENCES

Rowland LP (ed): Merritt's Textbook of Neurology, 7th ed. Philadelphia, Lea and Febiger, 1984.

Adams RD, Victor M: Principles of Neurology, 3rd ed. New York, McGraw-Hill, 1985.

Symposium on infections of the central nervous system: Medical Clinics of North America, 1985; 69:No.2.

Infectious diseases of the central nervous system: Neurol Clin, 1986;4:No.1.

Kieburtz K, Schiffer RB: Neurologic manifestations of human immunodeficiency virus infections. Neurol Clin 1989; 7(3):447–468.

Leehey M, Gilden D: Neurologic disorders associated with the HIV and HIV-1 viruses. *In* Current Neurology vol 10. Chicago: Year Book Medical Publishers, 1990, pp 1–63.

Tunkel AR, Wispelwey B, Scheld WM: Bacterial meningitis: Recent advances in pathophysiology and treatment. Ann Intern Med 1990; 1128(8):610–623.

Whitley RJ: Viral encephalitis. N Engl J Med 1990; 323(4):242–250.

Working Group of the American Academy of Neurology Aids Task Force: Nomenclature and research case definitions for neurologic manifestations of human immunodeficiency virus-type 1 (HIV-1) infection. Neurology 1991; 41:778–785.

Treatment of Lyme disease: Med Lett Drugs Ther 1992; 34(881):95–97.

The choice of antibacterial drugs: Med Lett Drugs Ther 1992; 34(871):49–56.

Drugs for AIDS and associated infections: Med Lett Drugs Ther 1993; 35(904):79–86.

Drugs for non-HIV viral infections: Med Lett Drugs Ther 1994; 36(919):27–32.

The choice of antibacterial drugs: Med Lett Drugs Ther 1994; 36(925):53–60.

16
Dizziness and Vertigo

The word *dizzy* derives from eddy, whirl. Dictionaries define *dizziness* as feeling giddy or unsteady, confused, bewildered, silly, and foolish. *Vertigo* is defined as a subjective sensation of dizziness in which an individual feels that he or she (or the surroundings) is whirling about sickeningly. Dizziness is the third most frequent complaint encountered in general clinical practice. Over 50% of the elderly are affected by dizziness and problems with balance at one time or another. Dizziness refers to the nonspecific and nonlocalizing complaints of light-headedness, faintness, giddiness, floating, swaying, or disorientation. Dizziness is not associated with specific signs. Many patients will also complain of dizziness when they have vertigo. Vertigo refers to any illusion of movement. This includes rotation of the environment about the subject, rotation of the subject, linear translation of subject or environment, and tilting or oscillation of the environment (oscillopsia). Vertigo is frequently associated with nystagmus and ataxia.

Dizziness may occur spontaneously without any precipitating event, only when the patient is moving, in certain positions (e.g., tilting the head back), or with increasing or decreasing barometric pressure. It may be acute, recurrent, or chronic. Vertigo is usually intermittent, precipitated or worsened by certain positions or movements, and often accompanied by nausea and vomiting.

Vision, hearing, vestibular activity, proprioception, and exteroception all orient a person about body position in space and body motion. These systems do not function independently but are interactive, and motion is guided by input from all. Impaired function of one system can be compensated for by another system to some degree. Any disturbance of function of sensory receptors (eye, ear, peripheral nerves), their connections to and within the CNS, and their respective CNS structures will lead to a mismatch between different, simultaneous inputs or inappropriate processing within the CNS and may produce the sensation of dizziness or vertigo or both. Thus, a great number of abnormalities may be accompanied by the complaint of dizziness and must be considered in the differential diagnosis and the work-up of a patient. Not infrequently, more than one sensory system is impaired in its functions, compounding a patient's problem.

The vestibular system is designed to detect angular and linear motion. The three semicircular canals respond to angular acceleration and the two otolith organs (utricle and saccule) to linear acceleration. Thus, disturbance of semicircular function may result in rotatory vertigo, whereas otolith dysfunction may be accompanied by a sensation of linear movement.

Most causes of dizziness and vertigo fall into one of the following categories: systemic disease, peripheral vestibular disease, or central vestibular disease. Systemic diseases tend to cause dizziness. Peripheral and central vestibular diseases tend to cause vertigo. There are exceptions, and diseases that cause vertigo may cause dizziness as well. Several specific questions need to be addressed when dealing with a dizzy patient. Is the problem related to end organ dysfunction (eye, ear, peripheral receptors), connections from receptor to the CNS (nerves), or CNS pathways and structures (central integrator)? Is the dysfunction the result of a primary insult, or is it secondary to a systemic or generalized disturbance? Some systemic causes of dizziness are listed in Table 16–1, peripheral causes of vertigo in Table 16–2, and central causes in Table 16–3.

HISTORY

The history should distinguish whether dizziness, vertigo, or both are occurring. Dizziness that occurs by itself may result from any number of systemic problems. This is usually not a primary neurologic problem but does require a neurologic examination. If there are no neurologic symptoms and no neurologic signs, a CT or MR scan, EEG, and further neurologic work-up are usually not required.

Vertigo is a neurologic symptom that always requires neurologic examination and work-up. Vertigo that occurs in isolation is frequently caused by peripheral vestibular problems. Unilateral deafness or tinnitus associated with vertigo usually indicates peripheral vestibular or eighth-nerve problems. Peripheral vertigo usually occurs in discrete or recurrent episodes but is rarely chronic. Severe vertigo associated with nausea and vomiting suggests a peripheral vestibular problem or cerebellar hemorrhage or infarction. Vertigo caused by loud noises, changes of barometric pressure, or increased pressure in the ear is usually due

TABLE 16–1. Systemic Causes of Dizziness

Drugs
  Sedatives
  Hypnotics
  Salicylates
  Anticonvulsants
  Tranquilizers
  Antihypertensives
  Diuretics
  Analgesics
  Ethanol
Decreased cardiac output
  Congestive heart failure
  Cardiomyopathy
  Valvular disease
  Constructive pericarditis
  Pulmonary hypertension
  Arrhythmias
Postural hypotension
Hyperventilation syndrome
Diabetes—hypoglycemia, hyperglycemia
Hypertension
Multiple sensory deficits
Dizziness of elderly
Hematological abnormalities
  Anemia
  Polycythemia
  Leukemia
  Paraproteinemias
Cervical osteoarthritis
Electrolyte abnormalities
Hepatic disease
Renal disease
Cancer
Collagen vascular disease
Chronic infection, meningitis
Hypothyroidism, hyperthyroidism
Eye problems (cornea, lens, retina)
Others (sarcoid, toxins, vitamin deficiencies)
Psychogenic disorders

to an inner ear fistula and is therefore peripheral. Vertigo precipitated by changes of head position (positional vertigo) can have peripheral or central etiology. Patients with oscillopsia complain that the horizon is unsteady and may not complain of spinning sensations. Oscillopsia is usually due to bilateral symmetrical peripheral vestibular disease—frequently from ototoxic drugs, metabolic problems, and otosclerosis, as well as other disorders that affect both labyrinths.

TABLE 16–2. Peripheral Causes of Vertigo

Acute labyrinthitis (presumed viral)
Recurrent labyrinthitis
Autoimmune vestibulopathy
Posttraumatic vertigo
    Perilymph fistula
    CSF leak
    Inner ear concussion
    Inner ear hemorrhage
    Eighth-nerve trauma
    Temporal bone fracture
Menière's disease
Benign paroxysmal positional vertigo
Microvascular compression syndrome
Dizziness of the elderly
Vestibulotoxic drugs
Ear disease
    Acute and chronic otitis media
    Otosclerosis
    Tumors of the inner and middle ear
    Eustachian tube dysfunction (infection)
    Cupulolithiasis
    Otolithiasis
Internal auditory artery occlusion
    Atherosclerotic
    Vasculitis
    Sinusitis, dental abscesses
Acoustic neuroma
Cerumen, foreign objects in external auditory canal
Motion sickness

Patients with central vestibular symptoms may have isolated instances of vertigo, or the complaints may be chronic or recurrent. Vertigo associated with brainstem symptoms or signs indicates central vestibular disease. Diplopia, visual field changes, dysarthria, focal weakness, focal numbness, dysphagia, or other focal symptoms indicate central disease. Alterations of consciousness, lethargy, or coma associated with vertigo always suggest central brain disease but may occur with metabolic (e.g. thyroid) or toxic (drugs, poisons) systemic disorders. Symptoms and signs of peripheral and central vestibular disorders are compared in Table 16–4.

Systemic diseases usually cause dizziness but not vertigo. Symptoms of dizziness may be intermittent or chronic. Virtually any medical, environmental, or psychic factor can cause patients to feel light-headed or dizzy. If dizziness is a persistent or aggravating problem, the following should be evaluated: drugs, toxic exposure, environmental situation,

TABLE 16-3. Central Causes of Vertigo

Vascular disease
  Microvascular compression syndrome
  TIAs of the vertebrobasilar system
  Strokes of posterior circulation
  Cerebellar hemorrhage
  Cerebellar infarction
  Subclavian steal syndrome
  Arteriovenous malformation
  Aneurysm
  Vasculitis

Posterior fossa lesions
  Primary brain tumor
  Ependymoma
  Metastasis
  Subdural hematoma
  Temporal bone cyst
  Hydrocephalus
  Syringobulbia
  Platybasia
  Arnold-Chiari syndrome

Basilar artery migraine

Demyelinating disease
  Multiple sclerosis
  Postinfectious demyelination
  Progressive multifocal leukoencephalopathy

Degenerative disease
  Friedreich's ataxia
  Olivopontocerebellar degeneration
  Ophthalmoplegia plus syndrome
  Refsum's disease

Temporal lobe epilepsy
  Vestibulogenic reflex epilepsy

Cranial neuropathies affecting the eighth nerve
  Sarcoid
  Cancer (meningeal carcinomatosis)
  Sjögren's syndrome, Vogt-Koyanagi-Harada syndrome
  Guillain-Barré syndrome
  Paget's disease
  Osteopetrosis

Infections
  Meningitis
  Syphilis
  Lyme disease
  Herpes zoster (Ramsay Hunt)
  Abscess—parenchymal, epidural, subdural

Trauma

---

head or ear trauma, hyperventilation, hypertension, cardiovascular disease, peripheral vascular disease, seizures, cervical disease, associated central or peripheral nervous system disease, infections, endocrine disorders including diabetes, electrolyte disorders, renal disease, hepatic

TABLE 16–4. Symptoms and Signs That May Distinguish Peripheral from Central Vestibular Dysfunction

Symptom or sign	Peripheral	Central
Direction of nystagmus	Mainly unidirectional	Bi- or unidirectional
Hallucination of movement	Definite	Less definite
Severity of vertigo	Marked	Mild
Autonomic nervous system symptoms	Definite	Less definite
Direction of falling	Toward slow phase	Variable
Influenced by head position	Frequent	Seldom
Effect of head turning	Present	No effect
Vertical nystagmus	Never present	May be present
Disturbance of consciousness	Rare	May be present
Duration of symptoms	Finite	Often chronic
Tinnitus or deafness	Often	Usually absent
Other neurological signs	Usually absent	Frequently present
Common causes	Labyrinthitis, positional vertigo, trauma	Vascular, MS, tumor

disease, hematologic disorders, pulmonary dysfunction, collagen vascular disease, cancer, and psychiatric disease. A very frequent complaint is dizziness on standing or getting up in the morning. Medications that produce orthostatic hypotension are a frequent cause of this problem. Causes of postural hypotension are listed in Table 16–5.

EXAMINATION

It is important to examine the heart and peripheral vascular system to determine specific causes of dizziness and vertigo. Arrhythmias and hypersensitive carotid sinuses cause abrupt onset of dizziness, vertigo, and syncope due to altered cerebral blood flow. Postural hypotension is a frequent medical problem; patients complain of dizziness and/or vertigo on standing or stooping. Hyperventilation may reproduce a patient's dizziness, but in the majority of these patients it is not the primary cause of their dizziness.

A neurologic examination should be performed on all patients, because almost any neurologic deficit can contribute to dizziness or postural instability. Hearing should be tested routinely, since it often accompanies peripheral dizziness. Because of the high prevalence of hearing loss in the elderly, asymmetrical hearing loss should be evaluated by audiometry. Any hearing loss in younger patients also requires

TABLE 16–5. Causes of Postural Hypotension

Antihypertensive medications
Diuretics
Antiarrhythmia drugs
Dehydration
Peripheral autonomic dysfunction
    Diabetes
    Guillain-Barré Syndrome
    Amyloidosis
    Familial dysautonomia
Central autonomic dysfunction
    Shy-Drager syndrome
    Hypothalamic disease
Peripheral venous disease
Central venous disease
Impaired cardiac output
    Aortic stenosis
    Constrictive pericarditis
    Congestive heart failure
    Atrial myxoma
Toxins
Idiopathic orthostatic hypotension

audiometry. Ear canals should be inspected, since wax impaction or foreign bodies can cause dizziness and vertigo.

Nystagmus is a rhythmic movement of the eyes with the fast component in one direction and the slow component in the other. The direction of nystagmus is named for the direction of the fast phase of the eye movements. The presence of nystagmus suggests peripheral or central vestibular disease and is only rarely pathognomonic of a particular disorder. Most systemic disturbances that cause dizziness do not cause nystagmus, with the exception of drugs, particularly analgesics, sedatives, stimulants, and anticonvulsants. In destructive peripheral vestibular disorders the slow phase occurs toward the lesioned labyrinth and the fast phase away from it. In central disorders, the slow phase may occur toward the lesioned or intact side.

There are two clinically relevant types of nystagmus: spontaneous and positional. In order to see spontaneous nystagmus, it is often necessary to remove fixation. This step can be accomplished by placing Frenzel glasses, which are magnifying glasses, in front of the patient's eyes or by ophthalmoscopy. The type of nystagmus present is often useful in distinguishing peripheral from central vestibular disorders. Vertical nystagmus, which is either primarily upbeating or downbeating, always suggests central disorders. Nystagmus, which is present in primary gaze that spontaneously changes direction or which changes direction when the direction of gaze changes, also suggests central disease. Prominent coarse nystagmus not associated with vertigo also suggests central disease. Nystagmus or vertigo of central origin is usually associated with other focal neurologic symptoms or signs.

Rotary nystagmus is usually associated with peripheral vestibular disorders. Unidirectional nystagmus, which is most prominent when looking away from the lesion, is commonly found in peripheral vestibular disorders. An acute destructive lesion of one labyrinth produces nystagmus to the opposite side, an illusion of movement opposite to the side of the lesion, with a tendency to fall and past-point to the side of the lesion. In peripheral vestibular disorders other focal neurologic signs are not present, with the exception of hearing loss. Nystagmus tends to parallel vertigo and is usually partially suppressed by visual fixation in peripheral vestibular disorders. Positional nystagmus and vertigo are most common in peripheral vestibular disorders but occur in central disease as well.

Several clinical tests are helpful in detecting peripheral and central vestibular lesions. In the head-shaking test the examiner or the patient rapidly moves the patient's head back and forth as fast as can be tolerated for about 20 cycles. When the head is stopped, the normal person does not have nystagmus. Patients with unilateral vestibular paresis may have nystagmus, which usually beats toward the normal ear. Positional nystagmus can be assessed using the Barany and Hallpike maneuvers. The patient is seated with the head turned to the right and then quickly placed in the supine position with the head 30 degrees below the horizontal. The procedure is repeated with the head straight ahead and then to the left. The position change needs to be accomplished within about 2 seconds. In each position the patient is observed for about 10 to 15 seconds. A normal response is no nystagmus or vertigo. In peripheral labyrinthine disorders there is generally a latency of 5 to 10 seconds followed by rotatory or horizontal nystagmus, and repetition produces fatigue of the response. The findings in central versus peripheral positional vertigo are listed in Table 16–6.

Caloric examination is particularly useful in comatose patients and in distinguishing peripheral from central vestibular disorders in awake patients. In the awake patient 0.2 to 0.5 ml of ice water (50 ml is needed in the comatose patient) is injected into the external ear canal; the patient's head is positioned 30 degrees above the horizontal, and the ear canals are checked to ensure that they are clear of wax and that the eardrums are not perforated. The time of onset and duration and direction of nystagmus are noted. After 5 minutes the procedure is repeated in the other ear. The normal response is nystagmus toward the opposite side of stimulation. Subtle amounts of vestibular paresis will

TABLE 16–6. Features of Positional Nystagmus That Help Distinguish Peripheral from Central Vestibular Causes

Feature	Peripheral	Central
Latency	2–40 seconds	None
Fatigability	Yes	No
Habituation	Yes	No
Intensity of vertigo	Severe	Mild
Reproducibility	Poor	Good

not be detected by this test. Nystagmus after caloric irrigation is seen only in awake patients. Absence of response is indicative of vestibular loss.

Other, more elaborate tests to evaluate vestibular function are available. These include electronystagmography (ENG), rotatory tests, electrocochleography (ECochG), and moving platform posturography. Currently available tests are unable to detect lesions of the otoliths or vertical semicircular canals. In addition, brainstem auditory evoked potentials (BAER) and gadolinium-enhanced MR scan are valuable in evaluating patients. A patient's specific problem will dictate what other tests to use.

SYSTEMIC CAUSES OF DIZZINESS

Many systemic diseases give rise to dizziness but not vertigo. Most systemic causes of dizziness can be diagnosed by history, examination, and laboratory tests. It is important to emphasize that patients with hypothyroidism may present with bilateral decreased hearing, gait ataxia, dementia, psychosis, coma, peripheral neuropathy, and myopathy. Systemic disorders may exacerbate or make apparent preexisting peripheral or central vestibular disease. Although systemic diseases usually cause dizziness, they may cause vertigo if decreased brain blood flow and ischemia occur. Some systemic disorders may only be apparent while the patient is dizzy. It is therefore helpful to examine patients when they are dizzy for cardiac arrhythmias, postural hypotension, episodic hypertension due to a carcinoid, hypoglycemia, episodic hypercapnea, and other conditions. It is important to determine whether symptoms have an abrupt onset (arrhythmia, TIA, seizure) or are related to posture, exercise, meals, environment, anxiety, hyperventilation, or drugs. Psychogenic disease and dizziness of the elderly are usually diagnoses of exclusion.

PERIPHERAL CAUSES OF VERTIGO

Disorders that affect the labyrinth or the extracranial portion of the eighth nerve are often referred to as peripheral causes of vertigo. Because the eighth nerve contains cochlear and vestibular fibers, and because the cochlea and labyrinth are adjacent in the temporal bone, peripheral vestibular disorders commonly have auditory symptoms and signs.

TREATMENT

Nonspecific dizziness often is not amenable to specific treatment unless an underlying systemic disorder can be successfully corrected. Explanation, a supportive attitude, and acceptance by the patient are frequently the only helpful means of management.

In dealing with a patient with vertigo, vegetative symptoms (nausea, vomiting, malaise) and distress from abnormal sensory function (motion-induced vertigo, imbalance, oscillopsia) need to be addressed. Unfortunately, measures to alleviate the vegetative symptoms, such as medication and bed rest, may delay the development of compensation for the vestibular deficit. The optimal approach is to use early ambulation and as little medication as possible. Anticholinergic drugs, such as scopolamine, prevent motion sickness but are ineffective in treating acute vestibular disorders. Promethazine and prochlorperazine suppress vomiting but not vertigo. Drugs such as diazepam sedate both the vestibular system and the patient. Any medication that is harmless can be used for its placebo effect. Management of permanent vestibular deficits is very difficult. Drug therapy is not useful because it suppresses more function in the face of function already lost. Formal vestibular rehabilitation programs may be tried to keep the patient active.

Surgical treatment of benign positional vertigo consists of cutting the nerve to the posterior semicircular canal. This procedure fails if the diagnosis is wrong and if the specific nerve is not properly identified. It may also be accompanied by significant hearing loss.

BENIGN PAROXYSMAL POSITIONAL VERTIGO

Benign positional vertigo is a syndrome, not a disease, that can be caused by several inner ear diseases. Positional vertigo, sometimes also seen with CNS disease, is the most common cause of vertigo in the elderly. Patients typically have brief (less than 30 seconds) episodes of vertigo when turning over in bed, getting in and out of bed, extending the neck, or bending over and straightening out. On the Hallpike maneuver a typical upbeat and torsional nystagmus develops and quickly fatigues. In some patients basophilic deposits, probably otoconia from a degenerating utricular macule, have been demonstrated on the cupula of the posterior circular canal. The syndrome may also be related to head trauma. It may be mild or severe and have slow or abrupt onset. Lasting days, weeks, or occasionally months, it virtually always improves, but there are recurrences. Drugs are not useful in treating this condition because a single episode is very brief. Positional exercises are effective in the majority of cases. The patient is instructed to sit on the edge of a bed and then rapidly to assume a lateral position to induce vertigo. After the vertigo subsides, the patient sits up again. This sequence is repeated until the vertigo is fatigued. Patients should have 3 sessions a day until vertigo no longer occurs or they learn to tolerate the symptoms. Recently, a "liberatory maneuver" has been proposed. This maneuver assumes that otoconia can be moved out of the posterior semicircular canal into the vestibule. A major drawback of this procedure is that patients have to remain upright for 72 hours after the maneuver.

ACUTE LABYRINTHITIS

In 20% of infants born deaf the cause is thought to be a congenital viral infection. Sudden deafness in children and adults is also thought to result from a viral infection in many cases. Vertigo, nausea, and vomiting without any neurologic or auditory symptoms usually develop over several hours. This syndrome is presumed to be of viral origin. Proof of viral etiology is difficult to obtain in an individual case. The disorder is often referred to as vestibular neuronitis, acute epidemic vertigo, or acute labyrinthitis. Symptoms usually reach their peak within 24 hours and then gradually subside over days or weeks. Acutely, patients are severely imbalanced and have difficulties with focusing because of nystagmus. Most patients recover completely within several months. In some patients intractable dizziness persists for years, and some 30% will have another bout of vertigo. Patients may require hospitalization for intravenous fluids because of persistent nausea and vomiting. Patients with multiple recurrent episodes will eventually develop persistent dysequilibrium and oscillopsia.

Menière's Disease

Menière's is an uncommon disease. The clinical syndrome includes recurrent bouts of tinnitus, vertigo, a sensation of fullness or pressure in the ear, and nystagmus associated with progressive hearing loss in the affected ear. In the beginning, hearing loss usually recovers completely, but with more episodes some hearing loss usually remains between attacks. The hearing loss should be of a cochlear pattern. The clinical picture does not differ markedly from that seen in some disorders of the eighth nerve and in perilymph fistula. Pathologically, the membranous labyrinth progressively dilates, and ruptures and herniations are common. Most cases have an unknown etiology. An acute attack may last minutes, hours, or days.

Initial work-up includes audiogram, ENG, BAER, CT or MR brain scan, serum FAT-ABS or CSF VDRL or both, glucose tolerance test, and thyroid function tests. Medical therapy for idiopathic Menière's is frequently disappointing. Acutely, the treatment is symptomatic. Long-term treatment is with diuretics and salt restriction (1 to 2 g of sodium per day). If medical therapy fails and symptoms are debilitating, surgical therapy is possible. This may involve labyrinth destruction, eighth-nerve section, or shunting and draining procedures for the endolymphatic hydrops.

Perilymph Fistula

The classic presentation of an acute perilymph fistula is with an audible pop, immediately followed by hearing loss, vertigo, and tinnitus. Changes of pressure in the external or middle ear may induce movement in the endolymphatic space in patients with perilymph fistula. These pressure changes that induce vertigo may occur with loud noises (Tullio's phenomenon), changes of barometric pressure in an airplane, or examiner-induced increases or decreases (Hennebert's sign) of pressure. Perilymph fistulae may occur after trauma, infection, and other causes. The great majority of fistulae heal spontaneously. For those with persistent and disabling symptoms, surgical exploration of the middle ear is recommended.

Autoimmune Vestibulopathy

This syndrome has been proposed in patients with autoantibodies to mesenchymal structures of the inner ear. These patients have sensorineural hearing loss, and many have gait ataxia thought to be due to bilateral vestibular paresis. The syndrome may occur in conjunction with other connective tissue disorders.

Syphilis and Lyme Disease

Syphilis is still a cause of deafness and vestibular dysfunction. Another spirochete, Borelia burgdorferi, can also cause vestibular paresis. Since both conditions are treatable with antibiotics, patients with undiagnosed vestibular syndromes should always have a Lyme titer and a fluorescein treponema antibody test.

Posttraumatic Vertigo

Head trauma may cause inner ear hemorrhage, inner ear concussion, temporal bone fracture with perilymph fistula, and eighth-nerve injury due to fracture or avulsion. There will often be hearing loss associated with vertigo. Some patients have positional vertigo. Although recovery usually occurs over weeks and months, it may be incomplete.

Acoustic Neurinoma

These are uncommon tumors that originate from the Schwann cells of the vestibular portion of the eighth cranial nerve in the internal auditory canal. Common complaints are dizziness, tinnitus, and progressive hearing loss, slowly increasing in severity. As the tumor enlarges, it may grow into the intracranial space in the cerebellopontine angle and compress adjacent cranial nerves and brainstem. There may be loss of the corneal reflex, facial weakness, and sometimes cerebellar signs ipsilateral to the tumor. Large neuromas may obstruct CSF flow, resulting in increased intracranial pressure. BAER is a sensitive, noninvasive screening test for these tumors. An MR scan is excellent in visualizing even very small tumors. Treatment is surgical.

Dizziness of the Elderly

A significant number of elderly patients complain of being dizzy, lightheaded, or off balance. The exact nature of this disorder is unclear. In some, dizziness is related to medications. In others, symptoms appear to be related to a combination of several subtle or severe sensory deficits, such as impaired vision, decreased hearing, and loss of peripheral sensory receptors. Otosclerosis affecting both the labyrinth and the cochlea may be accompanied by dizziness. Some patients have clear-cut strokes in the distribution of the anterior or posterior circulation and may never feel "right" again. Some patients may suffer from degenerative changes of the labyrinth related to aging. Dizziness of the elderly is not a specific syndrome, but the symptom of dizziness is usually the result of a multitude of dysfunctions in different systems.

Ear Disease

Examination of the ears may reveal evidence of otitis media, serous otitis media, herpetic involvement of the ear, blood behind the eardrum,

CSF leak, mastoiditis, fracture or rupture of the eardrum, or tumor in the external canal or behind the eardrum. These findings can point to causes of vestibular as well as cochlear dysfunction.

Ototoxic Drugs

Aminoglycoside antibiotics—including streptomycin, gentamicin, and many other antibiotics—are ototoxic and labyrinthotoxic in sufficient doses. Other drugs that may also temporarily or permanently affect the inner ear include aspirin, diuretics, alcohol, caffeine, quinidine, sulfonamides, analgesics, stimulants, and others.

Cervical Vertigo

Cervical vertigo is used by some authors to describe vertigo due to abnormal proprioceptive input from the neck, occlusion of the vertebral arteries, or compression of the brainstem by a craniocervical junction abnormality. Only the last one is an important cause of cervical vertigo. Vertigo is practically never due to vertebral artery occlusion in the neck.

Occlusion of the Internal Auditory Artery

The sudden onset of acute vertigo and deafness without change of consciousness or other neurologic signs can occur when the patient suffers an occlusion of the internal auditory artery. This artery either comes directly from the basilar artery or can be a branch of the anterior inferior cerebellar artery. Occlusion occurs in patients with vasculitis, atherosclerosis, or other arterial abnormalities.

CENTRAL CAUSES OF VERTIGO

Vertigo due to central causes is usually associated with other CNS symptoms or signs. If a central lesion is suspected from history and examination, EEG, audiogram, ENG, BAER, and CT and/or MR scan may be indicated in the work-up.

Vascular Disease

VERTEBROBASILAR SYNDROMES. TIAs and stroke in the vertebrobasilar perfusion territory are common causes of vertigo in patients over 60. Vertigo is often abrupt in onset, lasts several minutes, and is accompanied by nausea and vomiting. Vestibular symptoms are commonly part of the lateral medullary syndrome. The key to the diagnosis is to find other, nonvestibular symptoms or signs in the perfusion territory of the vertebrobasilar system. Some of these are diplopia, numbness, weakness, dysarthria, dysphagia, and drop attacks. Management is the same as that described for TIAs and stroke.

CEREBELLAR HEMORRHAGE. The acute onset of headache, nausea, vomiting, depressed consciousness, and ataxia suggests the possibility of a cerebellar hemorrhage. This syndrome may mimic acute labyrinthitis, except that patients with cerebellar hemorrhage often have a severe headache and become lethargic or comatose. In many cases of cerebellar hemorrhage there may be other signs—including diplopia, facial weakness and numbness, pupillary abnormalities, dysarthria, dysphagia, limb ataxia, and weakness. Cerebellar hemorrhage requires emergency CT brain scan and immediate surgical evacuation of the blood clot in the posterior fossa if it is endangering the patient's life.

SUBCLAVIAN STEAL SYNDROME. This rare syndrome is characterized by symptoms of brainstem ischemia produced by exercise or movement of the left arm, usually with a decreased or absent peripheral pulse and decreased blood pressure in the left arm. This syndrome is caused by a stenosis of the left subclavian artery proximal to the origin of the vertebral artery. Increased blood flow to the left arm, precipitated by various factors, results in retrograde flow down the vertebral artery, causing brainstem ischemia. Patients may experience TIAs with vertigo as one of the symptoms.

VERTEBROBASILAR MIGRAINE. Some patients with vertebrobasilar migraine experience recurrent episodes of vertigo or other brainstem symptoms prior to, during, or after their otherwise typical migraine headaches. Severe nausea, vomiting, and vertigo may occur. Vestibular symptoms may also occur without the typical headache. The syndrome occurs most often in children and young adults, particularly women. Rarely, loss of consciousness is associated with the syndrome. Management is as described for migraine.

Posterior Fossa Mass Lesions

Any posterior fossa lesion may produce vertigo or dizziness. There are usually cranial nerve or cerebellar symptoms or signs that may be associated with alterations of consciousness. Posterior fossa lesions can press directly on brainstem structures or compress the aqueduct and produce hydrocephalus. A tumor around the fourth ventricle can give rise to Brunn's syndrome. This syndrome includes vertigo, nystagmus, and vomiting, which is sometimes associated with loss of consciousness on head turning, freedom from symptoms until the head is turned, and maintenance of the head in a particular position in order to prevent attacks. A gadolinium-enhanced MR scan is optimal for demonstrating a posterior fossa mass lesion.

Multiple Sclerosis

MS can cause isolated vertigo or vertigo associated with other brainstem findings during an acute exacerbation. Hearing loss is unusual. The vertiginous symptoms usually resolve.

Seizure Disorder

Some patients have vertigo as the initial manifestation of a generalized seizure or a complex partial (psychomotor or temporal lobe) seizure. It is presumed that the seizure focus in these cases is located in the temporal lobe. Vertigo can be elicited by electrical stimulation of portions of the temporal and inferior frontal lobe in humans. Vestibulogenic epilepsy is a rare type of reflex epilepsy in which vestibular sensory input precipitates a generalized seizure.

REFERENCES

Drachman D, Hart C: An approach to the dizzy patient. Neurology 1972; 22: 323–334.

Spector M (ed): Dizziness and Vertigo. New York, Grune and Stratton, 1976.

Hybels RL: Drug toxicity of the inner ear. Med Clin North Am 1979; 63:309–319.

Brandt R, Paroll R: The multisensory physiological and pathological vertigo syndromes. Ann Neurol 1980; 7:195–203.

Troost BT: Dizziness and vertigo in vertebrobasilar disease. Stroke 1980; 11: 301–303, 413–415.

Jannetta PJ, Moller MB, Moller AR: Disabling positional vertigo. N Engl J Med 1984; 310:1700–1705.

Lechtenberg R, Shulman A: The neurological implications of tinnitus. Arch Neurol 1984; 41:718–721.

Baloh RW: Dizziness, Hearing Loss, and Tinnitus: The Essentials of Neurology. Philadelphia, FA Davis, 1984.

Baloh RW, Honrubia V, Jacobson K: Benign positional vertigo: Clinical and oculographic features in 240 cases. Neurology 1987; 37:371–378.

Semont A, Freyss G, Vitte E: Curing the BPPV with a liberatory maneuver. Adv Otorhinolaryngol 1988; 42:290–293.

Kroenke K, Mangelsdorff AD: Common symptoms in ambulatory care: Incidence, evaluation, therapy, and outcome. Am J Med 1989; 86:262–266.

Baloh RW: Modern vestibular function testing. West J M 1989; 150:59–67.

Baloh RW: The dizzy patient: Treatment options. *In* Hachinski VC (ed), Challenges in Neurology, 3rd ed. Philadelphia, FA Davis, 1992, pp 15–24.

Hain TC, Zee DS: The dizzy patient: Diagnostic approaches. *In* Hachinski VC (ed), Challenges in Neurology, 3rd ed. Philadelphia, FA Davis, 1992, pp 3–14.

Froehling DA, Silverstein MD, Mohr DN, Beatty CW: Does this dizzy patient have a serious form of vertigo? JAMA 1994; 271(5):385–388.

17
Tumors

Primary intracranial and intraspinal tumors are often slow and insidious in their growth and clinical presentation. Early detection is a worthwhile goal, since benign tumors, which comprise 40% of all brain and spinal neoplasms, can become impossible to remove if allowed to grow very large. Furthermore, the longer a tumor remains unrecognized, the more damage it does to the nervous system. Tumors of the CNS make up less than 1.5% of all malignancies. The incidence of primary intracranial neoplasms is estimated to be between 4 to 16 per 100,000 per year. Approximately 15,000 to 18,000 tumors of the CNS are diagnosed each year in the United States. Malignant gliomas are the most common tumors, and their peak incidence is in the sixth to eighth decades of life. Thus, with the rapid increase in the number of people over 65, a significant increase in malignant primary CNS tumors can be expected. Tumors may produce symptoms when their size reaches about 10g, and most tumors of 100g will produce an increase in intracranial pressure. Symptoms are based on tumor location and also relate to rate of growth. Slowly growing, infiltrating neoplasms may produce few symptoms early. Local cell destruction by invading tumors may produce focal neurologic signs, and deafferentation may cause a seizure focus. Brain function may be compromised by direct pressure or secondarily by interfering with arterial and venous blood flow. Hemorrhage into a tumor may precipitate neurologic signs and symptoms or aggravate preexisting ones. The most common distant effect of a tumor, increased intracranial pressure, may be caused by the tumor itself, hemorrhage into the tumor, surrounding edema, obstruction of cerebrospinal pathways, or venous occlusion. An MR scan with contrast has become the standard of diagnosing brain tumors. A CT scan with contrast enhancement is falsely negative in 3% to 5% of cases. Despite the excellent diagnostic yield of radiologic procedures, correlation between radiologic images and actual tumor pathology is still less than optimal. Therefore, precise histologic definition of tumor type is necessary to determine the choice of appropriate therapy. Depending on location, tumor tissue may be obtained by open or closed stereotactic biopsy.

CLINICAL PRESENTATION

The type of focal neurologic symptoms and signs, including partial and secondarily generalized seizures, depends on the location of the tumor. Seizures may occur with or without focal neurologic abnormalities. Headache, not caused by increased intracranial pressure, is common in patients with intracranial tumors but is often not a prominent symptom and lacks specificity. The possibility of a brain tumor should be considered in a patient with a headache in conjunction with a focal neurologic abnormality or when a new type of headache develops in a patient with preexisting chronic headache. Tumors, which are most likely to present initially with focal neurologic symptoms and signs, seizures, and headaches (or any combination thereof), include astrocytomas, glioblastomas, oligodendrogliomas, ependymomas, meningiomas, primary cerebral lymphomas, and metastatic carcinomas.

Tumors that frequently cause increased intracranial pressure in their initial manifestation include medulloblastomas, cystic astrocytomas of the cerebellum, papillomas of the choroid plexus, hemangioblastomas of the cerebellum, pinealomas, craniopharyngiomas, and colloid cysts of the third ventricle. When focal or lateralizing signs are present, they are often inconspicuous. Symptoms and signs of increased intracranial pressure are headache, nausea, vomiting, gait disturbance, and papilledema.

Tumors of the pituitary gland present with endocrine dysfunction and, often, compression of the optic chiasm.

HERNIATION

As a tumor growth or significant brain edema develops, brain herniation will occur. A tumor localized peripherally in the cerebral hemisphere will displace the cingulate gyrus under the semirigid falx to the opposite side. Clinically the patient may develop a hemiparesis, worse in the leg, on the same side as the tumor. Mass lesions in the temporal lobe force the medial part of the temporal lobe, usually the uncus, downward through the tentorial incisura and medially. The thalamus and midbrain are displaced to the opposite side, the ipsilateral third nerve is compressed between the posterior cerebral artery and the superior cerebellar artery, and the contralateral cerebral peduncle is pushed against the free edge of the tentorium. Clinically, this type of herniation is characterized by the development of a third-nerve paralysis and hemiparesis, both on the same side as the tumor. As this herniation progresses, hemorrhages in the midbrain, upper pons, and one or both occipital lobes can occur. Posterior fossa mass lesions produce herniation of the mesial parts of the cerebellum and medulla downward through the foramen magnum into the cervical spinal canal. Compression of the medulla leads to eventual respiratory arrest. An early sign may be a stiff neck, followed by coma and decerebrate posturing.

SPECIFIC PRIMARY CNS TUMORS

Gliomas

Gliomas (astocytomas, ependymomas, oligodendrogliomas) constitute approximately 50% of all intracranial tumors and are by far the most common neoplasm affecting the CNS. Several different systems of pathologic classification of these tumors exist. In this chapter astrocytomas will be subdivided into low-grade and malignant astrocytomas.

Low-Grade Astrocytoma

These tumors represent 5% to 8% of all primary brain tumors and 18% of all astrocytomas. In adults they most often present during the third to fifth decades of life and are usually supratentorial in location. In children, over 50% occur in the cerebellum, 18% in the cerebral hemispheres, 17% in the brainstem, and 2% in the optic chiasm. They are slow-growing lesions with insidious onset of symptoms. In adults, 60% to 90% of patients present with seizures. They are often difficult to separate histologically from other brain abnormalities (infarction, infection) associated with an increased number of glial cells. They arise in the white matter and grow by a most gradual insinuation of nearly normal-looking glial cells into the surrounding brain. They are impossible to remove totally because they lack a true, clearly visible tumor margin; and the surgeon lacks the option of resecting large amounts of brain around the tumor to insure total extirpation. However, when such lesions in the cerebellum occur in children and have a distinctly associated cyst (cystic cerebellar astrocytoma), total surgical cures can be achieved. The diagnosis is established by CT or MRI and biopsy. Survival following diagnosis is prolonged, usually at least 5 years and frequently decades. Treatment involves subtotal resection of the tumor, administration of anticonvulsants, and steroids if increased intracranial pressure exists; and most authorities recommend radiation therapy. In children radiation therapy is usually reserved for tumor recurrence.

Malignant Astrocytoma

These tumors include anaplastic astrocytomas and glioblastomas. Necrosis is an important feature differentiating anaplastic astrocytoma from glioblastoma. Focal motor deficits, headaches, seizures, and mental changes are the most common symptoms. Median survival in moderately anaplastic astrocytomas is 220 weeks, in highly anaplastic tumors 116 weeks, and in glioblastomas 66 weeks. A large tumor mass is usually found on CT or MRI and requires surgical intervention, not only to establish the diagnosis but also to debulk the lesion and prevent herniation. Surgery is followed by radiation therapy, which is the single most effective therapy. Dexamethasone (16 to 40 mg per day in divided doses) is usually begun upon radiographic demonstration of a sizable intracranial tumor and continued until surgery is accomplished and radiation therapy is well under way. Although not significantly affecting tumor growth, this glucocorticoid retards brain edema around the tumor, reduces increased intracranial pressure, and frequently improves neurologic function. A variety of chemotherapy protocols are being used and may add significant time to the survival period in these unfortunate patients. Radiosurgery is a technique suitable for patients with small tumors in surgically inaccessible areas. In this procedure a large radiation dose is administered in a single fraction.

Brainstem Glioma

Brainstem gliomas comprise 2% of all tumors in adults and 10% to 20% of those in children, usually between the ages of 3 and 9 years. Patients present with multiple cranial nerve palsies, most commonly involving the sixth and seventh nerve, and long tract signs. Symptoms of increased intracranial pressure occur in about one third of patients. Most brainstem gliomas are located in the pons, and up to 70% show malignant features histologically. MRI is the diagnostic procedure of choice. Biopsy of suspected brainstem tumors is controversial. Stereotactic biopsy has been reported to have a high diagnostic yield and low morbidity and mortality. Surgical intervention is rarely feasible, and standard treatment is fractionated radiation therapy. Five-year survival is approximately 20% to 30%.

Oligodendroglioma

Oligodendrogliomas make up 5% of all gliomas. Their peak incidence is between the third and fifth decades of life. Most tumors occur within the cerebral hemisphere. Seizures, headaches, and personality changes are the most common presenting symptoms. Up to 50% of these tumors have calcifications in them, and 20% to 30% are cystic. Treatment consists of total surgical removal. If total resection is not possible, radiation therapy is given after surgery.

Ependymoma

About 10% of all childhood brain tumors are ependymomas, while these tumors account for about 1% in adults. These tumors arise from the ventricular wall or from aberrant ependymal rests. Anaplastic features are seen in 1% to 8% of cases. More than 50% occur in the posterior fossa. Supratentorial tumors commonly present with hemiparesis, headache, and seizures. If an ependymoma is located in the posterior fossa, headache, nausea, and vomiting are frequent early symptoms. Because of their intraventricular location, metastasis through CSF occurs in about 5% to 30% of cases. Most tumors are subtotally resected, followed by radiation therapy.

Choroid Plexus Tumor

Choroid plexus tumors typically occur in neonates and infants and constitute a small percentage of all brain tumors. About 10% to 20% are malignant. They rarely occur in the third ventricle. Symptoms of increased intracranial pressure are common presenting features. Treatment is attempted total surgical removal.

Medulloblastoma

About 70% to 80% of all medulloblastomas occur in children under the age of 16 years. Overall, medulloblastomas account for 4% of all brain tumors in all ages. Classified as undifferentiated primitive neuroectodermal tumors, most of them are located in the cerebellum. The vast majority of children present with headaches, nausea, vomiting, ataxia, and papilledema. At the time of diagnosis 15% to 45% of patients will have CSF metastases. Treatment consists of dexamethasone, followed by surgical removal and radiation therapy. As a consequence of irradiation, growth hormone disturbances are common (60% to 70%), and intellectual deficits occur in 35% of patients.

Primary CNS Lymphoma

Primary CNS lymphoma accounts for approximately 1% to 3% of all brain tumors, significantly more than in the past because of increasing numbers of patients with compromised immune systems. In the non-immunocompromised patient, this condition is most common in those between 40 and 60 years of age. It is unusual for patients with focal primary lymphoma of the CNS to have coexisting systemic lymphoma. Presenting symptoms commonly are headache, focal weakness, and personality change. Most lesions are single, but multiple sites are involved in 30% to 50% of cases. The most frequent sites are basal ganglia, thalamus, and frontal and parietal white matter. Diagnosis is by biopsy. Treatment response to steroids and radiation is excellent, but median survival is still only 13 to 15 months.

Meningioma

These usually benign neoplasms constitute about 15% of intracranial tumors and arise from the dura mater. They are extremely slow growing and frequently achieve considerable size before the patient develops clinically detectable symptoms. The diagnosis is established by CT or MRI and angiography. Surgery is always indicated in these radioresistant lesions. Total resection can usually be accomplished because these lesions protrude into, but do not infiltrate, the brain. When the tumor intimately involves crucial structures such as the sagittal sinus or brainstem, only subtotal resection may be possible, but because regrowth is usually slow, long-term survival is usual.

Schwannoma (Acustic Neuroma)

This benign tumor group, which comprises about 10% of intracranial tumors, arises from cells that sheath the individual fibers of cranial nerves. Usually involving the eighth cranial nerve (occasionally the fifth or seventh), these tumors present with insidious loss of hearing in one ear, accompanied by tinnitus and, often, mild facial weakness. If the patient ignores the symptoms, or if the physician fails to recognize them, these neoplasms can reach considerable size, making total resection and cure—easy to achieve when the lesion is small—impossible without significant damage to the seventh cranial nerve or brainstem. The diagnosis is made by MRI. Even subtotal resections are associated with prolonged survival in these very slow-growing tumors.

Pituitary Tumor

These mostly adenomatous tumors are almost always benign and are associated with long survival. They make up about 10% of all intracranial tumors and present with gradual development of endocrine dysfunction and/or compression of the optic chiasm. When these tumors are small, total surgical removal via the transnasal, transsphenoidal route is possible. Some tumors are large and endocrinologically inactive but by their size destroy the pituitary and compress the optic chiasm.

Tumors that secrete excess adrenocorticotropic hormone produce truncal obesity, round face, hirsutism, striae, easy bruisability, glycosuria, amenorrhea, osteoporosis, muscle weakness, mental changes, and hypertension. The diagnosis can be established by measuring serum cortisol levels. Excess growth hormone production leads to gigantism before closure of the epiphyses takes place, and later results in acromegaly with enlargement of the jaw, feet and hands; arthritis; coarse features; emotional instability; and cardiac failure. Elevated serum growth hormone levels are diagnostic of this disorder, but the elevation may be minimal and cyclic during the day. Hyperprolactinemia (Forbes-Albright syndrome) is clinically marked by secondary (postmenarchal) amenorrhea and galactorrhea, with the latter often requiring manual expression to be demonstrated. Males may note decreased libido and impotence, gynecomastia and galactorrhea. A serum prolactin level usually establishes the diagnosis. Hyperthyroidism secondary to a pituitary neoplasm is extremely rare.

Other Primary Brain Tumors

Craniopharyngiomas are benign congenital neoplasms frequently present in childhood. Onset of symptoms in adult life is not rare. They arise in the region of the optic chiasm and hypothalamus and frequently present with visual field, endocrinologic, or pressure symptoms. They are detectable by CT or MR scan. Subtotal resection is the treatment of choice, and long survival is common. Radiotherapy is of questionable value.

Pineal tumors are usually benign in their growth characteristics and are generally inaccessible to the surgeon. Fortunately, many of them are radiosensitive and, following their symptomatic onset in a child or young adult, long-term survival after irradiation is common. Headache, caused by obstruction of CSF pathways and resultant hydrocephalus, and upward gaze paralysis usually are presenting features.

METASTATIC INTRACRANIAL TUMORS

Between 20,000 and 100,000 cases of brain metastases, are diagnosed annually, a figure considerably greater than for primary brain tumors. Approximately half of all brain metastases are single. Abdominal, pelvic, and renal malignancies produce single metastatic lesions with greater frequency than do other primary tumors. About 20% to 30% of patients with cancer have brain metastasis at autopsy, and approximately 65% to 75% of these are symptomatic during life. Most patients with brain metastasis die of their systemic cancer. The most common primary malignancies in patients with brain metastases are cancer of the lung and breast and malignant melanomas. Neurologic symptoms and signs may be the first manifestations of an underlying malignancy. The primary tumor can be identified in about 50% of cases but usually escapes detection in the remaining 50% of patients, even at detailed postmortem examination. Clinically, patients present like those with primary brain tumors. The best test is contrast-enhanced MRI. If MRI is not available, double-dose, delayed contrast CT scan should be done. If the primary tumor is unknown, biopsy of the brain lesion has to be done to confirm the diagnosis.

Symptomatic treatment with dexamethasone is started immediately (usually 16 mg per day in divided doses), regardless of whether single or multiple metastatic lesions are present. The majority of patients show marked clinical improvement within 24 to 72 hours. Headache and altered mental status improve more dramatically than do focal neurologic abnormalities. If no satisfactory response is apparent within 2 days, the dose should be increased. Some recommend doses as high as 100 mg of dexamethasone per day. Approximately one quarter of patients require long-term treatment, but most can be weaned off steroids within several weeks. Improvement may last for weeks and months. Seizures, most of which occur at the time of diagnosis, should be treated with anticonvulsants. The prophylactic use of anticonvulsants is controversial and does not appear to be effective in preventing seizures. Patients with metastases from melanoma may be an exception, because seizures occur in about 50% of cases. Surgery for single metastasis remains controversial, but some data suggest that surgery and irradiation of the whole brain are followed by longer survival. Whole-brain radiotherapy for single and multiple lesions is the treatment of choice after dexamethasone has been started. From 30% to 80% of all patients with brain metastasis have a favorable response. Most patients die from the disseminated systemic disease, which accounts for the relatively short median survival time of 3 to 6 months. Patients with relatively radio-resistant tumors, such as renal and colon carcinoma and melanoma, fare less well than those with breast and lung cancer. Headaches, nausea, and vomiting are common during radiation treatment and may be ameliorated somewhat by corticosteroids. Early delayed reaction to brain irradiation occurs weeks to months after completion of therapy. This reaction may resemble tumor progression, with reappearance or worsening of focal neurologic deficits. Lethargy, nausea, and vomiting are frequently present. Steroids can be useful, and most patients recover completely within a few weeks. This syndrome is thought to be due to demyelination. Because most patients do not survive long enough, delayed toxicity is infrequently seen. It usually develops about 1 year after completion of radiation therapy, but shorter and longer latency periods occur. Delayed toxicity may manifest as radionecrosis or dementia, the latter often associated with ataxia and urinary incontinence. Radionecrosis may mimic tumor progression, and biopsy may be necessary to establish the correct diagnosis. Dementia has been estimated to occur in 2% to 5% of all patients with brain metastasis, and its incidence increases with longer survival. In single metastatic lesions, radioactive seed implantation is used at times. Results of chemotherapy for brain metastases have been disappointing.

PRIMARY INTRASPINAL TUMORS

This group of neoplasms is made up of gliomas intrinsic to the spinal cord, meningiomas arising from the dura, and schwannomas originating from spinal nerves. Some gliomas (astrocytomas) are unresectable and radioresistant, whereas others (ependyomas) can be totally removed and are fairly radiosensitive. The meningiomas and schwannomas are all benign and can usually be totally resected. Spine pain may or may not be a clinical symptom with these tumors, but cord or spinal nerve dysfunction is always present. MRI establishes the diagnosis of intraspinal tumor. Surgery is indicated to attempt a cure, or at least to relieve pressure on the cord and nerves, and to establish tumor type to guide subsequent therapy.

METASTATIC INTRASPINAL TUMORS

These neoplasms present with radicular pain and extremity dysfunction secondary to compression of the cord. They are more common than primary intraspinal tumors. Fairly rapid onset is the rule, and paraplegia can occur rapidly unless the problem is diagnosed and treated early. Large-dose steroids may slow progression of cord dysfunction until diagnosis can be established and definitive therapy undertaken. The most common primary tumors are lung, breast, prostate, and lymphoma. Metastatic spinal tumors may be the first clinical presentation of the primary tumor. MRI is the diagnostic procedure of choice. Since these tumors grow in the epidural space, laminectomy and subtotal resection usually relieve the cord compression. Follow-up radiotherapy is given to control recurrence of cord compression. When the patient's primary tumor is known to be of the radiosensitive lymphoma group, steroids and immediate radiotherapy can be employed, and surgery withheld, unless neurologic deterioration continues.

REFERENCES

Sloff JL, Kernohan JW, MacCarty CS: Primary Intramedullary Tumors of the Spinal Cord and Phylum Terminalae. Philadelphia, WB Saunders, 1964.

Russell DS, Rubinstein L: Pathology of Tumors of the Nervous System, 4th ed. Baltimore, Williams and Wilkins, 1977.

LeChevalier T, Smith FP, Caille P, Constans JP, Rouesse JG: Sites of primary malignancies in patients presenting with cerebral metastases. Cancer 1985; 56: 880–882.

Delattre J-Y, Krol G, Thaler HT, Posner JB: Distribution of brain metastases. Arch Neurol 1988; 45:741–744.

Hochberg FH, Miller DC: Primary central nervous system lymphoma: Review article. J Neurosurg 1988; 68:835–853.

Asai A, Matsutani M, Kohno T, Nakamura O, Tanaka H: Subacute brain atrophy after radiation therapy for malignant brain tumor. Cancer 1989; 63:1962–1974.

DeAngelis LM, Delattre J-Y, Posner JB: Radiation-induced dementia in patients cured of brain metastases. Neurology 1989; 39:789–796.

Pollack IF, Lunsford LD, Flickinger JC, Dameshek HL: Prognostic factors in the diagnosis and treatment of primary central nervous system lymphoma. Cancer 1989; 63:939–947.

Shibata S: Sites of origin of primary intracerebral malignant lymphoma. Neurosurgery 1989; 25:14–19.

Harsh GR, Wilson CB: Neuroepithelial tumors of the adult brain. In Youmans JR (ed): Neurological Surgery, 3rd ed, vol 5. Philadelphia, WB Saunders, 1990, pp 3040–3136.

DeAngelis LM: The management of a single CNS metastasis. In Hachinski VC (ed): Challenges in Neurology, 3rd ed. Philadelphia, FA Davis, 1992, pp 257–267.

Dropcho EJ: Management of multiple brain metastases. In Hachinski VC (ed): Challenges in Neurology, 3rd ed. Philadelphia, FA Davis, 1992, pp 269–281.

McDermott MW, Wilson CB: Management of primary brain tumors. In Hachinski VC (ed): Challenges in Neurology, 3rd ed. Philadelphia, FA Davis, 1992, pp 215–255.

18

Craniospinal Trauma

Brain injury is one of the leading causes of disability and death in the United States. To understand head injury, it is necessary to understand cerebral structure and the dynamics of brain impact and motion. The structural characteristic of importance is brain consistency, which is similar to a semisolid gelatinous mass wrapped in a thin membrane (pia mater). The brain has an extremely rich network of cerebral blood vessels. The venous outflow occurs through thin-walled veins that leave the brain surface and cross the subdural space to empty into the dural sinuses. Brain impact is a prerequisite for brain injury. The point of impact is the skull, which is suddenly accelerated following external impact, so that the floating brain strikes the inner table of the skull. This contact can result in surface or subsurface cerebral petechial hemorrhages (cerebral contusion) and, if particularly severe, may cause large intracerebral hematomas. Once brain impact occurs, the hemispheral gelatinous ball (the brain) oscillates within the spinal fluid–filled skull—potentially distorting, stretching, and even rupturing the bridging veins and distorting or twisting the upper brainstem. As the brain is stressed, cerebral concussion occurs, and as the bridging veins are ruptured, a subdural hematoma begins to form. If the blow that accelerates the skull also fractures it, the fracture may tear the underlying dural meningeal vessels. The blood from the resulting hemorrhage collects and expands into the epidural space as an epidural hematoma. When the brain is struck by the skull, large populations of cerebral capillaries can lose their normal ability to retain serum within their lumina and begin to leak fluid into the brain substance, causing edema. Finally, a large population of impacted cerebral muscular arterioles may lose their normal constrictive tone and dilate in unison to create brain swelling.

Four different pathophysiologic mechanisms are responsible for brain injury: focal injury, diffuse axonal injury, superimposed hypoxia and ischemia, and diffuse microvascular injury resulting in loss of autoregulation. The most common structures to be contused are the anterior temporal and orbitofrontal cortices, in which case cognitive and behavioral abnormalities result. If delayed bleeding into contusions and hematomas occur, patients will present as normal when first seen after trauma and then develop neurologic deficits. Diffuse axonal injury may not become apparent until 12 to 24 hours after injury, but it occurs after even minor head trauma and in the absence of other pathologic changes. Diffuse axonal injury is probably responsible for the postconcussion syndrome. Superimposed hypoxic and ischemic damage occurs because the traumatized brain is particularly vulnerable. Comatose patients are often hypercarbic or hypoxic even though they appear to be ventilating normally. The significance of diffuse microvascular damage is still not certain. Trauma soon leads to dysfunction of the blood-brain barrier, which begins to recover after 6 to 7 hours. Later stages are characterized by endothelial changes, which peak 6 hours after injury but may persist for as long as 6 days. Secondary, delayed cellular injury is a major contributor to the ultimate outcome. Pathophysiologic mechanisms include increase of arachidonic acid metabolites, formation of oxygen-free radicals, excess amounts of naturally occurring neurotransmitters, alterations in calcium and magnesium metabolism, and activation of various enzyme systems.

The etiology of spinal cord injury is relatively simple to grasp. The cord lies within its own bony protective environment—the spinal canal—and the fit is a close one. Any significant distortion of the canal—either by extreme flexion or extension with narrowing of the canal—or the actual dislocation of the canal can result in compression of the spinal cord. The cord is immensely intolerant of such insult and can be expected immediately to lose part or, frequently, all of its functions. This physiologic transection and its unfortunate permanence is the rule. Pathophysiologic changes, acute and delayed, are similar to those described for the brain.

DIAGNOSIS

Cerebral Concussion

The distortion of the upper brainstem caused by brain motion usually results in cessation of function of those activating systems that maintain consciousness. The resulting unconsciousness has variable duration. When it is short-lived and followed by rapid return of awareness, concussion is the clinical designation. These patients are frequently awake or in a state of awakening at the accident scene or, certainly, by the time of arrival in the emergency room. Their examination shows no focal deficits, pupils are equal and reactive, and strength is symmetrical. Observation for several hours in the emergency room or an overnight stay is usually sufficient. Diagnostic studies in this situation are not really necessary, but a CT scan of the head is usually obtained anyway. No specific therapy is indicated.

With more severe brainstem distortion, long-term unconsciousness can result. Patients remaining comatose beyond the first hour are often designated as having sustained a brainstem contusion. The examination is nonfocal, pupils are equal, and movements are similar on both sides. These patients frequently exhibit decerebrate posturing spontaneously or in response to noxious stimuli, but the decerebration is always symmetrical. Such patients should have a CT scan of the head to detect a possible hematoma or brain swelling. Neither concussion nor brainstem contusion is a prerequisite for the occurrence of an intracranial hematoma, cerebral contusion, or skull fracture.

Cerebral Contusion

This form of cerebral trauma is caused by the impact between skull and brain and will become a threat only when the damaged vessels leak serum into the brain. The latter situation can cause edema, which overloads the capacity of the intracranial space. Significant swelling occurs only in a minority of contusions, but the function of the contused area is interrupted. Recovery is the rule, with time being the major healer. Clinical diagnosis is difficult and possible only if the patient is awake and can be tested. If the contusion involves the posterior frontal lobe, aphasia, gaze palsy, or hemiparesis may be seen. Receptive aphasia marks the posterior temporal lobe contusion, whereas hemianopsia signals the occipital lesion. Basal frontotemporal bruises are reflected in combative and vituperative behavior. The CT scan, usually done to rule out hematoma, accurately demonstrates most of these contusions, as well as many clinically silent lesions in the anterior frontal and temporal lobes.

Intracranial Subdural and Epidural Hematoma

These mass lesions, which are a direct threat to life and brain function, are usually amenable to clinical diagnosis. The posttraumatic patient who is experiencing a decreasing level of consciousness or who demonstrates even a minimal focal neurologic deficit (hemiparesis, dilated pupil) must be considered to have a hematoma. A Cushing response (hypertension, bradycardia) is suggestive of intracranial mass and can be a useful warning sign, particularly in the comatose patient. Patients who are rapidly deteriorating require immediate surgical evacuation of the hematoma. Those who are stable but whose status is questionable need to undergo a diagnostic study. The CT scan is the most efficient diagnostic tool. Skull radiographs are a waste of time and money. The immediate care of the patient with a suspected hematoma should include endotracheal intubation; hyperventilation; steroids (25 mg dexamethasone); and, if coma is present, mannitol (50 to 100 gm rapidly intravenously). If the patient is still communicative, close observation and steroids should suffice, and a CT scan should be rapidly obtained. Surgery to evacuate a significant hematoma should be carried out as soon as possible, because delay of more than 4 hours after injury results in poorer outcome.

MANAGEMENT

Besides evacuation of hematomas, acute management of the head trauma patient is directed toward prevention of secondary injury. Management of respiration and shock are the top priority. Patients in coma should be intubated and hyperventilated to a PCO_2 of 25 to 30. To prevent hypertension, morphine, (4 to 12 mg intravenously every 2 to 4 hours) is given. Patients requiring paralysis may be given pancuronium bromide (4 mg every 2 to 4 hours). Immobilization of the head in the plane of the body facilitates airway patency, prevents venous occlusion, and is the optimal position in patients suspected of having an associated cervical spine fracture. Elevation of the head may facilitate venous return. When a patient is in shock, a diligent search for bleeding elsewhere in the body is imperative. Patients should be overhydrated and be given lactated Ringer's solution or normal saline. Comatose patients should be managed in an intensive care unit. Monitoring of intracranial pressure in the severely injured patients is of utmost importance, because intracranial pressure has been shown to correlate significantly with outcome. Monitoring may be accomplished with a subarachnoid screw, fiber-optic epidural transducer, or an intraventricular catheter. Intracranial pressure should be kept below 20 mm Hg. If morphine sedation or paralysis does not control intracranial pressure, the patient should be hyperventilated. If that fails, ventricular drainage is instituted and the patient is given mannitol (initially 1 g/kg intravenously, followed by a bolus of 0.25 g every 4 hours for as long as necessary). If that fails, barbiturate coma is induced with pentobarbital (initially 10 mg/kg intravenously over a period of 30 minutes). Additional pentobarbital is given every hour for 3 consecutive doses (5 mg/kg). Ideally, serum levels of 3 to 4 mg/dl should be maintained. This usually requires about 1 mg/kilogram per hour. A major side effect of barbiturate coma is hypotension; blood pressure therefore needs to be closely monitored. After 24 hours, pentobarbital should be gradually decreased. Further management depends on response of intracranial pressure. Corticosteroids are widely used in patients with head trauma, but their beneficial effect has never been demonstrated. The use of nonglucocorticoid steroids is currently under investigation.

Many patients require long-term rehabilitation. Unfortunately, the plethora of various approaches available reflects the fact that none has ever been scientifically validated. In young patients the brain fortunately has a great capacity for restoration of function and compensation for many aspects of injury. Thus, the ultimate functional outcome may be better than anticipated. Recovery and compensation in the elderly patient are much less. Rehabilitation after significant brain injury is a long process, best managed by a physician who is experienced in using all potentially helpful services, e.g., social and psychological services, physical and occupational therapy, and neuropsychological testing.

Posttraumatic Seizure Disorder

The incidence of posttraumatic seizures is 2% to 5% overall in patients with closed head injury and 11% in those with severe injury. The incidence is considerably higher in patients with depressed skull fractures, hematomas, and penetrating brain injuries. The risk of developing seizures decreases with time. Patients with acute seizures should be treated with an anticonvulsant, but prophylactic use of phenytoin has been shown not to prevent the development of posttraumatic seizure disorder beyond the first week after brain injury. Acute use of phenytoin or phenobarbital for 2 to 4 weeks in severely injured, high-risk patients is probably justified.

Spinal Trauma

Any patient with spinal trauma who complains of pain or has a neurologic deficit should have an appropriate radiographic examination. Even in a relatively mild injury, spine pain can indicate an unstable fracture. Any injury severe enough to render the patient uncommunicative may very well have also fractured the neck, and this possibility needs to be confirmed or dismissed before beginning the movement of head and neck usually associated with caring for the critically ill. About 5% of patients in traumatic coma have an associated cervical fracture. Any patient who walks into the emergency department complaining of traumatically induced spine pain can safely be placed on a stretcher; if the neurologic examination is normal, routine transport to the radiology department and transfer to the x-ray table using the patient's own mobility is acceptable. If a fracture is seen, orthopedic or neurosurgical consultation is required. The patient who is carried into an emergency room with spine pain and whose examination is normal should be lifted to the x-ray table using the sheet on which he or she is lying; appropriate films should then be taken. When this kind of patient has an abnormal neurologic examination, he or she should not be moved without the supervision of a neurosurgeon. The treatment of spine fractures initially constitutes immobilization. For lumbar and thoracic fractures, merely lying in bed is adequate. The fractured cervical spine is initially immobilized with sandbags or rolled towels placed on either side of the head and neck. Adhesive tape running from the forehead to the sides of the stretcher will also assist immobilization. The orthopedic or neurologic surgeon may elect to use skeletal immobilization-traction by inserting skull tongs.

When a neurologic deficit is detected (paraplegia, quadriplegia), an unstable fracture is almost always present. The treatment of choice is intravenous methylprednisolone (initially 30 mg/kg, followed by infusion of 5.4 mg/kg) for 24 hours. This treatment, when begun within 8 hours of injury, has been shown to be beneficial both in complete spinal cord transection and in incomplete lesions. Surgery plays almost no role in the injured spinal cord, because cord contusion rarely responds to laminectomy. Operative stabilization of a fracture is almost always a delayed and elective procedure.

WHIPLASH AND MINOR HEAD INJURY

Whiplash

Whiplash injuries resulting from railway accidents were first described in the nineteenth century. The term *whiplash* was first used in 1928. Most often, neck injury follows a rear-end collision. Even in a low-velocity rear-end collision, the neck can extend to 120 degrees (normal maximum 70 degrees) and relative to the trunk the head can accelerate several g in the extension phase and even more in the flexion phase. The entire extension-flexion movement is completed within less than 500 milliseconds. Head restraints have not prevented cervical injuries, because the head is usually several inches in front of the restraint and flexion may be as important as extension as a mechanism for injury. Further, neck extension is followed by reflex contraction of neck flexors, which may add to the mechanical forward flexion of the head. As a result of this extension-flexion movement of the head and neck, muscle fibers may rupture, and ligaments may tear. Chronic pain may arise from musculoligamentous injury, which takes a long time to heal or heals only partially, and from abnormal movements of intervertebral joints as a result of incomplete or no healing of supporting ligaments and capsules.

A delay of symptoms from several hours to several days is typical. Some symptoms may not appear for several weeks. Initially, few if any physical findings are present on examination, but within days to weeks limitation of neck and head motion, tightness, muscle spasms, and tenderness will be present. Radiologically, the only abnormality is straightening of the cervical lordosis. Radionucleotide bone scanning may detect fractures of facet joints. Headache is also a common complaint and is often very disabling. Migraine or tension-type headaches frequently develop in patients without prior history of such. Dysphagia, the result of esophageal or pharyngeal injury, usually disappears within 1 week. Intermittent visual blurring, dizziness, vertigo, and tinnitus are frequent complaints, as are arm pains and paresthesias. The exact mechanism for these symptoms is not clear. Many patients will also complain of fatigue, irritability, memory and concentration problems, and difficulty in sleeping. Furthermore, 50% to 60% of patients also complain of low back pain. Psychological problems are extremely common.

Recovery from soft tissue injuries of the neck is a slow and tedious process. Few patients are symptom-free within a week. More than 50% continue symptomatic longer than 6 months, and about 40% do so longer than 1 year. Eventually, 80% to 90% of patients will achieve full functional recovery, but over 40% continue indefinitely with some intermittent discomfort. The longer disabling symptoms persist, the less the chance of functional recovery. Patients who have not returned to work or leisure activities after 18 months have a very poor prognosis. About 10% of patients remain functionally impaired even after 3 years.

One of the most important points to stress to the patient is that there are no quick fixes or cures. Another is that some injuries resulting in pain are not amenable to any form of therapy. While relative immobilization and avoidance of activities aggravating the pain are appropriate initially, in the long run this response may be self-defeating. Complete immobilization of the neck initially is optimal but practically impossible. A soft cervical collar, a compromise at best, should be worn in such a fashion as to avoid hyperextension of the neck. The use of such a collar beyond 2 weeks is probably not beneficial. Much has been written about proper posture, but the rationale behind it is mostly wishful thinking. The best posture is probably that in which the patient is comfortable. Physical therapy is of no scientifically proven value, but moist heat and gentle massage may temporarily relieve pain. Such therapy beyond 2 or 3 weeks is useless. Manipulation has no place in the treatment of patients with neck injury and may be injurious. Cervical traction, while beneficial in the treatment of cervical radiculopathies, does not benefit patients with whiplash injury. Medication has a limited role and is probably most beneficial in the acute stages. A tricyclic antidepressant may reduce the pain and may also help patients sleep.

Minor Head Injury

Symptoms following minor head injuries are probably related to diffuse axonal damage. In the postconcussion syndrome, headaches, fatigue, decreased energy, dizziness, instability, poor concentration, and difficulty in sleeping are common complaints. Abnormalities on neuropsychological testing have been demonstrated even after minor injuries. The most important aspect of managing patients with minor head injuries is to recognize that there is usually an organic basis to the complaints and to convey this to the patient. Management is supportive and symptomatic, minimizing the use of drugs. Patients should probably return to work in a graded fashion over a period of 4 to 8 weeks. Most patients improve after 3 months, but some continue to have significant, disabling symptoms for months and even years. Older patients have a less favorable prognosis than young patients.

REFERENCES

Voris HC: Craniocerebral trauma. *In* Baker AB (ed), Baker LH (asst ed), Clinical Neurology, 3rd ed, vol 2, chapter 23. New York, Harper, 1975.

Plum F, Posner JB: The diagnosis of stupor in coma. *In* Contemporary Neurology. Philadelphia, FA Davis, 1980.

Alksne JF, Ignelzi RJ, Marshall LF: Acute brain injury. *In* Rosenberg, R (ed), The Science and Practice of Clinical Medicine: Neurology. New York, Grune and Stratton, 1979.

Wilson CB, Hoff JT (eds): Current Surgical Management of Neurological Disease. Edinburgh, UK, Churchill Livingstone, 1980.

Youman JR (ed): Trauma. *In* Neurological Surgery, vol 4. Philadelphia, WB Saunders, 1982.

Norris SH, Watt F: The prognosis of neck injuries resulting from rear-end vehicle collisions. J Bone Joint Surg 1983; 65B:608–611.

Weiss G, Salazar A, Vance S, Grafman J, Jabbari B: Predicting posttraumatic epilepsy in penetrating head injury. Arch Neurol 1986; 43:771–773.

Feeney DM, Sutton RL: Pharmacotherapy for recovery of function after brain injury. CRC critical review in Neurobiology 1987; 13:135–197.

Levin H, Mattis S, Ruff R, Eisenberg H, Marshall L, Tabaddor K, High WJ, Frankowski R: Neurobehavioral outcome following minor head injury: A three-center study. J Neurosurg 1987; 66:234–243.

Yarnell PR, Rossie GV: Minor whiplash head injury with major debilitation. Brain Inj 1988; 2:255–258.

Klauber MR, Marshall LF, Luerssen TG, Frankowski R, Tabaddor K, Eisneberg HM: Determinants of head injury mortality: Importance of the low risk patient. Neurosurgery 1989; 24:31–36.

Drugs for acute spinal cord injury: Med Lett Drugs Ther 1993; 35:72–73.

Katz DI, Alexander MP: Traumatic brain injury: Predicting course of recovery and outcome for patients admitted to rehabilitation. Arch Neurol 1994; 51: 661–670.

Teasell RW: The whiplash patient: A sympathetic approach. *In* Hachinski VC (ed), Challenges in Neurology, 3rd ed. Philadelphia, FA Davis, 1992, pp 29–52.

Salazar AM: Traumatic brain injury: The continuing epidemic. *In* Hachinski VC (ed), Challenges in Neurology, 3rd ed. Philadelphia, FA Davis, 1992, pp 55–67.

19

Congenital Anomalies and Inherited Disorders

A variety of problems can occur during intrauterine development. The nervous system is differentiating and growing at an extremely rapid rate, and anything that produces even a small aberration may result in a major alteration of brain development. Drugs such as diphenylhydantoin and warfarin may damage the developing fetus. Certain infections that cause relatively mild problems in adults can cause devastating damage to the fetal nervous system. Toxins such as ethanol also cause fetal maldevelopment. Many disorders of brain development have not as yet been linked with an identifiable event or toxin. A congenital abnormality is a defect present at birth and secondary to some intrauterine mishap. Many neurologic disorders are inherited in a clearly defined manner. Some are clinically apparent during the neonatal period, while many more become clinically manifest in later infancy, early or late childhood, or adulthood. Several typically start in midlife. There are variations in age of onset, clinical manifestations, and severity of expression. Advances in biochemistry and molecular genetics have opened the door to the discovery and definition of well over 100 inherited diseases of the central and peripheral nervous system. It is beyond the scope of this book to attempt comprehensive coverage of all known inherited disorders of the nervous system. Several important inherited disorders are discussed in other chapters.

EMBRYOLOGICAL DEVELOPMENT OF THE NERVOUS SYSTEM

The nervous system develops from the embryonic ectoderm. Between the twenty-first and twenty-ninth day of gestation, thickened ectodermal cells fold over the midline notochord to form the neural tube. The neural tube then develops cavities, which eventually form the cerebral ventricles. The most rostral part becomes the prosencephalon, the midportion becomes the mesencephalon, and the caudal part becomes the rhombencephalon. The prosencephalon undergoes further division into the telencephalon, which will become the cerebral hemispheres, and the diencephalon, which will differentiate into eyes and optic nerves. The midportion, or mesencephalon, will become the midbrain. The rhombencephalon divides into the metencephalon, which will become the pons and cerebellum, and the myelencephalon, which eventually forms the medulla. An aberration in any of these phases of development will result in a congenital anomaly of the nervous system.

CONGENITAL ANOMALIES

Cerebral Malformations

ANENCEPHALY. This is a massive malformation in which there is virtually no brain, although the brainstem and cerebellum may be present. The incidence of this congenital defect in the United States is 1 per 1000 live births. A large bony defect is apparent in the skull, and a major portion of the cranial vault may be absent. The skin over the surface of the cranium may also be absent, leaving the malformed brain remnants exposed. The hindbrain is usually well preserved, but there is no recognizable forebrain. The cause of anencephaly is not known. Although there is an increased risk of occurrence (4% to 5%) in mothers who have had one anencephalic pregnancy and a further increase in risk (10% to 15%) after two affected children, there is no clear hereditary pattern. A combination of genetic and environmental factors is likely. Diagnosis of this and other dysraphic states can be made prenatally by amniocentesis. Alpha-fetoprotein concentrations in the amniotic fluid are elevated.

HOLOPROSENCEPHALY. In this disorder the prosencephalon fails to differentiate normally into separate cerebral hemispheres, and a single large cerebrum remains. With complete failure of segmentation, there is a single medially placed eye (cyclopia), a proboscis that is displaced above the orbit, and a small head. This extreme degree of holoprosencephaly is incompatible with life. In less complete forms, there may be some degree of separation into cerebral hemispheres. These infants have varying degrees of hypotelorism, a flat nose with absent nasal septum, and a cleft upper lip. They are usually microcephalic and may have optic atrophy. Severe mental retardation is common.

GYRAL MALFORMATIONS. These may manifest as unusually wide (macrogyria) or extremely small and numerous (microgyria) gyri. In either case, normal convolutional markings are distorted. Neurons may be abnormally placed (heterotopias) or be abnormal in appearance. Both conditions are usually associated with mental retardation and spasticity. Microgyria has been associated with maternal cytomegalovirus infection and with maternal carbon monoxide poisoning.

Macrocephaly

Many different disorders cause macrocephaly. Hydrocephalus is the most common cause of enlargement of the head. Enlargement of the cerebral ventricles is due to a block in normal outflow of CSF (noncommunicating hydrocephalus) or to a defect in reabsorption through the arachnoid villi (communicating hydrocephalus). Noncommunicating or obstructive hydrocephalus is usually the result of a congenital defect. Causes include aqueductal stenosis, Arnold-Chiari malformation, and Dandy-Walker syndrome. Posterior fossa tumors, meningoencephalitis, and intraventricular hemorrhage may also result in obstruction of CSF flow. Communicating hydrocephalus may occur as a sequel to meningoencephalitis (especially tuberculous and fungal diseases), subarachnoid hemorrhage, and severe head trauma. The clinical presentation of acute hydrocephalus is that of increased intracranial pressure. Head size increases rapidly, and sutures spread in infants and children. Papilledema may be present, especially in older children. With chronic hydrocephalus, an unusually large head is the most prominent clinical feature. Headache, vomiting, and irritability may also develop. The increased intracranial pressure produces compression of optic nerves, with gradually decreasing vision and optic atrophy. Sixth-nerve palsy is common, as is downward deviation of the eyes ("setting sun" sign). Spasticity and hyperreflexia of the lower extremities may be found.

Examination of an infant with an enlarged head should include transillumination, looking for focal or generalized increases in the spread of light around the beam of the flashlight, percussion of the head, testing for a "cracked pot" sound (Macewen's sign), and auscultation of the head for unusually loud or asymmetrical bruits (suggesting the possibility of vein of Galen aneurysm or other vascular malformation). In children over 1 year of age, transillumination is not helpful. The diagnosis can be confirmed by CT or MR scan demonstrating dilated ventricles. In communicating hydrocephalus, the lateral and third ventricles, the aqueduct of Sylvius, and the fourth ventricle are large. In obstructive hydrocephalus the aqueduct is small and the fourth ventricle is of normal size. Treatment consists of a surgical procedure to drain excess spinal fluid and release pressure. For obstructive hydrocephalus, a ventriculoperitoneal or ventriculoatrial shunt is usually performed. A lumboperitoneal shunt may be effective for communicating hydrocephalus.

In some patients hydrocephalus becomes compensated, and there is no progression of neurologic deficit. Often, the deficit is so subtle that it cannot be detected in infancy and is easily missed later. Only a careful developmental history and neurologic examination, which includes measuring head circumference, will demonstrate that the patient has hydrocephalus. These patients are often intellectually normal and lead a normal life. An example is the famous mathematician C. F. Gauss, the inventor of the logarithmic tables, who had hydrocephalus. Often the diagnosis is made incidentally in adulthood. Unless a neurologic deficit develops or there is definite worsening of a preexisting deficit, such patients may not benefit from a shunt procedure, which carries considerable risk because of possible intracranial bleeding.

Microcephaly

Head size reflects brain size. Thus, if the brain fails to grow, the head will be smaller than normal. If head circumference is less than two standard deviations below the normal mean for age, the child is microcephalic. Genetic forms of microcephaly include familial microcephaly, maternal phenylketonuria, and chromosomal anomalies. Familial microcephaly is an autosomal recessive disorder associated with moderate mental retardation, hyperactivity, and seizures in approximately one third of cases. Facial appearance is normal except for a receding forehead. In other identifiable genetic disorders, such as Cornelia DeLange's syndrome and Prader-Willi syndrome, microcephaly is associated with other anomalies. Several chromosomal abnormalities are associated with microcephaly, which also occurs as a result of various intrauterine or postnatal insults to the brain. These acquired causes of microcephaly include fetal alcohol syndrome, fetal irradiation, congenital viral infections, anoxia, and neonatal meningoencephalitis. Most of these children have mental retardation, and many have seizures and spasticity.

Porencephaly

Porencephaly refers to an abnormal cystic cavity within the cerebral hemispheres that communicates with the ventricles or subarachnoid space. This cavity forms after destruction of normal brain tissue. Causes include cerebral infarctions, intracranial hemorrhage, and meningitis. There is usually some atrophy of the brain on the side of the porencephaly. At times this cyst is under tension and may produce abnormal enlargement of the head and pressure on the surrounding brain. A shunt from cyst to peritoneum or right atrium may be necessary to relieve pressure. Children with porencephaly may have hemiparesis on the side opposite the cyst and focal motor seizures that are difficult to control.

Craniosynostosis

Premature closure of one or more cranial sutures is a developmental disorder of unknown cause. Multiple suture involvement can result in compression of the underlying brain, increased intracranial pressure, and inhibition of brain growth. Premature closure of only one suture produces an asymmetrical head and is primarily a cosmetic problem. Surgical treatment of craniosynostosis is required to prevent increased intracranial pressure and possible brain damage and to improve facial or head appearance. Surgery consists of a craniectomy to reopen the sutures.

Encephalocele

An encephalocele is a congenital anomaly in which part of the brain protrudes through a midline bony defect in the skull (cranium bifidum). The extent of displacement can vary from only meninges to a large part of the brain and ventricular system. In the latter case, the entire brain may be malformed. In many cases encephaloceles are obvious as large, soft, midline pulsating tumors. Others are more subtle and may look like a hemangioma over the scalp. Still other encephaloceles are located anteriorly and may present as a nasal mass. Encephaloceles may grow after birth. One serious complication is rupture of the sac, leading to introduction of bacteria producing meningitis. Hydrocephalus is another possible complication. If any midline defect is detected on examination of an infant, a CT scan should be obtained to look for cranium bifidum. Treatment consists of a shunt procedure for hydrocephalus, and, if possible, closure of the bony defect. Prognosis depends on the extent of brain involvement in the defect.

Spina Bifida and Related Anomalies

Failure of the neural tube to close during embryogenesis may result in midline defects of the spine. The simplest malformation is spina bifida, in which the vertebral arches fail to fuse. There is usually a cutaneous defect over the bifid spine, (e.g., a tuft of hair, pilonidal dimple, or hemangioma). The meninges may protrude through the bifid spine, producing a meningocele. In more extensive forms, part of the spinal cord and nerve roots as well as meninges protrude through the bony defect, forming a myelomeningocele. These defects may occur anywhere along the spine but are most common in the lumbosacral area. An estimated incidence of 2 to 3 myelomeningoceles per 1000 live births has been reported. In some instances the anomaly has a genetic basis, with an autosomal recessive transmission. The disorder can be diagnosed prenatally by determination of elevated alpha-fetoprotein concentrations in amniotic fluid.

Spina bifida occulta, which has only vertebral involvement, may be asymptomatic, at least in early life. A midline cutaneous defect should alert the physician to the possibility of an underlying problem. Spina bifida occulta may be associated with tethering of the spinal cord to surrounding bony structures. When this occurs, progressive neurologic deficits may arise as the child grows and the tethered cord is stretched. These include gait disturbances, leg weakness, hyporeflexia, and poor bladder and bowel control.

Meningocele is usually obvious on examination, with a soft, fluctuant sac protruding from the spine. It may not be associated with any neurologic abnormality. However, rupture of the sac may result in meningitis. Myelomeningocele is associated with neurologic impairment related to the spinal cord level involved. Lumbosacral lesions may cause paraplegia, urinary and fecal incontinence, and profound sensory deficits. These deficits are usually present at birth. Both meningocele and myelomeningocele are associated with an increased incidence of aqueductal stenosis, Arnold-Chiari malformation, and hydrocephalus. Treatment is multifaceted. Surgery to close the defect should be performed in the first 24 hours of life, primarily to reduce the risk of meningitis. Ventriculoperitoneal shunts may also be needed to treat hydrocephalus. Infants with the disorder then require physical therapy, orthopedic assistance, and urological care.

Syringomyelia and Hydromyelia

In syringomyelia, a cavity is present within the spinal cord, usually in the cervical region. If the cavity is the result of dilatation of the central canal, it is known as hydromyelia. The cause is unknown. Other congenital anomalies may coexist with syringomyelia, including spina bifida, platybasia, and kyphoscoliosis. Syringomyelia may be present in conjunction with a spinal cord tumor. Symptoms typically appear in the second or third decade, beginning with loss of pain and temperature sensation in the hands, followed by weakness and atrophy of the hands and arms and subsequent progressive spasticity of lower extremities. Spinal CT will demonstrate the defect. Laminectomy and decompression of the cavity may retard progression of symptoms.

Diastematomyelia

In this congenital anomaly a calcified or bony septum, usually located at the lumbar or lower thoracic level, bisects the spinal cord for a small distance, producing distortion of the cord and neurologic impairment below the level of the defect. The cause of this anomaly is not known. Diastematomyelia is often associated with congenital malformations of the vertebrae (spina bifida occulta, hemivertebrae) and skin (midline lipomas, hemangiomas, or hair tufts). Clinical manifestations of this problem occur because of stretching of the impaled spinal cord and include progressive weakness, atrophy, and areflexia of one or both legs. Diagnosis is made by radiographic evidence of an area of calcification within the spinal canal. Treatment consists of surgical removal of the bony septum. This procedure may not improve the neurologic deficit but may prevent further progression of symptoms.

Klippel-Feil Malformation

This disorder consists of fusion of the cervical vertebrae and a reduction in the number of vertebrae. There may be associated platybasia as well. Children with Klippel-Feil malformation have short necks with limitation of lateral movement. In mild cases the child may have torticollis, short stature, kyphoscoliosis, and incoordination with mirror movements. More severely affected children may develop progressive paraplegia from cervical cord compression. The diagnosis is made radiographically. If cord compression occurs, decompressive laminectomy may relieve symptoms and prevent progression.

Sacral Dysgenesis

In this malformation the lower part of the vertebral column fails to develop. The entire sacrum may be absent, and the lumbosacral cord may be displaced or malformed. Spina bifida, club foot, arthrogryposis, dislocated hips, and renal anomalies may be associated with sacral dysgenesis. Clinical features include weakness, atrophy, areflexia, and sensory disturbances in the lower extremities, particularly below the knees. Bowel and bladder incontinence may be a complication. Lumbosacral spine films demonstrate the vertebral malformation. There is no corrective treatment for this disorder, but physical therapy may aid gait.

Cerebellar malformations

CEREBELLAR DYSGENESIS. This is a rare congenital malformation in which the entire cerebellum, vermis only, or one cerebellar hemisphere may be missing. The cause of these malformations is unknown. Some children with cerebellar dysgenesis are asymptomatic; others are hypotonic and ataxic, with nystagmus and intention tremors.

DANDY-WALKER MALFORMATION. In this malformation, cystic dilatation of the fourth ventricle and obstructive hydrocephalus are present. The cerebellum is hypoplastic and is displaced upward. Clinical symptoms include hypotonia, developmental delay, large head with prominent occiput, and nystagmus. Intermittent apnea from medullary dysfunction can be a fatal complication. Diagnosis is established by a CT scan demonstrating a cystic dilatation of the fourth ventricle with hydrocephalus. Treatment consists of drainage of the cyst and ventriculoperitoneal shunt to control the hydrocephalus. These steps may prevent further progression of symptoms but may not reverse the developmental delay and other problems already present, especially if associated cerebral anomalies coexist.

ARNOLD-CHIARI MALFORMATION. This is a congenital anomaly of the posterior fossa in which the cerebellum is displaced downward through the foramen magnum and in which the pons and medulla are also elongated and displaced. There are three main types of Arnold-Chiari malformation. In type 1, the mildest form, the cerebellar tonsils are displaced downward into the spinal canal and the medulla is somewhat elongated but not displaced. Type 2, the most common form, consists of cerebellar and medullary displacement into the spinal canal, with elongation of pons and medulla. This type is frequently associated with other congenital anomalies, including myelomeningocele and Klippel-Feil malformation. Type 3 is really an occipital myelomeningocele, with protrusion of the cerebellum through a cervical spina bifida defect. Clinical symptoms result primarily from compression of displaced structures. Progressive hydrocephalus develops from compression of the fourth ventricle. Nystagmus, ataxia, and lower cranial nerve dysfunction eventually appear. In type 1, the malformation may be asymptomatic until the second or third decade, when symptoms gradually appear. Type 2 often presents early in life with progressive hydrocephalus. If a patient with myelomeningocele develops hydrocephalus, Arnold-Chiari malformation should be suspected. Diagnosis can usually be made by CT or MR scan. Surgical decompression of the cervical area will often alleviate at least some of the symptoms and may prevent progression. A ventriculoperitoneal shunt may be necessary to control hydrocephalus.

CONGENITAL INFECTIONS

Some infectious agents that produce relatively mild problems in children and adults are devastating to the nervous system of the developing fetus. The most notable of these are cytomegalovirus (CMV), toxoplasmosis, rubella, and syphilis. The primary treatment for these is prevention of maternal infection.

Cytomegalovirus

Intrauterine infection during the second and third trimesters may result in severe neurologic impairment. Symptoms and signs are often apparent in the neonatal period and include prematurity, smallness for gestational age, hepatosplenomegaly, hyperbilirubinemia, thrombocytopenia, anemia, chorioretinitis, microcephaly, intracranial calcifications, mental retardation, and hydrocephalus. Diagnosis can be established by presence of intracranial calcifications, elevated umbilical cord blood IgM (greater than 20mg%), elevated CMV titers in serum and CSF, and isolation of virus from urine. Infected infants may shed virus for more than 2 years after birth.

Rubella

Maternal rubella infections, especially in the first and second trimesters, can produce a variety of neurologic impairments. Clinical manifestations include smallness for gestational age, microcephaly, deafness, microphthalmia, cataracts, chorioretinitis, congenital heart disease, psychomotor retardation, hypotonia, seizures, elevated CSF protein, cord blood IgM greater than 20mg%, and elevated rubella antibody titer in serum. The degree of impairment is variable, but in general, the earlier in pregnancy the infection occurs, the greater the damage to the fetus. To prevent fetal infection, women should be immunized with rubella vaccine prior to pregnancy. Rubella syndrome has been reported following immunization of pregnant women.

Toxoplasmosis

Toxoplasma Gondii is a protozoan that can produce mild upper respiratory symptoms in adults. It crosses the placenta and infects the fetus in the second and third trimesters. Clinical features are hepatosplenomegaly, jaundice, anemia, hydrocephalus, chorioretinitis, seizures, intracranial calcifications, and microcephaly. Overall prognosis for infants with congenital toxoplasmosis is poor. Mortality is 12%, and 90% of survivors have significant neurologic impairment—including seizures, mental retardation, impaired vision, spasticity, and deafness. Diagnosis can be established by the presence of elevated toxoplasma titers in serum and CSF. Treatment with a combination of sulfadiazine and pyrimethamine may arrest the progress of the disease in some cases.

Syphilis

Maternal transmission of syphilis to the fetus can occur at any time during gestation. Infants usually appear normal at birth. Lethargy, restlessness, anemia, and failure to thrive may develop in the first few weeks or months. Clinical features include chorioretinitis, malformed (Hutchinson's) teeth, saddle nose, interstitial keratitis, deafness, frontal bossing, saber shins (from persistent periostitis), swollen (Clutton's) joints, ragades (scars from mucocutaneous lesions), persistent rhinitis ("snuffles"), rash involving palms and soles, and pseudoparalysis (Parrot's paralysis). If untreated, the infection persists and may lead to syphilitic meningitis in the first few months of life. Symptoms of acute meningitis—vomiting, lethargy, seizures, and bulging fontanel—may then appear, or a more chronic inflammation may present as evolving hydrocephalus from thickening and fibrosis of meninges, with obliteration of the subarachnoid space. Tertiary syphilis can occur in children with untreated congenital syphilis, usually after the age of 6, causing progressive deterioration of intellectual functions. Seizures, spasticity, and optic atrophy may also develop. The disease is fatal within 5 years.

Diagnosis is made by finding a positive VDRL or fluorescent treponemal antibody absorption test (FTA-ABS) in serum and CSF. VDRL may be negative if the infant was partially treated. Pleocytosis may be present in CSF, with elevated protein concentration. Antibiotic therapy will stop disease progression. Procaine penicillin G (100,000 units/kg intramuscularly for 10 days) or benzathine penicillin G (50,000 units/kg as a single injection) are the drugs of choice. Erythromycin (6–8 mg/kg every 6 hours for 10 days) may be used in children with penicillin allergies. Serologic tests should be followed for 2 years after treatment to ensure that the infection is eradicated.

Congenital Hypothyroidism

Congenital diseases of the thyroid gland include complete absence of the gland and several biochemical blocks that prevent production of thyroxine. Some infants with hypothyroidism are already symptomatic at birth, whereas others appear normal in the neonatal period and begin to develop symptoms during the first few months of life. Signs of congenital hypothyroidism are large head, persistent patent posterior fontanel, delayed bone age, hoarse cry, large tongue, umbilical hernia, hypotonia, muscular hypertrophy, and delayed development. Any infant with a large head, hypotonia, and developmental delay should have a serum thyroxine level determination. Treatment with desiccated thyroid to maintain a euthyroid state will prevent progression of neurologic problems. If the infant already has psychomotor retardation by the time treatment has been initiated, it is unlikely that this will completely reverse. The prognosis is best for those children diagnosed and treated prior to the development of symptoms and signs.

HEREDITARY DISORDERS

Chromosome defects

With the advent of refined techniques for chromosome analysis, numerous minor and major defects in chromosomes (deletions, translocations, etc.) have been described. Virtually all are associated with some degree of impairment in intellectual function. Only three will be briefly described here: trisomy 21, trisomy 18, and fragile X syndrome.

TRISOMY OF CHROMOSOME 21. Known as Down's syndrome or mongolism, this condition is the result of an extra number 21 chromosome caused by the failure of normal cell division in meiosis or by the translocation of one chromosome to another (usually 21 to 14) so that, effectively, there is a third chromosome 21. Translocation defects are independent of maternal age, whereas true trisomies are increasingly frequent with advanced maternal age. The primary neurologic manifestations of Down's syndrome are mental retardation and hypotonia. Dementia can occur as early as the first or second decade of life. Most patients with Down's syndrome will become demented during the fourth decade of life, and on autopsy the brain shows the typical changes of Alzheimer's disease. Systemic problems associated with Down's syndrome include major congenital heart defects (most commonly ventricular septal defect and patent ductus arteriosus) and gastrointestinal anomalies (duodenal atresia). The numerous clinical manifestations of Down's syndrome include low birth weight, short stature, mental retardation, hypotonia, hyperextensible joints, epicanthal folds, brushfield spots on the iris, low-set ears, fissured and protruding tongue, transverse palmar crease (simian fold), and incurving little fingers. Life expectancy is shortened because of complications from cardiac and gastrointestinal defects, increased susceptibility to infection, and increased incidence of leukemia. Few patients live into the fifth decade of life.

TRISOMY OF CHROMOSOME 18. This relatively common condition occurs in about 1 in 4500 births. Infants with trisomy of chromosome 18 have profound psychomotor retardation, spasticity, webbed neck, and low-set ears. The most characteristic feature is the position of the fingers, in which the second finger overlaps the third. The great majority of these infants die in the first year of life.

FRAGILE X SYNDROME. This condition is thought to be the most common inherited form of mental retardation. It is estimated to be the cause of retardation in 1 out of 1500 males. The pattern of inheritance is neither dominant nor recessive. The characteristic presentation in males is mental retardation; a long, thin face; prominent jaw; protuberant ears; macroorchidism; and autistic features, but the expression is quite variable. Intelligence levels range from severely retarded to normal. Women are affected about half as often as males, and clinical expression in females is less severe.

Neurocutaneous Syndromes

The neurocutaneous syndromes are a group of inherited disorders with characteristic cutaneous anomalies in association with abnormalities of the nervous system.

NEUROFIBROMATOSIS. Also known as von Recklinghausen's disease this is the most common of the neurocutaneous syndromes, occurring with a frequency of approximately 1 in 2000 births. Patients with neurofibromatosis may have a range of manifestations in one or multiple systems. Besides the neurologic and cutaneous problems, these individuals may have skeletal anomalies, including scoliosis and absence of the sphenoid wing. The latter can produce a pulsating exophthalmos. Subperiosteal neurofibromas may produce pathologic fractures. Monohypertrophy of a limb is the result of a bony overgrowth or plexiform neuroma with obstruction of lymphatic drainage. Hypertension may result either from an increased incidence of pheochromocytomas or from renal artery stenosis. Various types of tumors are common. Neurofibromas may arise along any peripheral nerve, including autonomic nerves innervating the viscera. Malignant degeneration may occur but is rare. Intraspinous tumors, particularly neurofibromas and meningiomas, may also arise in either single or multiple manifestations. The most common intracranial tumors are optic gliomas and acoustic neuromas, but other gliomas may occur as well. The diagnosis is based on the presence of at least 5 café-au-lait spots 1 cm in diameter or larger. These lesions may be small and subtle in infants but enlarge as the child gets older. Biopsy confirmation of neurofibromata can make the diagnosis in the absence of café-au-lait spots. Treatment is symptomatic. Intracranial and intraspinal tumors that can be removed are treated surgically. Removal of peripheral nerve neurofibromas must be weighed carefully, since significant damage to the nerve may be incurred.

TUBEROUS SCLEROSIS. This disorder occurs with a frequency of 1 in 30,000 births. Two thirds of patients are mentally retarded. In some, intelligence is normal initially but regression occurs over the course of several years. Seizures are the most common presenting symptoms and may be difficult to control with anticonvulsants. Tuberous sclerosis is a major cause of infantile spasms with hypsarrhythmia. Tumors of various organs may arise at any time. Rhabdomyomas of the heart, embryonal cell tumors of the kidney, and hamartomas of multiple other organs can develop. Intracranial tumors occur in approximately 15% of patients with tuberous sclerosis. In addition, periventricular and intracerebral calcifications develop as the child gets older. These calcifications consist of sclerotic brain tissue. Treatment is symptomatic. Seizure control should be attempted and tumors removed when feasible.

STURGE-WEBER SYNDROME. This disorder has a variable inheritance pattern. The cutaneous anomaly is a port-wine nevus over the face in the distribution of the first division of cranial nerve V. The primary neuropathologic abnormality is a leptomeningeal angioma over one cerebral hemisphere, with a predilection for the occipital lobe. Cortical calcifications are present beneath the vascular malformation and appear as parallel lines on skull radiographs ("railroad track" in appearance). Contralateral hemiparesis and homonymous hemianopsia are common. Focal and generalized seizures and mental retardation are also found frequently. Seizures may be difficult to control with anticonvulsant medications and may require partial or complete hemispherectomy of the affected side. Intellectual deterioration can occur because of progression of the intracranial lesion. Glaucoma secondary to angiomatous malformations of the eye occurs congenitally or develops over the course of several years.

ATAXIA TELANGIECTASIA. This condition is characterized by multiple cutaneous and conjunctival telangiectasias, progressive neurologic symptoms, and immunologic deficiencies. Symptoms begin between 3 and 6 years of age with ataxia, choreoathetosis, abnormal arm movements, nystagmus, hypotonia, generalized weakness, hyporeflexia, and progressive intellectual deterioration. Immunologic incompetence is manifested by diminished IgA and IgE activity and impaired delayed hypersensitivity reaction. There is a high rate of malignancy, and tumors of the lymphatic system in particular commonly occur.

VON HIPPEL-LINDAU DISEASE. This condition is characterized by retinal hemangiomas in association with cerebellar hemangioblastoma. Symptoms usually appear in late childhood with progressive ataxia and signs of increased intracranial pressure. Intra-ocular hemorrhages may occur. Many patients with this disorder have polycythemia as a result of the cerebellar lesion. Diagnosis is made by CT scan.

INHERITED METABOLIC DISEASES

Inherited metabolic defects are usually the result of an enzyme block in a metabolic pathway. Compounds present in the reaction chain at steps prior to the enzyme defect accumulate in abnormally large quantities, whereas substances that are formed in reactions taking place after the enzyme block are absent or diminished. These metabolic imbalances eventually lead to impairment in brain function. Those metabolic diseases with early onset are almost all transmitted as autosomal recessive traits. The fetus is protected by the mother's normal metabolism, and the disease does not become clinically manifest for a variable amount of time after birth. If a disease is identified early in life, preventive measures can be taken.

In the neonatal period the usual manifestations of inherited metabolic diseases are poor feeding, unstable temperature, hyperventilation, reduced alertness and responsiveness, hypo- or hypertonia, seizures, absence of support reaction of body and neck, lack of Moro and startle responses, quivering, and disturbance of eye movements. During the neonatal period the following diseases are most likely to became evident: maple syrup urine disease, galactosemia, hyperglycinemia, hyperammonemia, B^6 dependency, cretinism, sulfide oxidase deficiency, lactic acidemia, and cretinism.

During early infancy the hallmark of inherited diseases is regression from already achieved milestones. Common manifestations include loss of interest, regression of motor development, loss of head control, loss of vision, and seizures. During this period lysosomal storage diseases, e.g., Tay-Sachs disease, Gaucher's disease, Niemann-Pick disease, and Pompe's disease, are the most important group.

During late infancy and early childhood, milder forms of amino acid disorders become clinically manifest, as do later-onset lysosomal storage diseases (gangliosidosis, Gaucher's disease, and Niemann-Pick disease), other lysosomal storage diseases (metachromatic, globoid and sudanophilic leukodystrophies, mucopolysaccharidoses, mucolipidoses, fucosidosis, mannosidosis, lipofuscinosis), and others.

During late childhood and adolescence, late-onset variants and other inherited disorders become clinically apparent. At this age many patients present with regression of cognitive functions and behavioral disturbances, but other neurologic abnormalities invariably appear. Some of the diseases affecting cognition are Hallervorden-Spatz disease, Wilson's disease, juvenile Gaucher's disease, late-onset ceroid lipofuscinosis, Schilder's disease, metachromatic leukodystrophy, Lafora's body myoclonic epilepsy, and childhood Huntington's chorea. Cortical blindness, deafness, and bilateral hemiparesis are frequently the presenting symptoms in leukodystrophies. Other diseases appearing during this period are Friedreich's ataxia, ataxia-telangiectasia, Bassen-Kornzweig acanthocytosis, Refsum's disease, Lesch-Nyhan disease, lipofuscinosis, cherry-red-spot myoclonus syndrome, dyssynergia cerebellaris myoclonica, adrenoleukodystrophy, Fabry's disease, and homocystinuria.

Friedreich's ataxia may be transmitted in either autosomal dominant or autosomal recessive forms. Cardiomyopathy also develops. The first clinical symptom may be a pes cavus deformity of the foot. This is followed by progressive ataxia and nystagmus. Sensory impairments consist primarily of absent vibratory and position senses. Muscle stretch reflexes are absent. Loss of bladder and bowel control occurs. Intellectual deterioration is not uncommon. Death occurs from cardiac failure or intercurrent infection.

Several of the diseases mentioned may first become clinically manifest during adulthood or, rarely, present in a mild and chronic form.

Amino Acid Disorders

Most of the hereditary disorders of amino acid metabolism are associated with some degree of mental retardation or other neurologic deficit. Infants may appear normal at birth, but as abnormal metabolites accumulate over a period of days to weeks, neurologic symptoms appear. Untreated, some of the disorders are fatal within a few months. Others may stabilize with some neurologic deficit. The most common amino acid disorders producing significant neurologic problems are phenylketonuria, maple syrup urine disease, and homocystinuria.

PHENYLKETONURIA. This is an inherited autosomal recessive disorder with a frequency of 1 in 1400 births. The metabolic defect is in the conversion of phenylalanine to tyrosine, with a block in the enzyme phenylalanine hydroxylase. Symptoms typically begin at between 2 and 6 months of age. Projectile vomiting may be the first symptom and may be so severe that pyloric stenosis is suspected. The infants usually have dry skin and eczema. Seizures develop, most often infantile spasms. Psychomotor retardation is apparent by 6 months of age. Untreated, most children are moderately mentally retarded and hyperactive. They typically have blond hair, blue eyes, fair skin, and a musty odor due to excess accumulation of phenylacetic acid, a breakdown product of phenylalanine.

Screening tests for phenylketonuria are performed routinely in the newborn period. The screening test most commonly used is the Guthrie test. A positive Guthrie test should be followed by quantification of phenylalanine and tyrosine in serum. In normal infants, the concentrations of these amino acids are generally less than 1 mg%. In this way, transient tyrosinemia and hyperphenylalaninemia of other causes can be distinguished. One pitfall in newborn screening is that the test may be performed too early, before phenylalanine accumulates significantly. Phenylalanine is an essential amino acid that comes from dietary sources, so that the infant must receive a protein diet for several days before phenylalanine begins to accumulate. Thus, any infant who develops hypsarrhythmia and has delayed milestones should have an amino acid screen, even if a Guthrie test in the neonatal period was negative. Treatment consists of a low phenylalanine diet and maintenance of serum phenylalanine at levels less than 12 mg%. If treatment is begun prior to the onset of neurologic problems, psychomotor development may proceed normally.

HOMOCYSTINURIA. This disorder of methionine metabolism is inherited in an autosomal recessive fashion. The primary neurologic complication of homocystinuria is recurrent thromboembolic events in cerebral vessels. At between 6 and 12 months of age, infants develop seizures, mental retardation, spasticity, and pseudobulbar palsy as a result of multiple strokes. Ectopia lentis and Marfanoid features, including arachnodactyly, develop as the child gets older. Thromboembolic episodes also occur in other vessels and may cause fatal pulmonary or renal infarctions. Treatment with dietary restriction of methionine (a precursor of homocystine) results in decreased serum concentrations of methionine and decreased urinary excretion of homocystine. High doses of vitamin B^{12}, pyridoxine, and folate appear to benefit some patients.

MAPLE SYRUP URINE DISEASE. This autosomal recessive disorder is caused by a defect in the metabolism of the branched-chain amino acids valine, leucine, and isoleucine. Symptoms may begin in the first week of life with lethargy, respiratory difficulties, and opisthotonus. There may be rapid deterioration and death within a few weeks, or survival with severe mental retardation and spasticity. In other infants the disease is less rapidly progressive and is characterized by episodes of ataxia, drowsiness, and behavioral disturbances. Children have a characteristic maple syrup odor due to excretion of the keto-acid derivatives of the branched-chain amino acids. Treatment in the first few days of life must first aim toward stabilization of life-threatening problems. Exchange blood transfusions may be necessary. Once initial stabilization is achieved, a diet containing restricted amounts of leucine, isoleucine, and valine should be instituted.

UREA CYCLE DEFECTS. The urea cycle is the mechanism for detoxification of ammonia by its conversion to urea. Ornithine transcarbamylase (OTC) deficiency is an X-linked recessive disorder and is rapidly fatal in male infants. Symptoms begin in the first days of life (soon after protein feedings are initiated) with seizures, coma, and respiratory abnormalities. Females with OTC deficiency and infants with other hyperammonemia syndromes have common clinical features of vomiting, seizures, lethargy, mental retardation, and intermittent episodes of coma. Diagnosis can be suspected by finding elevated blood ammonia concentrations. Serum and urine amino acids and organic acids are helpful in differentiating each of the defects. Treatment in the acutely ill patient consists of exchange transfusions to decrease serum ammonia concentrations.

ORGANIC ACID DISORDERS

Several abnormalities of intermediary metabolism are recognized. They share the clinical features of intermittent vomiting, lethargy or coma, ketosis, and acidosis.

Disorders of Carbohydrate Metabolism

GALACTOSEMIA. This autosomal recessive disorder of carbohydrate metabolism is caused by an enzymatic block in galactose-1-phosphate uridyltransferase, which catalyzes the conversion of galactose-1-phosphate to galactose uridine diphosphate, a step in the metabolism of galactose to glucose. Thus, such infants become hypoglycemic when fed lactose or galactose. Infants with galactosemia are usually normal at birth, but soon after the introduction of lactose-containing formula, symptoms develop. These include vomiting, lethargy, jaundice, hepatosplenomegaly, and failure to thrive. Cataracts appear within the first few weeks. Neurologic symptoms include hypotonia, developmental delay, and cerebral edema. Seizures result from hypoglycemia. If untreated, these infants develop mental retardation, hepatic cirrhosis, and growth failure. Diagnosis is suspected from the clinical features of persistent jaundice, hepatomegaly, and seizures and from documentation of hypoglycemia and the presence of reducing substances in the urine. The diagnosis can be confirmed by documenting reduced enzyme activity in erythrocytes. Treatment consists of a galactose-free diet.

GLYCOGEN STORAGE DISEASES. These disorders are expressed in at least nine types, in each of which an enzymatic block in glycogen breakdown results in an abnormal accumulation of glycogen in tissues. Most of these are associated with hypoglycemia and seizures. Glycogen accumulation in muscle results in muscle cramps and weakness. Pompe's disease is an autosomal recessive disorder in which glycogen accumulates in virtually every tissue. Symptoms usually begin in the first few months of life with hypotonia, progressive weakness, and feeding difficulties. Cardiomegaly and muscular hypertrophy appear. The disease is progressive, and death may occur in the first year from intercurrent infections. Diagnosis can be made by muscle biopsy, which demonstrates extensive accumulation of glycogen, and by assay of acid maltase activity in leukocytes.

MUCOPOLYSACCHARIDOSES. These disorders are characterized by accumulation of mucopolysaccharides in virtually all tissues. Several disorders of mucopolysaccharide metabolism are recognized. Because patients typically have coarse facial features, the term *gargoylism* is used to describe such patients. Bony abnormalities, dwarfism, intellectual impairment, cardiac involvement, and cloudy corneas are also common features. Diagnosis is made by identification of mucopolysaccharides in the urine.

Disorders of Lipid Metabolism

Abnormalities of lipid metabolism in the brain result in storage of lipid materials within cells. These disorders involve all major lipid classes (neutral, polar, and very polar lipids). As these substances accumulate, the symptoms become progressively worse and lead to neurologic deterioration. GM_2-gangliosidoses are classified by phenotype, genetic locus, and allele involved. Progressive infantile encephalopathy used to be the most common clinical presentation, but successful carrier screening programs and prenatal diagnosis have reduced the incidence dramatically. These hexosaminidase deficiencies present with different phenotypes from infancy to childhood, including the classic infantile Tay-Sachs disease. In this disease infants develop normally until about 4 to 6 months of age and then become weak, floppy, and hyperreflexic and gradually lose vision. An exaggerated startle response, seizures, and myoclonus are prominent, and the macular cherry-red spot is present. The disease is fatal within 2 to 3 years. GM_1-gangliosidoses present as infantile and late-infantile forms. In the infantile variant the disease starts early and progresses rapidly. It is characterized by hypotonia soon after birth, poor sucking ability, slow weight gain, frontal bossing, coarsened features, large and low-set ears, gum hypertrophy, macroglossia, and peripheral edema. Half of these patients develop the macular cherry-red spot. At the age of about 6 months liver and spleen are enlarged, and the skin is coarse and thickened. Infants die before the age of 2.

Gaucher's disease includes several autosomal recessive sphingolipidoses in which glucocerebroside is stored due to deficiency of glucocerebroside beta-glucosidase. The reticuloendothelial system and brain are involved. In the adult form, neuronal structures are not involved. In the infantile form, symptoms begin at 4 to 6 months of age and include progressive spasticity, intellectual deterioration, anemia, and splenomegaly. The diagnosis is made by identifying Gaucher cells in the bone marrow. In Niemann-Pick disease several clinical types have been described. In this disorder lysosomal storage of glycosphingolipid sphingomyelin occurs. In the classic form the disease appears in infancy with symptoms of persistent jaundice and retarded psychomotor development. Seizures, including infantile spasms, are common. Hepatomegaly and anemia occur. The clinical course is variable, but the disease is usually fatal within a few years. Diagnosis is made by identification of vacuolated storage cells in the bone marrow.

Refsum's disease, also known as heredopathia atactica polyneuritiformis, is unique because the lipid stored is exclusively dietary in origin. Phytanic acid alphahydroxylase is deficient, leading to accumulation of phytanic acid. Onset is usually in early childhood but may be delayed well into the fifth decade in some patients. Progressive nightblindness is followed by weakness and ataxia. Symptoms are progressive, but exacerbations and gradual remissions occur. The peripheral neuropathy is manifested by weakness and muscle atrophy, distal sensory loss, and absence of muscle stretch reflexes. Retinitis pigmentosa is usually present. CSF protein is elevated. Sudden death may occur from cardiac arrhythmias. Treatment consists of limiting phytanic acid and its precursor, phytol, in the diet.

Leukodystrophies

The leukodystrophies are a heterogeneous group of disorders. In some, abnormal metabolism of myelin constituents appears to be the major factor. Krabbe globoid cell leukodystrophy is characterized by extensive, progressive CNS demyelination and the presence of globoid cells containing cerebroside. The deficient enzyme is galactocerebroside beta-galactosidase. Symptoms begin in the first few months of life with repetitive vomiting, irritability, progressive spasticity, loss of developmental milestones, blindness with optic atrophy, and loss of muscle stretch reflexes. CSF protein is elevated. Assays of the deficient enzyme in cultured skin fibroblasts confirm the diagnosis. Metachromatic leukodystrophy is characterized by decreased activity of the enzyme arylsulfatase A. The disease produces diffuse demyelination in the CNS. Symptoms and signs are progressive and include ataxia, spasticity, loss of muscle stretch reflexes, and intellectual deterioration. Cerebrospinal protein is elevated, and peripheral nerve conduction velocities are slowed. Symptoms usually begin during the second and third year of life, and the disease is fatal within 4 to 5 years. Diagnosis is confirmed by assay of the enzyme in leukocytes. A juvenile form begins between 5 and 7 years of age and has a slower progression.

HEREDITARY DISEASES OF THE BASAL GANGLIA

HUNTINGTON'S CHOREA. This autosomal dominant disorder has a chronic progressive course characterized by a movement disorder and intellectual deterioration. For more details, see Chapter 14.

DYSTONIA MUSCULORUM DEFORMANS. This progressive movement disorder has both autosomal dominant and recessive patterns of inheritance. Initial symptoms are intermittent involuntary postures (e.g., writer's cramp in the hand or pes cavus posture of the foot). These symptoms worsen with stress. Eventually, more permanent involuntary postures develop, as well as torsion spasms of the neck and trunk. Intellect remains intact. Death occurs from intercurrent infection. Diagnosis is difficult to make in the absence of a positive family history. Laboratory studies are all normal. Other causes of dystonia, e.g., Wilson's disease, encephalitis, and carbon monoxide poisoning, must be ruled out. See also Chapter 14.

WILSON'S DISEASE. This is an autosomal recessive disorder of copper metabolism in which excessive copper is deposited in the brain and liver. Symptoms may begin in childhood with progressive hepatic dysfunction or in young adults with neurologic symptoms, including dysarthria, dysphagia, tremors, dystonia, rigidity, and emotional lability. Liver involvement may be subclinical. Copper deposited in the cornea produces a Kayser-Fleischer ring that may require slit-lamp examination to detect. Without treatment, death occurs in 2 to 3 years, usually from hepatic failure. Laboratory abnormalities include elevated serum copper levels, increased urinary excretion of copper, decreased serum ceruloplasmin levels, and evidence of hepatic dysfunction. Diagnosis can be made on the basis of Kayser-Fleischer ring. Chemical confirmation may require measurement of hepatic copper content. Treatment is aimed at decreasing dietary intake of copper and removing copper from organs with penicillamine (1 to 2 gm per day in divided doses) or zinc acetate or trientine.

REFERENCES

Adams RG, Lyon G: Neurology of Hereditary Metabolic Diseases of Children. New York, Hemisphere, 1982.

Optiz JM, Sutherland GM: Conference report: International workshop on the fragile X and X-linked mental retardation. Am J Med Genet 1984; 17:5–94.

Scriver CR, Beaudet AL, Sly WS, Valle D (eds): The Metabolic Basis of Inherited Disease, 6th ed. New York, McGraw-Hill, 1989.

Shapiro LR: The fragile X syndrome: A peculiar pattern of inheritance. N Engl J Med 1991; 325:1736–1738.

INDEX

NOTE: Page numbers in *italics* indicate illustrations; page numbers followed by t indicate tables.

Abdominal reflexes, 40, 125
Abscess, 249, 257
  brain, bacterial infections and, 259, 260
    cerebrospinal fluid in, 45
    headache with, 60, 259
    radiological studies of, 60
    seizures and, 212
    vertigo and, 273t
  spinal epidural, 260
Absence seizures, 215–216
Acoustic neuroma, 272t, 281, 292
Acquired immunodeficiency syndrome (AIDS), 121, 253–254, 262. See also *Human immunodeficiency virus (HIV-1)*.
Acquired immunodeficiency syndrome (AIDS) dementia, 104, 253–254
Acquired (non-Wilsonian) hepatolenticular degeneration, 144
Adrenocorticotropic hormone (ACTH), in multiple sclerosis, 117–118
  in myoclonus, 244
  in seizure disorders, 215, 227t
  pituitary tumors and, 293
Adrenoleukodystrophy, 321
Adversive seizures, 217
Aging. See *Elderly*.
Akinetic seizures, 216
Alcohol and alcoholism, 168
  central pontine myelinolysis in, 138–139
  dementia and, 104–105
  developmental defects and, 310
  dizziness and, 271t, 282
  hypomagnesemia and, 140t
  peripheral neuropathy and, 196–197

Alcohol and alcoholism (*continued*)
  seizures and, 213, 219t, 222
  thiamine deficiency and, 142
Allodynia, 181
ALS. See *Amyotrophic lateral sclerosis*.
Alzheimer's disease, 95–96, 98, 99t, 100–103, 105
  with Parkinson's disease, 237
  seizures with, 213
Amino acid disorders, 321–323
Amnesia, 217, 228, 252
Amyotrophic lateral sclerosis (ALS), 127–130, 171t
Amyotrophy, focal, 129
Anatomy, 1–22
  cellular elements of, 1–2
  of basal ganglia, 18–19
  of brainstem, 11–16
    medulla, 12–13
    mesencephalon, 15–16
    pons, 13–15
  of cerebellum, 16–17
  of cerebral hemispheres, 19–20
  of internal capsule, 19
  of peripheral nervous system, 2–6
  of pineal gland, 19
  of spinal cord, 6–11
  of thalamus and hypothalamus, 17–18
  of visceral nervous system, 17
  of visual system, 20–22
Anencephaly, 308
Aneurysm(s), cerebrovascular disease and, 83, 84
  congenital, 90–91
  in stroke patient, 87, 88

329

Aneurysm(s) (*continued*)
  radiological studies for, 52
  seizures and, 213
  subarachnoid hemorrhage and, 90–91, 92
  vertigo and, 273t
Angiography, 51–52
  for sinus thrombophlebitis, 260
  in cerebrovascular disease, for arterial lesions, 93
    for stroke, 86, 87
    for subarachnoid hemorrhage, 74, 92
    for TIAs, 85–86
  in dementia evaluation, 101t
  risks of, 52
Anoxia. See *Ischemia; Oxygen deficits.*
Anoxic encephalopathy, 135–136
Anterior horn cell disease, 46–47
Anterior horn cells, 125, 189
Anticoagulant therapy, 86, 87–88, 89
Anticonvulsants, 226t–227t, 228
  causing dizziness, 271t
  prophylactic, for posttraumatic seizure disorder, 228, 301
Antidepressants, 152, 213, 238
Antihypertensives, 88, 275t
Aphasia, 85, 252
  evaluation of, 28, 29t
Apraxia, 15, 27, 37
Arachnoiditis, 43, 45
Argyll-Robertson pupils, 195, 264
Arnold-Chiari malformation, 116, 273t, 309, 312, 314
Arrhythmias, 87, 274, 277
Arterial occlusion. See *Cerebrovascular disease; Infarcts; Thromboembolism.*
Arteriosclerosis. See *Cerebrovascular disease.*
Arteriovenous malformation. See *Vascular malformations.*
Arteritis, 93–94
  giant cell, 74
  headache with, 58, 59, 63t, 74
  intracranial hemorrhage and, 83
  seizures and, 213
Astrocytomas, 52, 289–290, 295
Ataxia, Friedreich's, 273t, 321
  in multiple sclerosis, 112, 114
  vertigo with, 269, 273t
Ataxia-telangiectasia, 319, 321
Atherosclerosis. See *Cerebrovascular disease.*
Athetosis, 19, 36, 233–234, 244–245
Auditory evoked responses, 50–51
Auditory system, 15. See also *Hearing; Vestibular system.*
Aura, 66, 216
Autoimmune disorder(s). See also *Collagen vascular diseases.*
  multiple sclerosis as. See *Multiple sclerosis.*

Autoimmune disorder(s) (*continued*)
  myasthenia gravis as, 171–175
  vestibulopathy as, 280

Babinski sign, 40, 114, 125
Bacterial endocarditis, 88
Bacterial infection(s), 255–261. See also *Infection(s).*
  brain abscess due to, 259
  cerebral thrombophlebitis due to, 260–261
  coma with, 155
  meningitis due to, 255–258
  seizures and, 212
  spinal epidural abscess due to, 260
  subdural empyema due to 259–260
Balo's concentric sclerosis, 109
Barany maneuver, 276
Barbiturate coma, induced, 89, 300
Basal ganglia, 7, 11, 17, 18–19
Basal ganglia disorders, dystonia with, 241
  hereditary, 326
  in lymphomas, 292
  movement abnormalities with, 233–234
Basilar artery, 12, 20. See also *Vertebrobasilar syndromes.*
Basilar artery migraine, 66, 220, 283
Bassen-Kornzweig acanthocytosis, 321
Becker dystrophy, 161t, 164
Behavioral neurology, 54
Bell's palsy, 187–188
Benign familial neonatal convulsions, 212
Benign febrile convulsions, 212, 218–219
Benign paroxysmal positional vertigo, 272t, 278–279
Birth control pills, 65, 76, 81
Blepharospasm, 241
Blood flow. See also *Ischemia.*
  dizziness and, 227
  radiographic studies of, 51, 53
Blood pressure, high. See *Hypertension.*
  in head trauma management, 300–301
  in subarachnoid hemorrhage, 92
  low. See *Hypotension.*
Blood supply, to brainstem, 12
  to forebrain, 19–20
  to spinal cord, 8–9
Bone scans, 53
Borrelia burgdorferi, 264, 280
Botulinum toxin, 242
Botulism, 171t, 176
Brain. See specific parts.
Brain abscess. See *Abscess, brain.*
Brain death, 50, 156
Brain edema. See *Cerebral edema; Increased intracranial pressure.*
Brain scans. See *Computed tomography; Magnetic resonance imaging; Radiology.*

INDEX   331

Brainstem, anatomy of, 2, 3, 7, 8, 11–16, 17
   in toxic metabolic encephalopathies, 134
Brainstem auditory evoked potentials (BAEP), 51, 277
Brainstem glioma, 290
Brainstem lesions, 13
   in motor system diseases, 125–132
   movement abnormalities with, 234
   speech abnormalities with, 27
Brain tumors. See *Mass lesions; Tumor(s)*.
Brain waves, 48
Breath-holding spells, 220–221
Bromism, 150–151
Bruits, 32, 85–86, 309
Bulbar palsy, 128, 129

Calcium, 140–142, 213
California encephalitis, 250
Caloric irrigation, 276–277
Cancer, 141t. See also *Metastasis; Tumor(s)*.
   dizziness and, 271t, 274
   motor neuron disease and, 132
   peripheral neuropathies and, 187, 198–199
Carbohydrate metabolism, 137–138, 150, 271t
   brain reqirements and, 133
   diabetes mellitus and. See *Diabetes*.
   in hepatic encephalopathy, 144
   inherited disorders of, 323–324
Carbon monoxide poisoning, 309
Carcinomatosis, meningeal, 43, 45
Cardiac abnormalities, 32, 87, 274, 277
   in dermatomyositis, 155
   with myotonic dystrophy, 163
Cardiac arrest, 156
Cardiac murmur, 32
Cardiovascular disorders, Alzheimer's disease and, 102
   cerebrovascular disease and, 82t, 87, 88
   dizziness and vertigo with, 271t, 273, 275t, 283
   increased intracranial pressure and, 45
Cardiovascular system, physical examination, 32
Carotid artery, 20
   bruits, 32, 85–86
   dilation of, 52
   in TIAs, 85–87
   radiographic studies, 51, 52
Carotid artery dissection, 81, 82, 212
Carotid bifurcation, 32, 52
Carotid endarterectomy, 86–87, 88
Carotid sinus, 219, 274
Carotidynia, 74–75
Carpal tunnel syndrome, 182–183

Castelman disease, 194
Causalgia, 181
Central pontine myelinolysis, 138–139
Cerebellar astrocytoma, cystic, 289
Cerebellar dysgenesis, 313–314
Cerebellar hemangioblastoma, 319
Cerebellar hemorrhage, and vertigo, 270, 273t, 283
Cerebellar tremor, 234
Cerebellum, anatomy, 8, 12, 14, 16–17
   astrocytoma of, 289
   congenital malformations of, 313–314, 319
   development of, 308
   motor system function in, 36
   movement disorders in, 234
   speech abnormalities in, 27
Cerebral aqueduct, 15
Cerebral arteries, 12, 20
Cerebral arteritis, and seizures, 213
Cerebral atherosclerotic disease. See *Cerebrovascular diease*.
Cerebral concussion, 298–299
Cerebral contusion, 299
Cerebral dysfunction, language abnormalities with, 28
Cerebral edema. See also *Increased intracranial pressure*.
   brain herniation and, 288
   CT imaging of, 52
   rehydration and, 139
   with encephalopathies, 133
      anoxic, 135, 136
      diabetic, 138
      hepatic, 145
   with infections, tuberculous, 262
   with lead poisoning, 149
   with tumors, 290
Cerebral hemispheres, anatomy of, 19–20
   development of, 308
Cerebral hemorrhage. See also *Hemorrhage*.
   cerebrospinal fluid in, 45
   headache and, 59
   hypertensive, 84
   stroke and, 87, 89
Cerebral hypoxic ischemia, 156
Cerebral infarction, 82
   after subarachnoid hemorrhage, 92
   cerebrovascular disease and, 84
   CT imaging of, 52
   EEG abnormalities in, 49
   infections and, 249
   seizures and, 212, 213
   stroke and, 87–89
Cerebral malformations, 308–309
Cerebral palsy, 131
Cerebral peduncles, 15, 16

Cerebral perfusion pressure (CPP), 133
Cerebral thrombophlebitis, 260–261
Cerebritis, 249
Cerebrospinal fluid (CSF), 45, 53
  in hydrocephalus, 105–106. See also *Hydrocephalus.*
  leakage of, 73, 76, 272t, 282
  pressure of, 75
  shunting of, 106, 310, 311, 312
  xanthochromia of, 45, 92
Cerebrospinal fluid pressure, and headache, 75–76
Cerebrovascular disease, 81–94
  arteritis, 93–94. See also *Arteritis.*
  coma and, 153
  dizziness and vertigo in, 272t, 282
  headache and, 63t
  hypertension and, 81
  ischemic. See also *Ischemia; Transient ischemic attacks.*
    causes of, 82t
  multiple sclerosis vs., 116
  pathophysiology of, 81–84
  seizures vs., 220
  stroke as, 87–89, 90
  subarachnoid hemorrhage as, 90–93
  venous thrombosis as, 90
Ceroid lipofuscinosis, 320
Cervical radiculopathy, 183, 205t, 206. See also *Radiculopathy(ies).*
Cervical spine disease. See *Spine abnormality(ies).*
Cervical vertigo, 282
Charcot-Marie-Tooth disease, 199–200
Cherry-red spot myoclonus, 212, 321
Childhood dystonia, 241
Childhood Huntington's chorea, 320
Children. See *Infants; Pediatric patients.*
Chin-chest maneuver, 206
Chorea, 242–243
  basal ganglia lesions and, 19
  motor system lesions and, 36
Chorea gravidarum, 242
Choreiform movements, characteristics of, 233
  l-dopa therapy and, 238
Choroid plexus tumor, 291
Chromosome defects, 317–318
Chronic inflammatory demyelinating polyneuropathy (CIDP), 194
Chronic paroxysmal hemicrania, 72–73
Chvostek sign, 140
Cingulate gyrus, 17, 19
Cisternogram, 105
Clonazepam, 215, 216, 244, 227t
Clonus, 221
Cluster headaches, 58, 59, 61, 71–72
Coccidiomycosis, 104, 262–263

Collagen vascular diseases, dizziness in, 271t, 274
  multiple sclerosis vs., 116, 117
  peripheral neuropathies in, 190
Coma, 150, 152–156
  barbiturate-induced, 89, 300
  causes of, 153
  with metabolic/toxic encephalopathies. See also *Metabolic encephalopathy(ies).*
    anoxic, 135–136
    barbiturate poisoning and, 151
    diabetic, 138
    hepatic, 144
    pulmonary, 147
    Reye's syndrome and, 149
  with stroke, 84
  with vertigo, 272
  with viral encephalitis, 251
Comatose patient, 152–156, 221
  brain death of, 156
  EEG abnormalities of, 48, 49, 50
  examination of, 40–41
  management of, 152–155
  mental status evaluation of, 27, 154
  nystagmus in, 276
  prognosis for, 155–156
  respiration in, 134
Communicating hydrocephalus, 105, 106, 309
Completed stroke, 84, 87–90
Compression neuropathy, 181, 182t. See also *Radiculopathy(ies).*
Computed tomography (CT), 49, 50, 52
  in Alzheimer's disease, 102
  in bacterial meningitis, 256
  in comatose patient, 154
  in hematoma, 300
  in hydrocephalus, 92, 106
  in seizures, 222
  in subarachonid hemorrhage, 74
  in subhyaloid hemorrhage, 91
  of spine, 53
Concussion, 298–299
Conduction studies, 45–47, 129
Conduction velocity, 3, 129
Congenital aneurysm, 90–91
Congenital anomaly(ies), 308–314
  anticonvulsants and, 225
  cerebral malformations as, 308–309
  cranial neuropathy and, 187
  craniosynostosis as, 311
  development of nervous system and, 307–308
  encephalocele as, 311
  macrocephaly as, 309–310
  microcephaly as, 310

Congenital anomaly(ies) (*continued*)
of cerebellum, 313–314
of spinal cord and vertebral column, 311–313
porencephaly as, 310–311
Congenital hypothyroidism, 147, 316–317
Congenital infection(s), 309, 310, 314–317
Congenital myasthenia, 171t, 175
Congenital myopathy(ies), 161t, 165
Congenital myotonia, 163
Congenital neoplasm(s), 293
Connective tissue diseases. See *Collagen vascular diseases.*
Contusions, head trauma and, 297, 299
Convulsions. See also *Seizures.*
benign febrile, 218–219
Corneal reflexes, 34, 35
Cornelia DeLange's syndrome, 310
Costen's syndrome, 77
Coxsackieviruses A and B, 126
Cranial nerve(s), examination of, 26, 59
testing of, 32–36
Cranial nerve II. See *Optic nerve.*
Cranial nerve III, 234
anatomy and function of, 15–16, 17, 20, 22
neuropathies of, 186
Cranial nerve IV, anatomy and function of, 15, 20
neuropathies of, 186, 187
Cranial nerve V, anatomy and function of, 13, 14, 15, 18
trigeminal neuralgia involving, 58, 59, 78–79, 187. See also *Trigeminal neuralgia.*
tumors of, 292
Cranial nerve VI, anatomy and function of, 14, 15, 20
neuropathies of, 186, 187
tumors of, 290
Cranial nerve VII, 14
Bell's palsy involving, 187–188
herpes zoster neuropathy of, 188
Lyme disease affecting, 264
tumors of, 290, 292
Cranial nerve VIII, 11, 13, 278, 292
Cranial nerve IX, 12, 17, 36, 61, 79
Cranial nerve X, 12, 17, 36
Cranial nerve XI, 36
Cranial nerve XII, 12, 13, 36
Cranial neuralgias. See specific cranial nerves.
Cranial neuropathy(ies), 186–188, 290
headaches and, 64t–65t, 77–79
hydrocephalus with, 309
infections with, 249
bacterial meningitis and, 255–256

Cranial neuropathy(ies) (*continued*)
herpes zoster and, 77–78, 188
Lyme disease and, 264
tubercular meningitis and, 261
pain with, 58
vertigo with, 273t, 281
Craniopharyngiomas, 293
Cretinism, 147
Cryptococcal meningitis, 262
CSF. See *Cerebrospinal fluid; Lumbar puncture.*
CT. See *Computed tomography.*
Cushing response, 299
Cushing's syndrome, 169–170
Cystic cerebellar astrocytoma, 289
Cysticercosis, 168, 212, 266
Cystic necrosis, 81
Cytomegalovirus, 212, 250, 309, 315

Dandy-Walker syndrome, 309, 314
Deafferentiation pain, 77–79
Decorticate/decerebrate posturing, 156, 221
Delta waves, 48–49
Dementia(s), 95–106, 252
AIDS, 253–254
alcoholism and, 104–105, 142
Alzheimer's disease and, 100–103
with amyotrophic lateral sclerosis, 128
causes of, 99t–100t
definition of, 95
dialysis encephalopathy and, 146
electrolyte disturbances and, 140t
epidemiology of, 95–96
evaluation and diagnosis of, 97–98, 100, 101t
with hydrocephalus, 105–106
hypercalcemia and, 141
with hypothyroidism, 148
infection and, 103–104. See also specific infections.
intoxication and, 105
manifestations of, 96–97
with multiple sclerosis, 112
old age vs., 96
with Parkinson's disease, 237
with spastic paraplegia, 132
with subdural hematoma, 103
trauma and, 104
with vitamin deficiencies, 142, 143–144
Demyelinating diseases, central, 109–122
acute disseminated encephalomyelitis as, 121
central pontine myelinolysis as, 139
chronic inflammatory demyelinating polyneuropathy with, 194
CSF in, 45
diffuse cerebral sclerosis as, 121

Demyelinating diseases (*continued*)
  multiple sclerosis as. See *Multiple sclerosis.*
  necrotizing hemorrhagic encephalitis, 122
  nerve conduction studies with, 46
  vertigo and, 273t
Demyelination, peripheral. See *Peripheral neuropathy(ies).*
Dermatomyositis, 159, 161t, 166–167
Developmental disorders. See *Congenital anomaly(ies); Familial disorders.*
Devic's neuromyelitis optica, 109
Dexamethasone, 290, 291, 294
Diabetes, 137–138
  dizziness and, 271t, 273, 275t
  neuropathies with, 187, 190–191, 194–195
Diabetic ketoacidosis, 138, 140t
Diagnosis. See *Examination; Radiography;* specific disorders.
Dialysis encephalopathy, 146
Diastematomyelia, 313
Diffuse axonal injury, 298, 304
Diffuse cerebral sclerosis, 110t, 121
Digital subtraction angiography, 52
Diphenylhydantoin, 197–198, 216, 225, 226t, 228, 230
Disc disorders. See *Radiculopathy(ies).*
Disequilibrium syndrome, 146
Disseminated encephalomyelitis, acute, 110t, 121
Distal muscular dystrophy, 161t, . 165
Diuretics, 275t, 282
Dizziness and vertigo, 269–284
  causes of, 270, 271t, 272t, 273t, 277t, 278
  dizziness, 219
    causes of, 271t, 277t
    diffuse axonal damage and, 304
    history taking for, 24
    vs. seizures, 220
  examination in, 274–277
  history taking for, 270–274
  treatment of, 278
  vertigo, and basilar migraine, 66
    causes of, 272t, 273t
    definition of, 269
    medullary lesions and, 13
    Menière's disease and, 279–280
Dopamine, Parkinson's syndrome and, 235
Dopamine-receptor antagonist neuroleptics, 152
Dorsal nerve roots. See *Radiculopathy(ies).*
Double vision, 33. See also *Vision.*
Down syndrome, 317
Drug-induced chorea, 242

Drug therapy. See specific disorders.
Drug toxicity, 242
  coma and, 153
  dementia and, 97, 100, 105
  EEG activity in, 50
  myopathies and, 168
  neuroleptics and, 152
  of aminoglycosides, 171t, 177, 282
  of barbiturates, 50, 100, 105, 151, 213
  of bromides, 150–151
  Parkinsonism and, 235
  peripheral polyneuropathy due to, 197–198
  salicylism from, 150
  seizures vs., 220t
  tardive dyskinesias from, 234–235, 245–246
Drug withdrawal, 64t
  l-dopa, 238
  seizures and, 213, 222
Drugs, dizziness and vertigo and, 271t, 272, 274, 282
  headache and, 58, 59, 61, 63t–64t
  seizures and, 213, 219t, 222
Duchenne dystrophy, 132, 161t, 163–164
Dysautonomia, primary. See *Primary dysautonomia.*
Dysimmune multiple mononeuropathy, 191
Dyssynergia cerebellaris myoclonica, 321
Dystonia, 233, 241–242
Dystonia musculorum deformans, 326
Dystonic posturing, 241
  athetosis and, 234
  with basal ganglia lesions, 19
  motor system lesions and, 36
  phenothiazines and, 221

Ear disease, of otitis media, 59, 61, 272t
  vertigo and, 271, 272t, 281–282
Ear examination, 32, 35–36
Eastern equine encephalitis, 250
Eaton-Lambert syndrome, 171t, 175–176
Echoviruses, 126
Edema, brain. See *Cerebral edema; Increased intracranial pressure.*
Edrophonium test, 172, 173
EEG. See *Electroencephalography.*
Efferent nuclei, 2
Elderly, anticonvulsant metabolism in, 224
  dementias in, 95–96, 101–103, 105. See also *Alzheimer's disease.*
  dizziness and vertigo, causes of, 271t, 272t, 277, 281
    in benign paroxysmal positional vertigo, 278–279

INDEX   335

Elderly (continued)
  EEG evaluation of, 50
  tardive dyskinesias in, 245
Electrocardiography (ECG), 47, 101t
Electrocochleography (ECochG), 277
Electroencephalography (EEG), 47–50
  in brain death, 156
  in completed stroke, 87
  in dementias, 98, 101t, 102
  in headache, 60
  in hydrocephalus, 105
  in infections, viral encephalitis, 251
  in pyridoxine deficiency, 143
  in seizure disorders, 222–223
    akinetic, 216
    petit mal/absence, 215–216
    tonic-clonic, 214–215
  in toxic-metabolic encephalopathies, 135,
    anoxic, 136
    barbiturate poisoning and, 151
    hepatic, 144
    thyroid disorders and, 148
    uremic encephalopathy, 146
Electrolyte abnormalities. See *Fluid and electrolyte balance.*
Electromyography (EMG), 45–47, 160, 195
  in amyotrophic lateral sclerosis, 129
  in congenital myopathies, 165
  in Fazio-Londe disease, 132
  in hypothyroidism, 148
  in juvenile motor neuron disease, 131, 132
  in median neuropathy, 183
  in muscular dystrophies, 163, 164, 165
  in myotonic dystrophy, 162
  in radiculopathies, 207
Electronystagmography (ENG), 277
Embolism. See *Infarct(s); Thromboembolism.*
Embryological development, 307–308
Emery-Dreifuss dystrophy, 161t, 164
EMG. See *Electromyography.*
Empyema, subdural, 259–260
Encephalitis, 244, 249
  cerebrospinal fluid in, 45
  dementia and, 99t
  lumbar puncture indications for, 43
  movement disorders and, 251, 254
    dystonia, 241
    Parkinsonism, 235
  necrotizing hemorrhagic, 122
  viral, 250–252
Encephalocele, 311
Encephalomyelitis, acute disseminated, 110t, 121
Encephalopathies. See *Metabolic encephalopathy(ies).*

Endocrine functions. See also *Thyroid disorders.*
  regulation by hypothalamus, 18
  pituitary tumors and, 288
Endocrine myopathies, 161t, 169–170
Eosinophilia-myalgia syndrome (EMS), 168, 198
Ependymoma, 291, 295
Epidural abscess, spinal, 260
Epidural hematoma, diagnosis, 299–300
Epilepsia partialis continua, 217
Epilepsy. See also *Seizure(s).*
  EEG in, 48, 49
  posttraumatic, 50, 104, 228, 301
  seizure classification in, 213–219
  vertigo with, 273t, 284
Epstein-Barr virus, 250
Erythema chronicum migrans, 264
Essential tremor, 234, 240–241
Evoked potentials, 50–51, 114–115
Examination, 23–41
  in cerebrovascular disease, TIAs, 85
  in dementia, 97–98
  in radiculopathy, 205–207
  in vertigo, 270
  of carotid arteries, 51
  of comatose patient, 40–41
  of cranial nerves, 26, 32–36, 59
    for facial sensation and movement, 35
    for hearing and vestibular function, 35–36
    for olfaction, 32
    for vision, 32–35
  of headache patient, 59–60
  of mental status, 25, 26–29, 30–31
  of motor system, 36–38
  of muscles, 25, 26
  of muscle stretch reflexes, 39
  of reflexes, 25, 26, 40
  of sensory system, 38–39
  sequence/order of, 26
Extensor digitorum brevis, 26
Eye, 16, 17, 18, 20, 21. See also *Ocular; Optic* entries; *Vision; Visual Fields.*
  development of, 308
  examination of, 33–35, 41
  in galactosemia, 323
  hypertensive retinopathy of, 88
  Kearns-Sayre syndrome and, 161t, 165
  motor function and. See *Eye movement.*
  neuropathies of, 187
  subhyaloid hemorrhage and, 91
Eye movement, 20–22. See also *Nystagmus.*
  assessment of, 32–33, *34,* 174, 175
  central lesions affecting, of mesencephalon, 16

Eye movement (continued)
    of optic pathway, 21–22
    of pons, 15
    in multiple sclerosis, 111
    vestibular function and, 35

Fabry's disease, 321
Facial muscles, assessment of, 35
    in amyotrophic lateral sclerosis, 128
    in comatose patient, 41
Facioscapulohumeral dystrophy, 132, 161t, 164
Familial chorea, 242
Familial disorders, 317–319
    Alzheimer's disease as, 102
    amyotrophic lateral sclerosis as, 127–130
    of basal ganglia, 326
    chromosome defects in, 317–318
    congenital myasthenia gravis as, 175
    development of nervous system and, 307–308
    dystonia as, 241
    hereditary neuropathies as, 199–200
    infantile muscular atrophy as, 130–131
    metabolic diseases as, 320–323
    metabolic myopathies as, 168
    microcephaly as, 310
    muscular dystrophies as, 162–165
    myasthenia gravis as, 171–175
    myoclonus in, 244
    neurocutaneous syndromes as, 212, 318–319
    organic acid disorders as, 323–326
    pyridoxine dependency in, 143
    seizures in, 212, 218–219
    spastic paraplegia and, 132
Familial dysautonomia, 275t
Familial spastic paraplegia, 132
Familial tremor, 234
Fasciculations, 36, 38, 46, 125, 129–130, 131
Fazio-Londe disease, 132
Febrile seizures, 218–219
Femoral cutaneous neuropathy, 186
Femoral nerve stretch test, 207
Fetal alcohol syndrome, 310
Fever, in multiple sclerosis, 112
    seizures triggered by, 218–219
    subarachnoid hemorrhage and, 74
Fibromyalgia, 161t, 170
Fistula, perilymph, 280
Fluid and electrolyte balance, 138–142
    dizziness and, 271t, 273
    in anoxic encephalopathy, 136
    in hyperthyroidism, 148
    in renal failure, 145, 146

Fluid and electrolyte balance (continued)
    postural hypotension, causes of, 275t
    seizures and, 213
Focal amyotrophy, 129
Focal seizures, causes of, 213
Foramen of Monroe, 105
Foramina, 2, *3*
Forbes-Albright syndrome, 293
Fractures. See *Trauma.*
Fragile X syndrome, 318
Freznel glasses, 275
Friedreich's ataxia, 273t, 321
Fundus, examination of, 34, 59, 111
Fungal infection(s), 262–263
    cerebrospinal fluid in, 45
    dementia and, 99t, 104
    lumbar puncture in, 43, 93–94
    seizures and, 212, 222

Galactosemia, 213, 323
Galen aneurysm, 309
Gangliosidoses, 324
Gargoylism, 324
Gaucher's disease, 320, 324–325
Generalized seizures, 213, 214–216
Generalized status epilepticus, 229–230
General paresis, 264
Genetic disorders. See *Familial disorders.*
Giant cell arteritis, 74, 93
Gilles de la Tourette syndrome, 245
Glasgow coma scale, 154
Glioblastomas, anaplastic, 290
Gliomas, 287, 289
    brainstem, 290
    multiple sclerosis vs., 116
    spinal cord, 295
Globus pallidus, 18, 244
Glossopharyngeal neuralgia, 61, 79
Glucose, cerebrospinal fluid, 45
Glucose metabolism, brain requirement and, 133
    disorders of, 136–137
    seizures and, 213
Glycogen storage diseases, 323–324
Guillain-Barré syndrome, 160, 176, 191–194
    lumbar puncture indications for, 43
    vertigo, 273t, 275t

Hallervorden-Spatz disease, 320
Hallpike maneuver, 276, 279
Hallucinations, 217–218, 274t
Headache(s), 57–79, 288
    classification of, 60, 62t–65t
    benign, 73
    chronic paroxysmal hemicrania, 72–73
    cluster, 71–72
    migraine, 61, 62t, 65–67, 68t, 69–70
    tension-type, 70–71

Headache(s) (*continued*)
  Costen's syndrome and, 77
  drug use and, 58, 59
  electroencephalography evaluation and, 50
  examination of, 59–60
  history of, 57–59
  in pulmonary encephalopathy, 147
  lumbar puncture sequelae and, 43, 44, 75, 76
  nausea and vomiting with, 61
  postherpetic neuralgia and, 77–78
  subarachnoid hemorrhage and, 74–75
  treatment of, 60–61. See also specific types of headaches.
  trigeminal neuralgia and, 78
  unassociated with structural lesion, 73
  with brain abscess, 259
  with brain tumors, 291, 293
  with head trauma, 73
  with hydrocephalus, 309
  with metabolic disorders, 77
  with nonvascular intracranial disorders, 75–76
  with substance use or withdrawal, 76
  with vascular disorders, 74
Head trauma. See *Trauma.*
Hearing, 35–36
  bacterial meningitis and, 258
  with dizziness and vertigo, 274–275
  medullary lesions and, 13
  Ménière's disease and, 279–280
  with multiple sclerosis, 120
Heart. See *Cardiac abnormalities; Cardiovascular disorders.*
Hemangiomas, 319
Hematologic disorders, 82t, 271t, 274
Hematoma, 228. See also *Subdural hematoma.*
  intracerebral, 90, 91
    CT in, 52
    headache with, 63t
    head trauma and, 297
    stroke and, 89
  subdural. See *Subdural hematoma.*
Hemiballismus, 19, 36, 234, 244
Hemicrania, chronic paroxysmal, 72–73
Hemorrhage, anticoagulant therapy and, 86
  cerebellar, vertigo with, 270, 273t, 283
  from aneurysm, in completed stroke, 87
  head trauma and, 297
  imaging techniques for, 53, 60
  inner ear, and vertigo, 272t
  into tumor, 287
  intraventricular, 309
  subarachnoid. See *Subarachnoid hemorrhage.*
  subhyaloid, 91
  subthalamic nucleus, hemiballismus with, 244

Hennebert's sign, 280
Hepatic disease, dizziness and, 271t, 273–274
  with galactosemia, 323
Hepatic encephalopathy, 144–145
Hepatolenticular degeneration, 144
Hereditary disorders. See *Familial disorders.*
Hereditary neuropathies, 199–200
Heredopathia atactica polyneuritiformis, 325
Herniated intervertebral disc. See *Radiculopathy(ies).*
Herniation, brain, 44, 52, 84, 288–289
Herpes simplex encephalitis (HSE), 250, 251
Herpes virus, and seizures, 212
Herpes zoster. See *Varicella zoster virus.*
Holoprosencephaly, 308
Homocystinuria, 321, 322
Hormone therapy. See *Adrenocorticotropic hormone.*
Horner's syndrome, 35, 66, 71, 73
Human immunodeficiency virus (HIV-1), causing AIDS, 104, 121, 253–254, 262
  disorders associated with, 194, 255t
Human T lymphotrophic virus type 1 (HTLV-1), 254
Huntington's chorea, 242, 326
Huntington's disease, 243
Hydrocephalus, brain tumors and, 293
  communicating, 105, 106, 309
  congenital disorders and, 309–310, 312, 314, 315
  dementia with, 98, 100t, 105–106
  imaging studies for, 60, 92, 106
  normal pressure, 98, 105
  subarachnoid hemorrhage and, 92
  vertigo and, 273t, 283
  with infections, 249, 256, 258, 262
Hydromyelia, 312
Hypercalcemia, 141–142
Hyperglycemia, 137–138, 150, 271t
Hyperkalemia, 145
Hypermagnesemia, 140t
Hypernatremia, 139
Hyperparathyroidism, 141
Hyperphosphatemia, 145
Hypertension, cerebrovascular disease and, 81
  cranial neuropathies with, 187
  dizziness and, 271t, 273, 277
  subarachnoid hemorrhage and, 74
  with completed stroke, 88
Hypertensive encephalopathy, 88, 136
Hypertensive retinopathy, 88
Hyperthyroidism, 129, 148, 293

Hyperventilation, dizziness and, 271t, 274
EEG and, 49
in anoxic encephalopathy, 136
in toxic metabolic encephalopathies, 134
pseudoseizures and, 221
Hypocalcemia, 140, 141t, 145, 213
Hypoglossal nerve, 12, 13, 36
Hypoglycemia, 150
cerebrospinal fluid in, 45
comatose patient, 41
dizziness and, 271t, 277
encephalopathy and, 136–137
in hepatic encephalopathy, 144
in Reye's syndrome, 149
seizures and, 213, 220, 222
Hypokalemic periodic paralysis, 169
Hypomagnesemia, 139–140
Hyponatremia, 138, 139
Hypophosphatasia, 141t
Hypotension, orthostatic. See *Orthostatic hypotension.*
poststenotic ischemia and, 83
Hypothalamus, 8, 11
anatomy of, 17–18
disorders with dizziness and vertigo, 275t
tumors of, 293
visceral pathways of, 8
Hypothyroidism, 147
Hypoventilation, 221
Hypoxia. See *Ischemia; Oxygen deficits.*

Idiopathic orthostatic hypotension, 235, 275t
Idiopathic Parkinson's disease, 236–237
Idiopathic transverse myelitis, 116
Immunization. See *Vaccination.*
Immunocompromised patients
AIDS in, 104, 121, 253–254, 262
infections in, 253–254, 262, 267–268
Impotency. See *Sexual dysfunction.*
Inborn errors of metabolism. See *Metabolic disorders, inherited.*
Increased intracranial pressure, 288, 309. See also *Cerebral edema.*
causes of, 45
cranial neuropathy and, 187
headache and, 75
in pulmonary encephalopathy, 147
in tubercular meningitis, 261
ischemia and, 133
with coma, 155
Infantile muscular atrophy, 130–131
Infantile spasms, 143, 215
Infants, breath-holding spells of, 220–221
choroid plexus tumors in, 291
motor diseases of, 130–131

Infants (*continued*)
newborn, bacterial meningitis and, 249, 257
cerebrospinal fluid of, 45
choroid plexus tumors in, 291
congenital cytomegalovirus infection and, 315
meningoencephalitis in, 310
myasthenia gravis in, 175
perinatal insults in, 211–212
of diabetic mothers, 213
pyridoxine dependency of, 143
seizures of, 213, 215
Infarct(s). See also *Cerebral infarction.*
dementia and, 103
intracranial, venous thrombosis and, 90
radiological studies for, 60
subthalamic nucleus, hemiballismus with, 244
vertigo and, 273t
Infection(s), 249–268
bacterial. See *Bacterial infection(s).*
cerebrospinal fluid in, 45
congenital, 309, 310, 314–317
dementia and, 99t–100t, 103–104
dizziness and, 271t, 273
encephalomyelitis after, 121
fungal. See *Fungal infection(s).*
headache and, 63t, 64t, 76
in immunocompromised patients, 267–268
in stroke patient, 88
leprosy, 266–267
lumbar puncture complications and, 44
lumbar puncture contraindications and, 43
Lyme disease and, 264–265
motor neuron disease and, 132
myoclonus with, 244
parasitic, 266
peripheral neuropathies and, 191. See also *Cranial neuropathy(ies).*
radiculopathies and, 203
Reye's syndrome and, 149
seizures and, 212, 219t, 222
spirochetes and, 263–265, 266–267
syphilis, 263–264
toxoplasmosis, 265
tuberculosis, 261–262
vertigo and, 272t, 273t
viral. See *Viral infection(s).*
Infectious myopathies, 161t, 167–168
Inferior olive, 13, 234
Inflammatory diseases. See also *Autoimmune disorders.*
headache with, 63t, 64t
vascular. See *Arteritis; Vasculitis.*
Inflammatory myopathies, 161t, 166–167

INDEX   **339**

Inflammatory neuropathies, peripheral, 194
Inherited disorders. See *Familial disorders.*
Injury. See *Trauma.*
Internuclear ophthalmoplegia, 21, 111, 114
Intervertebral disc disease. See *Radiculopathy(ies).*
Intoxication, 41, 241. See also *Drug toxicity; Metabolic disorders; Metabolic encephalopathy(ies); Toxins.*
Intracerebral hemorrhage. See *Cerebral hemorrhage.*
Intracranial pressure. See also *Increased intracranial pressure.*
　cerebral perfusion pressure and, 133
　head trauma management and, 300
Intraventricular hemorrhage, 309
Ischemia. See also *Transient ischemic attacks.*
　bilateral occipital lobe, 66
　brain injury and, 297–298
　cerebral hypoxic, coma prognosis, 156
　cerebrovascular disease and, 81, 82t, 85–87
　dizziness and, 277
　encephalopathy and, 133
　perinatal, 211–212
　poststenotic, 83
　reversible deficits and, 90

Jacksonian march, 217
Jakob-Creutzfeld disease, 98, 100t, 104, 244, 253
Juvenile ceroid lipofuscinosis, 212
Juvenile Gaucher's disease, 212, 320
Juvenile hypothyroidism, 147
Juvenile motor neuron disease, 131–132
Juvenile myoclonic epilepsy, 212

Kayser-Fleischer rings, 98, 99t
Kearns-Sayre syndrome, 165
Ketoacidosis, diabetic, 138, 140t
Kidney disease. See *Renal disease.*
Klippel-Feil malformation, 313, 314
Korsakoff syndrome, 104–105, 142, 143
Krabbe globoid cell leukodystrophy, 325
Kugelberg-Welander disease, 131–132

Labyrinth disorders, 271, 272t, 278, 279–282
Lafora's body disease, 244, 320
L-dopa, 237–238
Lead poisoning, 133, 149–150, 198, 213
Leigh's syndrome, 213
Leprosy, 191, 266–267
Lesch-Nyhan disease, 321

Leukodystrophies, 110t, 122, 213, 320, 325–326
Leukoencephalopathy, multifocal, 104, 121
Levodopa. See *L-dopa.*
Lewy bodies, 102, 235, 237
Lhermitte's phenomenon, 112
Limb girdle dystrophies, 161t, 164
Lipid metabolism disorders, 321, 324–325
Lumbar puncture, 43–45, 150
　complications of, 60
　contraindications to, 87
　dementia evaluation by, 101t
　in acute viral encephalitis, 251
　in acute viral meningitis, 250
　in bacterial meningitis, 256
　in comatose patient, 154
　in completed stroke, 87
　in demyelinating diseases, 121, 122
　in hepatic encephalopathy, 145
　in hypothyroidism, 148
　in multiple sclerosis, 114, 115
　in ocular dystrophies, 165
　in poliomyelitis, 127
　in spinal epidural abscess, 260
　in seizure disorders, 222
　in subarachnoid hemorrhage, 74, 91–92, 91
　in temporal arteritis, 93–94
　intracranial pressure related headache with, 75
　with intervertebral disc protrusion, 209
Lumbosacral root damage, 205t, 206, 208
Lyme disease, 264–265, 273t, 280–281
Lymphocytic choriomeningitis, 250
Lymphoma, 45, 121, 199
　primary CNS, 291–292
　spinal metastases from, 293
Lymphomatoid granulomatosis, 191

Macewen's sign, 309
Macrocephaly, 309–310
Magnesium, 139–140
Magnetic resonance imaging (MRI), 50, 52–54, 277
　in Alzheimer's disease, 102
　in amyotrophic lateral sclerosis, 129
　contraindications to, 53
　focal lesion on, 49
　in radiculopathies, 207, 209
　in seizures, 222
Malignancy. See *Cancer; Metastasis; Tumor(s).*
Malignant astrocytoma, 290
Malignant gliomas, 287
Manual cervical traction test, 206
Maple syrup urine disease, 213, 322
McArdle disease, 161t, 169

Measles, 253, 254
Median neuropathy, 182–183
Medications. See *Drug intoxication; Drugs; specific disorders.*
Medulla, anatomy of, 8, 11, 12–13
  Arnold-Chiari malformation and, 314
  development of, 308
  hypothalamus and, 18
Medulloblastoma, 291
Mee's lines, 198
Ménière's disease, 272t, 279–280
Meningeal carcinomatosis, 43, 45
Meningeal lesions, cranial neuropathy and, 187
  headache with, 58
Meninges, in spina bifida, 311
Meningiomas, 292, 295
Meningitis, 249
  bacterial, 255–258
  cerebrospinal fluid in, 45
  cranial neuropathy and, 187
  cryptococcal, 262
  cerebrospinal fluid leakage and, 73
  dizziness and, 271t
  fungal, 93–94, 262
  headache and, 76
  lumbar puncture in, 43, 93–94
  seizures and, 212
  tuberculous, 261–262
  vertigo and, 273t
  viral, 250
Meningocele, 312
Meningococcal meningitis, 256, 257
Meningoencephalitis, 309
  developmental defects and, 310
  Lyme disease and, 264
  viral, 250–252
Mental status evaluation, 25, 26–29, 30–31
  in coma patient, 27, 154
  in dementia, 97–98
Meralgia paresthetica, 186
Metabolic disorders, amyotrophic lateral sclerosis vs., 129
  congenital myasthenia gravis and, 175
  dementia and, 99t
  dizziness and, 271t
  encephalopathies with. See *Metabolic encephalopathy(ies).*
  headache and, 64t, 77
  inherited, 320–326
    amino acid, 321–323
    leukodystrophies, 325–326
    lipid, 324–325
    organic acid, 323–324
  nerve function and, 4
  peripheral neuropathies and, 192t, 194–196
  seizures and, 213, 222

Metabolic encephalopathy(ies)
  acquired, 148–152
    barbiturate poisoning and, 151
    bromism and, 150–151
    lead poisoning and, 149–150
    methanol poisoning and, 151
    neurologic malignant syndrome and, 152
    Reye's syndrome and, 148–149
    salicylism and, 150
  causes of, 135–136
    from cofactor deficiencies, 142–144
    from fluid and electrolyte disorders, 138–142
    from glucose disorders, 136–138
    from hypertension, 88, 136
    from organ failure, 144–147
    from thyroid disorders, 147–148
  coma in, 152–156. See also *Coma.*
  EEG in, 48, 49–50, 60, 135
  seizures and, 213
  symptoms and signs of, 134
Metabolic myopathies, 161t, 168–169
Metachromatic leukodystrophy, 320, 325
Metal toxicity, 102, 198
Metastasis, intracranial, 293–295
  intraspinal, 295
  of spine, CT imaging, 53
  radiculopathies and, 203
  vertigo and, 273t
Methyl alcohol, 151
Microcephaly, 310
Migraine, 58, 60, 61, 62t, 65–70
  age of onset, 59
  with carotidynia, 75
  vs. cluster headache, 71–72
  vs. seizures, 220
  treatment of, 61, 67, 68–70, 71
  and vertigo, 273t
Monoamine oxidase (MAO) inhibitors, 152, 238
Mononeuropathies, 181–191. See also *Periperal neuropathy(ies), mononeuropathy(ies) as.*
Motor function. See also *Demyelinating diseases.*
  basal ganglia lesions and, 19
  cerebellar lesions and, 17
  eye, 20–22, 34. See also *Eye movement.*
  physical assessment of, 25, 26, 31, 32, 36–38
Motor neurons, 2, 3, 4.]. See also *Motor system diseases.*
  degeneration of, 125
  motor system function and, 36
  myasthenic phenomena with, 177
  physical findings of, 38
  spinal tract organization of, 7

INDEX	341

Motor polyneuropathies, 192t
Motor symptoms, partial elementary seizures with, 217
  peripheral neuropathies and, 181, 192t
Motor system diseases, 125–132
  amyotrophic lateral sclerosis, 127–130
  infantile muscular atrophy, 130–131
  juvenile motor neuron disease (Kugelberg-Welander disease), 131–132
  poliomyelitis, 126–127
  Werdnig-Hoffmann disease, 130–131
Motor unit potential, 46–47
Movement disorders, 233–246
  abnormalities of movement and, 233–235
  athetosis and, 244–245
  basal ganglia lesions and, 19
  cerebellar lesions and, 17
  chorea, 242–243
  dystonia, 241–242
  essential tremor, 240–241
  Gilles de la Tourette syndrome, 245
  hemiballismus, 244
  hereditary, 326
  in AIDS, 254
  in viral encephalitis, 251
  myoclonus, 244
  Parkinson's syndrome, 235–240
  spasmodic torticollis, 242
  tardive dyskinesia, 245–246
Moving platform posturography, 277
MRI. See *Magnetic resonance imaging.*
Mucopolysaccharidoses, 324
Multifocal leukoencephalopathy, 104, 121
Multifocal seizures, causes of, 213
Multi-infarct dementia, in 98, 99t
Multiple mononeuropathies, 160, 181, 190–191
Multiple myeloma, 45, 199
Multiple sclerosis, 109–121
  cerebrospinal fluid in, 45
  clinical diagnosis of, 114
  course of, 113
  differential diagnosis of, 116–117
  evoked potentials in, 51, 114–115
  laboratory examinations in, 45
  lumbar puncture indications for, 43
  MRI in, 53
  pathology of, 109
  precipitating and exacerbating factors in, 112–113
  seizures in, 213
  speech and, 27
  symptoms and signs of, 110–112
  treatment of, 117–121
  trigeminal neuralgia in, 78
  vertigo with, 273t, 284
Mumps virus, 250

Muscle, 3
  electromyography, 45–47
  examination of, 25, 26, 37
    cranial nerve function and, 33, *34*, 35
    motor system assessment and, 36, 37–38
    stretch reflexes and, 39
  eye. See *Eye movement.*
  innervation of, *4*, 6
  respiratory, 130, 146
Muscle atrophy, electrical tests for, 46
  in muscle diseases, 159
  infantile, 130–131
Muscle contraction headache, 70–71
Muscle diseases, 159–177
  classes of, 161t
  congenital myopathies as, 165
  diagnosis of, 159–160, 162, 162t
  infectious, 167–168
  inflammatory myopathies as, 166–167
  juvenile motor neuron disease vs., 131–132
  muscular dystrophies as, 46, 162–165
  neuromuscular transmission disorders as, 171–177
    botulism and, 176
    myasthenia gravis and, 171–175
    myasthenic syndrome and, 175–176
    tick paralysis and, 176
  toxic, metabolic, and endocrine myopathies as, 168–170
  electromyography use in diagnosis for, 45
Muscle strength, assessment of, 36–37
  in motor system disorders, 125, 126t, 131
  in multiple sclerosis, 111
  in muscle diseases, 159
  in neuromuscular junction disorders, 171
  lower vs. upper motor neuron and, 126t
  physical examination of, 25
  testing of, 37
Muscle stretch reflexes, anatomy and physiology of, 6
  in muscle diseases, 159
  innervation of, 39t
  motor neuron abnormalities and, 38
  physical examination of, 25
  testing of, 39
Muscle tone, abnormalities of, 233–234, 241–242. See also *Dystonic posturing; Movement disorders.*
  physical assessment of motor system and, 36
Muscular dystrophies, 161t, 162–165
  electromyography in, 46
  juvenile motor neuron disease vs., 131–132

Myasthenia gravis, 171–175
    amyotrophic lateral sclerosis vs., 129
    classification of, 172t
    electromyography in, 45
    treatment of, 174t
Myasthenic syndrome, 175–176
Myclonus, postanoxic, 136
Myelin/myelinated fibers, 1, 2–3, 4, 6, 8.
    See also *Demyelinating diseases,
    central; Peripheral neuropathy(ies).*
    leukodystrophies and, 325
    peripheral neuropathies and, 179
Myelography, 209
    CT of spine vs., 116
    in spinal epidural abscess, 260
    plain radiographic, 53
Myelomeningoceles, 312, 314
Myoclonus, 221, 234, 244, 254
Myopathies. See *Muscle diseases.*
Myophosphorylase deficiency, 161t, 169
Myotonic dystrophy, 131, 161t, 162–163
    electromyography for, 46
    Fazio-Londe disease vs., 132

Nausea and vomiting, 288
    with brain tumors, 291, 294
    with hydrocephalus, 309
    with migraine, 65, 66, 69
    with vertigo, 270, 278
Neck, examination of, 32
Necrotizing hemorrhagic encephalitis, 110t, 122
Neonatal meningoencephalitis, 310
Neonatal myasthenia gravis, 175
Neonates. See *Infants, newborn.*
Neoplasm. See *Cancer; Tumor(s);* specific neoplasm.
Nerve conduction studies, 45–47, 183, 195
Nerve roots. See *Radiculopathy(ies).*
Nerve trunk pain, 77–79
Neural foramina, 6
Neuralgias, cranial. See under specific cranial nerves
Neurocutaneous syndromes, 212, 318–319
Neurofibromatosis, 191, 318
Neuroleptic malignant syndrome, 152
Neurologic examination. See *Examination.*
Neuromuscular function. See *Demyelinating diseases.*
Neuromuscular junction, in amyotrophic lateral sclerosis, 130
    in movement disorders, 233
    motor system function and, 36
Neuromuscular junction disorders, 171–177
    Eaton-Lambert syndrome as, 175–176
    electromyography in, 45–47
    myasthenia gravis as, 171–175
    toxins in, 176, 177

Neurons, general features of, 1–2
Neuropathies, peripheral. See *Cranial neuropathy(ies); Peripheral neuropathy(ies).*
Neuropsychological evaluation procedures, 31, 54
Neuroradiology. See *Radiology.*
Neurosyphilis, 43, 45, 263–264
Neurotoxins. See *Intoxication; Toxins.*
Newborns. See *Infants, newborn.*
Niemann-Pick disease, 320, 325
Normal pressure hydrocephalus, 98, 105
Nystagmus, 35, 269, 274t, 279
    evaluation of, 275–276, 277t
    in Menière's disease, 279–280
    in multiple sclerosis, 111, 112, 114

Obstructive hydrocephalus. See *Hydrocephalus.*
Occipital lobes, 19, 20, *21*
Occipital myelomeningocele, 314
Ocular dystrophies, 161t, 165
Ocular mononeuropathies, 187
Ocular muscle. See *Eye movement.*
Ocular myasthenia, 172, 173
Ocular plethysmography, 32
Oculogyric crises, in Parkinson's syndrome, 235
Olfactory region, brain anatomy, 18
Olfactory sense, testing of, 32
Oligdendroglia, 1
Oligodendroglioma, 290–291
Olivopontocerebellar degeneration, 273t
Opthalmoplegia, internuclear, 21
Ophthalmoplegia plus syndrome, 273t
Ophthalmoplegic migraine, 66
Optic atrophy, in congenital syphilis, 316
    methanol poisoning and, 151
    with spastic paraplegia, 132
Optic chiasm, 20, *21.*, 288, 293
Optic disc, examination of, 34–35
    in multiple sclerosis, 111
Optic gliomas, 318
Optic nerve, 20, *21*
    development of, 308
    in multiple sclerosis, 111
    tumors, 293, 318
Optic neuritis, 116
    arteritis and, 93
    in multiple sclerosis, 111, 114
Optic tracts, 18, 20, *21*
Oral contraceptives, 65, 76, 81
Organic acid disorders, 323–326
Organophosphate insecticides, 132, 171t, 177
Ornithine transcarbamylase (OTC) deficiency, 322

INDEX

Orthostatic hypotension, 274
  causes of, 275t
  dizziness and, 271t, 275t, 274, 277
  idiopathic, 235
  in stroke patient, 88–89
  sinemet and, 238
  syncope and, 219
Oscillopsia, 269, 271
Otitis media, 59, 61, 272t
Otosclerosis, 271, 272t, 281
Ototoxic drugs, 271, 281
Oxygen, brain requirements for, 133
  in pulmonary encephalopathy, 147
Oxygen deficits, anoxic encephalopathy and, 135–136
  brain injury due to, 297–298
  cerebral hypoxic ischemia due to, 156
  developmental defects and, 310
  myoclonus and, 244
  seizures and, 212, 215, 222

Paget's disease, 273t
Pain sensation, 13, 15
  anatomic pathways of, 3, 8, 9, 10
  testing of, 38
Palsy, bulbar, 128, 129
  cranial nerve, 187–188, 309
  progressive supranuclear, 235
  pseudobulbar, 125, 128
Papilledema, 34
  in pulmonary encephalopathy, 147
  from pseudotumor cerebri, 75
  lumbar puncture contraindications for, 43
  with hydrocephalus, 309
  with increased intracranial pressure, 288
  with subhyaloid hemorrhages, 91
Papillitis, in multiple sclerosis, 111
Parainfectious encephalitis, 254–255
Parasite infections, cerebrospinal fluid in, 45
  muscle disorders from, 167–168
  seizures and, 212, 222
Paratonia, 234
Parietal lobes, 19, 21., 31, 37
Parkinsonian tremor, 234
Parkinsonian-type symptoms, antipsychotic drugs and, 245–246
Parkinson's disease, basal ganglia lesions and, 19
  dementia in, 98, 99t
  idiopathic, 236
  speech and, 27
  with ALS syndrome, 128
Parkinson's syndrome, 235–240
Paroxysmal hemicrania, 61, 72–73
Partial seizures, 216–218, 221

Pediatric patients. See also *Infants*.
  anticonvulsant metabolism and, 224
  bacterial meningitis in, 257
  brain tumors in, 289–290, 291, 292, 293
  breath-holding spells in, 220–221
  dystonia in, 241
  Huntington's chorea in, 320
  infantile muscular atrophy in, 130–131
  lead poisoning in, 149–150
  migraine in, 66
  Reye's syndrome in, 148–149
  seizure disorders in, 213, 215, 216, 218–219
Periarteritis nodosa, 190
Perilymph fistula, 280
Perinatal insults, 211–212, 244–245
Periodic paralyses, 169
Peripheral nervous system, anatomy of, 2–6
  assessment of, 36, 39t
Peripheral neuropathy(ies), electromyography use in diagnosis for, 45
  extensor digitorum brevis in, 26
  hereditary, 199–200
  infections and, herpes zoster and, 188–189
    Lyme disease and, 264
  lumbar puncture indications, 43
  mononeuropathy(ies) as, 181–191
    cranial, 186–188
    extremities and, 181–186
    multiple, 190–191
    postherpetic, 188–189
    traumatic, 189–190
  motor unit potentials and, 46–47
  of cranial nerves, 186–188
  of extremities, 181–186
  pathology, symptoms, and diagnosis of, 179–181
  polyneuropathy(ies), 160, 181, 191–199
    alcoholic, 196–197
    causes of, 192t
    chronic inflammatory demyelinating (CIDP), 194
    diabetic, 194–195
    drug- and toxin-induced, 197–198
    Guillain-Barré syndrome and, 191–194
    laboratory tests for, 193t
    malignancy and, 198–199
    metabolic, 194–197
    uremic, 195–196
    with spastic paraplegia, 132
  radiculopathy(ies) as, 203–209
  speech abnormalities in, 27
  traumatic, 189–190
Peripheral vertigo, 270
Peripheral vision, testing of, 32–33

Peroneal neuropathies, 181, 185
Peroneal-type progressive muscular atrophy, 199–200
Pesticide toxicity, 132, 171t, 177, 198
Petit mal epilepsy, 212, 215–216
Phenylketonuria, 213, 215, 321–322
Physical examination. See *Examination.*
Pick's disease, 98, 99t, 100–101, 102, 213
Pineal gland, 19, 293
Pituitary gland, 18, 288
Poliomyelitis, 126–127, 203, 252
Polyarteritis nodosa, 93, 190
Polymyalgia rheumatica, 74, 93
Polymyositis, 129, 171t, 177, 264
Polyneuropathies. See *Peripheral neuropathy(ies), polyneuropathy(ies) as.*
Pompe's disease, 320
Pons, anatomy of, 12, 13–15, 20
   Arnold-Chiari malformation in, 314
   central pontine myelinolysis of, 138–139
   development of, 308
Porencephaly, 310–311
Positional nystagmus, 276, 277t
Position sense, 3, 31, 38–39
Postconcussion syndrome, 298, 304
Posterior fossa mass lesions, 283–284, 309
Postherpetic neuralgia, 61, 77–78, 188
Post-polio syndrome, 127
Posttraumatic epilepsy, 50, 104, 228, 301
Posttraumatic vertigo, 281
Postural hypotension. See *Orthostatic hypotension.*
Potassium, 169
Prader-Willi syndrome, 310
Pregnancy. See *Congenital anomalies.*
Primary dysautonomia, 235
Primary lateral sclerosis, 128, 129
Prochlorperazine, 235
Progressing stroke, 82, 84, 90
Progressive bulbar palsy, 128
Progressive multifocal leukoencephalopathy (PML), 100t, 253, 273t
Progressive rubella panencephalitis (PRPE), 45
Progressive supranuclear palsy, 235
Proprioception, 3, 31, 38–39
Pseudobulbar palsy, 125, 128
Pseudobulbar speech, 27
Pseudohypertrophy, muscle, 159, 163
Pseudoradicular pain, in multiple sclerosis, 112, 119
Pseudoseizures, 221
Pseudotumor cerebri, 43, 60, 75
Psychogenic disorders, dizziness and, 277
   headache and, 70–71
Psychogenic seizures, 221
Psychomotor seizures, 217
Pulmonary encephalopathy, 146–147

Pupil reflex, 16, 33, 35, 187
Pyramidal system, 7, 12, 13, 15
   motor system function and, 36
   movement abnormalities and, 233
Pyridoxine, 133, 143, 197, 238

Radial neuropathy, 184–185
Radicular arteries, spinal cord blood supply, 8–9
Radicular nerves, 3, 4, 5
Radiculopathy(ies), 203–209
   anatomy, pathophysiology, and etiology of, 203–204
   carpal tunnel syndrome vs., 183
   clinical examination of, 205–207
   clinical presentation of, 204, 205t
   electromyography in, 46
   in multiple sclerosis, pseudoradicular pain and, 112, 119
   radiologic imaging of, 55, 207
   symptoms and signs of, 205t
   treatment of, 207–209
Radiography. See *X-ray studies.*
Radioisotope bone scans, 53
Radiology, 51–54
   before lumbar puncture, 43
   in cerebrovascular disease, 84, 87
   in dementias, 98
      evaluation of, 101t
      vascular, 103
   in headache, 60, 67
   in hydrocephalus, 60, 92, 106, 106
   in multiple sclerosis, 114, 115, 116
   in radiculopathies, 207
   in completed stroke, 87
   in viral encephalitis, 251
   techniques of, 51–54. See also specific techniques.
   tumors and, 287–288
Red nucleus, 16, 17
Reflex sympathetic dystrophy (RSD), 189–190
Reflex testing, 25, 33, 34, 35, 36, 40. See also specific disorders.
   for comatose patient, 41
   for muscle stretch. See *Muscle stretch reflexes.*
   sequence of, 26
Refsum's disease, 273t, 321, 325
Renal disease, 45
   dizziness and, 271t, 273
   renal failure in, 145–147, 197
   uremic encephalopathies from, 48, 145–146, 213
   uremic polyneuropathy from, 195–196
Respiration. See also *Hyperventilation.*
   in amyotrophic lateral sclerosis, 129, 130
   in comatose patient, 41
   sleep apnea and, 48

INDEX 345

Respiratory alkalosis, 150
Retina. See also *Papilledema*.
    anatomy of, 18, 20, *21*
    in spastic paraplegia, 132
Retinitis pigmentosa, 325
Retinopathy, hypertensive, 88
Retrobulbar neuritis, 111
Reversible ischemic neurologic deficit (RIND), 82, 84, 90
Reye's syndrome, 133, 148–149, 213
Rheumatic disorders, 93, 190
Rigidity, 36, 37, 233
Rotary nystagmus, 276, 277
Rubella, 212, 315
Rubral tremor, 234

Sarcoid myopathy, 161t, 167
Sarcoidosis, 191
    cerebrospinal fluid in, 45
    cranial neuropathy and, 187
    dizziness and, 271t
    multiple sclerosis vs., 116, 117
    vertigo and, 273t
Scanning speech, 27
Scapuloperoneal muscular dystrophy, 161t, 164
Schilder's disease, 109, 121, 320
Schilling test, 144
Schwann cells, 1, 2, 179
Schwannomas, 292, 295
Sclerosis, primary lateral. See *Primary lateral sclerosis*.
Segmental demyelination, 179–180
Segmental dystonias, 242
Segmental innervation, 4, 39t
Seizure(s), 211–230, 252, 288, 315
    after rehydration, 139
    causes of, 211–213
    classification of, 213–219
        benign febrile convulsions, 218–219
        generalized, 214–216
        partial, 216–218
    differential diagnosis of, 219–221
    EEG in, 49, 50, 60, 221–222
    electrolyte disturbances and, 140
    in AIDS, 254
    in anoxic encephalopathy, 136
    in dementias, 97
    medication for, 226t–227t
    patient evaluation and, 221–222
    porencephaly and, 311
    posttraumatic, 50, 104, 228, 301
    status epilepticus, 229–230
    Sturge-Weber syndrome lesions and, 319
    treatment of, 223–230
    vertigo with, 284

Seizure(s) (*continued*)
    with infections, bacterial meningitis, 255–256, 258
        syphilis, congenital, 316
        tubercular meningitis, 261
        tuberculous, 262
        viral encephalitis, 251
    with inherited metabolic disorders, 320
    with lead poisoning, 149, 150
    with metabolic disorders, 323
    with migraine, 65
    with pulmonary encephalopathy, 147
    with pyridoxine deficiency, 143
    with tumors, 287, 294
Sensorimotor polyneuropathies, 192t
Sensory axons, 1, 3
Sensory function, anatomy of, 1, 3, 8, 13, 14, 15
    assessment of, 25, 26, 32, 35, 38–39
Sensory input, 2
Sensory neurons, 1, 3, 8
    motor system function and, 36
    neuropathies and, 189, 192t
Sensory stimulation, evoked potentials, 50–51, 114–115
Sensory symptoms, partial complex seizures with, 218
    with migraine, 66
    with multiple sclerosis, 112
    with peripheral mononeuropathies, 181
    with vertigo and dizziness, 268–270, 271t
Sepsis, and headache, 76
Septic venous sinus thrombosis, 260–261
Sexual dysfunction, history taking, 25
Shunts, CSF, 106, 310, 311, 312
Shy-Drager syndrome, 235, 275t
Sinemet, 237–238, 239
Sinusitis, 58, 59, 60, 272t
Skin, 2, 4, *5*
    electrical test contraindications for, 46
    lateral femoral cutaneous neuropathy and, 186
    neurocutaneous syndromes and, 212, 318–319
Skull, 2
    congenital anomalies of, 309–310, 311
    cranial defects of, 26
    plain films of, 51
Sleep apnea, 48
Sleep myoclonus, 221
Smell sense, 32
Smoking, 61, 81
Sodium, 138, 139
Somatosensory evoked potentials (SSEP), 50–51
Somatosensory symptoms, partial elementary seizures with, 217
Spasmodic torticollis, 242

Spastic dysphonia, 242
Spasticity, characteristics of, 233
　in syphilis, congenital, 316
　motor system lesions and, 36–37, 125
　with hydrocephalus, 309
　with spinal cord transection, 9
Spastic paraplegia, familial, 132
Speech, aphasias of, 28, 29t, 85, 146, 252
　in multiple sclerosis, 112
　in Parkinson's disease, 236
　mental status evaluation of, 26, 27
Spina bifida, 311–312, 313, 314
Spinal canal, 2
Spinal cord, 116
　abscess, epidural, 260
　anatomy of, 2, 3, 6–11, 13, 17, 18
　congenital anomalies of, 311–313
　motor system diseases and, 125–132
　poliovirus and, 126
　radiological studies of, 53–54
　tumors of, 295
Spinal cord compression, lumbar puncture complications of, 43–44
　lumbar puncture contraindications for, 43
　with intervertebral disk protrusion, 209
Spinal cord injury, 9–10, 298
　in lumbar puncture, 44
　management of, 301–302
Spinal muscle atrophy, juvenile, 131–132
Spinal muscular atrophy, 128
Spinal nerves. See also *Radiculopathy(ies)*.
　anatomy of, 9, 10
　infections and, 249
Spinal tap. See *Lumbar puncture*.
Spine abnormality(ies), 116, 117, 129
　congenital, 311–313
　disk protrusion as, 208. See also *Radiculopathy(ies)*.
　dizziness and vertigo with, 271t, 282
　headache with, 60, 66
　whiplash causing, 302–304
Spontaneous nystagmus, 275–276
Status epilepticus, 48, 49, 229–230
Status migrainosus, 67, 69
Stokes-Adams attacks, 190
Straight-leg raising test, 206–207
Strauss syndrome, 190
Streptococcus pneumoniae, 256, 257
Stress, headache and, 58, 65, 67, 70–71
　seizures and, 219t
Stress headache, 70–71
Stretch reflexes, 6, 39. See also *Muscle stretch reflexes*.
Striated muscle, 1, 2, 3

Stroke, 81
　cerebral angiography complications in, 52
　coma prognosis and, 156
　completed, 87–90
　dementia and, 98, 103
　EEG abnormalities in, 49
　headache and, 59
　migraine and, 65
　progressing, 90
　vertigo and, 273t
　white blood cells in, 45
Sturge-Weber syndrome, 212, 319
Subacute encephalitis, AIDS, 253–254
Subacute necrotizing encephalomyelopathy, 213
Subacute sclerosing panencephalitis (SSPE), 45, 244, 253
Subarachnoid hemorrhage, 44, 90–93, 309
　headache and, 58, 59, 74–75
　imaging for, 58, 59
　lumbar puncture in, 43, 45, 91
Subarachnoid space, porencephaly, 310
Subclavian steal syndrome, 273t, 283
Subdural empyema, 259–260
Subdural hematoma, dementia and, 103
　diagnosis of, 299–300
　headache with, 63t, 73
Substantia nigra, 16, 18, 235
Subthalamic nucleus, 18, 234
Sucking reflex, 40
Superior colliculi, 15, 19
Swallowing, testing of, 36
Sydenham's chorea, 242
Sympathetic nervous system anatomy, 2, 17, 18
Syncope, 219–220
Syphilis, 263–264
　congenital, 316
　dementia and, 100, 103
　seizures and, 212
　vertigo and, 273t
　vestibular syndromes, 280–281
Syringomyelia, 129, 312
Systemic diseases. See also *Metabolic disorders; Metabolic encephalopathy(ies)*.
　cancer, brain metastases and, 294
　cerebrospinal fluid in, 45
　dizziness and, 270, 271t, 272–273
Systemic lupus erythematosis, 93, 190, 194

Tabes dorsalis, 263–264
Tactile perception, 8, 10, 14, 38
Tapeworm, 266
Tardive dyskinesias, 234–235, 245–246
Tay-Sachs disease, 212, 213, 215, 320, 324
Temperature sensation, 3, 8, 10, 13, 15

INDEX

Temporal arteritis, 58, 59, 93–94
Temporal lobe, 19, 20, *21*
Temporal lobe epilepsy, 217–218, 273t
Temporomandibular joint disease, 58, 77
Tensilon test, 172
Tension-type headache, 58, 59, 60, 70–71
Thalamus, 3, 8, 11, 14, 17–18, 19, 20, 292
Thiamine, 104, 105, 133, 142–143, 196
Thromboembolism, 82t
    cerebral infarction and, 83
        stroke and, 87–90
        TIAs and, 85–86
        venous and venous sinus thrombosis and, 83, 90
Thrombophlebitis, cerebral, 260
Thymoma, 173–174
Thyroid crisis, 148
Thyroid disorders, 141, 147–148, 187, 175
    congenital hypothyroidism as, 316
    dizziness and, 271t
    myopathic changes in, 170
    pituitary tumor and, 293
Thyrotoxicosis, 141
TIAs. See *Transient ischemic attacks.*
Tic douloureux, 78–79. See also *Trigeminal neuralgia.*
Tick paralysis, 176
Tinnitus, 66, 274t, 279–280
Todd's paralysis, 217
Tolosa Hunt syndrome, 66
Tonic-clonic seizures, 214–215
Torsion spasms, 326
Torticollis, spasmodic, 242
Touch sense, 8, 10, 14, 38
Tourette syndrome. See *Gilles de la Tourette syndrome.*
Toxic ischemic brain damage, perinatal, 211–212
Toxic metabolic disturbances. See *Metabolic disorders; Metabolic encephalopathy(ies).*
Toxic myopathies, 161t, 168
Toxins, dizziness and, 271t, 272
    hypotension, causes of, 275t
    organophosphates as, 132, 171t, 177
    Parkinsonism and, 255
    peripheral polyneuropathy from, 197–198
    pesticides as, 132, 171t, 177, 198
    seizures and, 213
    tick paralysis from, 176
    with dementia, 100t, 105
Toxoplasmosis, 212, 265, 315
Transient ischemic attacks (TIAs), 81, 82, 85–87
    definition of, 84
    dizziness and, 277
    headache and, 59

Transient ischemic attacks (TIAs) (*continued*)
    seizures vs., 220
    vertigo and, 273t, 283
Trauma, 297–304, 309
    Alzheimer's disease and, 102
    coma and, 153, 154
    cranial neuropathy and, 187
    CSF leakage and, 73
    diagnosis of, 298–300
    diffuse axonal injury in, 298, 304
    EEG in, 50
    headaches and, 73
    hyponatremia and, 138
    imaging studies of, 50, 52
    management of, 301–302
    multiple sclerosis and, 112
    pathophysiology of brain injury and, 297–298
    seizures and, 212, 228
        CT in, 54
        lumbar puncture and, 44
    stroke and, 81
    subdural hematoma and, 103
    vertigo and, 272t, 273, 273t, 281
    whiplash and, 302–304
Traumatic mononeuropathy, 189–190
Tremors, essential, 240–241
    in AIDS patients, 254
    in multiple sclerosis, 120
    types of, 234
Trichinosis, 167
Tricyclic antidepressants, 152, 213
Trifluoperazine, 235
Trigeminal neuralgia, 58, 59, 78–79, 187
    multiple sclerosis and, 112, 119
    treatment of, 61
Trihexyphenidyl (Artane), 239
Tropical spastic paraparesis, 254
Trousseau sign, 140
Tryptophan, 168, 198
Tuberculous (TB) meningitis, 261–262, 309
Tuberous sclerosis, 212, 215, 318–319
Tullio's phenomenon, 280
Tumor(s), 52, 191, 287–295
    amyotrophic lateral sclerosis vs., 129
    cerebrospinal fluid with, 45
    clinical presentation of, 288
    dementia and, 99t
    headache with, 59, 63t, 75
    histologic characterization of, importance of, 288
    metastatic, 293–295
        seizures with, 213
    neurofibromatosis and, 318
    primary intracranial, 287–293
    primary intraspinal, 295

Tumor(s) (*continued*)
  radiological studies of, 51–52, 53, 60
  with tuberous sclerosis, 319
Typical absence, 215–216

Ulnar neuropathies, 181, 183–184
Ultrasonography, 51
Unverricht-Lundborg progressive myoclonic epilepsy, 212
Urea cycle defects, 322–323
Uremia. See *Renal disease.*

Vaccination, complications of, 121, 191, 254
  meningitis prevention, 257–258
Valproic acid, 215, 216, 226t, 228, 244
Varicella zoster virus, 78, 252–253
  parainfectious encephalitis from, 254
  peripheral mononeuropathy from, 188–189
  postherpetic neuralgia and, 61, 77–78, 188
  radiculopathies and, 203
  Reye's syndrome and, 149
  vertigo and, 273t
Vascular dementias, 103
Vascular disorders. See also *Cerebrovascular disease; Ischemia.*
  amyotrophic lateral sclerosis vs., 129
  cerebral thrombophlebitis as, 260–261
  dementia and, 99t
  dizziness and, 271t, 274
  extracranial, 32
  headaches with, 63t, 74
  imaging, MRI for, 53
  peripheral neuropathies and, 190–191
  physical examination and, 32
  seizures and, 213
  vertigo and, 273t, 282–283
Vascular malformations, 32, 83, 319. See also *Aneurysm(s).*
  angiography of, 51–52
  congenital, 90–91, 309
  dementia with, 99t
  headache with, 63t, 74
  in cerebellum, 319
  seizures with, 213
  vertigo with, 273t
Vasculature. See *Blood flow; Blood supply.*
Vasculitis. See also *Arteritis.*
  cranial neuropathies with, 187
  dementia and, 99t
  motor neuron disease and, 132
  vertigo and, 272t, 273t
Vasovagal syncope, 219
Venous and venous sinus thrombosis, 83, 90

Ventral nerve roots. See *Radiculopathy(ies).*
Ventricles, cerebral, 309, 310
Vertebral artery dissection, 81, 82
Vertebrobasilar migraine, 283
Vertebrobasilar syndromes, 220, 273t, 282–283
Vertigo. See *Dizziness and vertigo.*
Vestibular paresis, 280
Vestibular system, 11, 13, 292
  dizziness and vertigo and, 269, 270, 271, 274t, 278. See also *Dizziness and vertigo.*
  evaluation of, 35–36, 275–277
Vibration sense, 8, 10, 38
Viral infection(s), 250–255
  acute encephalitis as, 250–252
  acute meningitis as, 250
  cerebrospinal fluid in, 45
  congenital, 212, 309, 310, 313
  encephalomyelitis after, 121
  Guillain-Barré syndrome and, 191–194
  headache and, 76
  herpes zoster. See *Varicella zoster virus.*
  herpes zoster neuropathy as, 188–189
  in AIDS patients, 253–254
  parainfectious encephalitis as, 254–255
  poliomyelitis as, 126–127, 252
  postherpetic neuralgia as, 77–78
  Reye's syndrome and, 149
  subacute infection, 253
  tropical spastic paraparesis as, 254
Viral myositis, 168
Visceral innervation, 2, 3, 6–7, 8, 17, 18
Vision. See also *Eye.*
  arteritis and, 93, 94
  assesment of, 32–35
  blindness and, 85, 93, 94
  cerebrovascular disease and, 85
  cranial neuropathies and, 186
  dizziness and, 271t
  in multiple sclerosis, 111, 113, 114, 120
  in myasthenia gravis, 171, 172, 173
  methanol poisoning and, 151
  migraine and, 66, 67
  papilledema and, 75
Visual evoked potentials (VEPs), 51, 114–115
Visual fields, 21, 66, 272
Visual system anatomy, 15, 20, *21.*, 18
Vitamin B_1, deficiency of, 104, 105, 133, 142–143
Vitamin B_6, dopa interactions, 238
  deficiencies of 133, 143, 197
Vitamin deficiencies, 10, 142–144, 271t
  pyridoxine (vitamin B_6), 133, 143, 197
  thiamine (vitamin B_1), 104, 105, 133, 142–143

Vomiting. See *Nausea and vomiting.*
Von Hippel-Lindau disease, 319

Waldenstrom's macroglobulinemia, 199
Wallerian degeneration, 179
Wegener's granulomatosis, 191
Werdnig-Hoffmann disease, 130–131
Wernicke-Korsakoff syndrome, 104–105, 142, 143

Western equine encephalitis, 250
Whiplash, 302–304
Wilson's disease, 98, 99t, 320, 326
Writer's cramp, 241

X-ray studies, 53
   in bacterial meningitis, 256
   in headache, 60

ISBN 0-7216-4191-1

90038